MOLECULAR CARDIOLOGY
IN
CLINICAL PRACTICE

BASIC SCIENCE FOR THE CARDIOLOGIST

1.   B. Levy, A. Tedgui (eds.): *Biology of the Arterial Wall.* 1999
                                                    ISBN 0-7923-8458-X
2.   M.R. Sanders, J.B. Kostis (eds): *Molecular Cardiology in Clinical Practice.* 1999.   ISBN 0-7923-8602-7
3.   B. Swynghedauw (ed.): *Molecular Cardiology for the Cardiologist.* Second Edition. 1998.   ISBN: 0-7923-8323-0

MOLECULAR CARDIOLOGY
IN
CLINICAL PRACTICE

edited by

Michael R. Sanders
John B. Kostis

Department of Medicine
University of Medicine and Dentistry of New Jersey
Robert Wood Johnson Medical School

KLUWER ACADEMIC PUBLISHERS
Boston / Dordrecht / London

Distributors for North, Central and South America:
Kluwer Academic Publishers
101 Philip Drive
Assinippi Park
Norwell, Massachusetts 02061 USA
Telephone (781) 871-6600
Fax (781) 871-6528
E-Mail <kluwer@wkap.com>

Distributors for all other countries:
Kluwer Academic Publishers Group
Distribution Centre
Post Office Box 322
3300 AH Dordrecht, THE NETHERLANDS
Telephone 31 78 6392 392
Fax 31 78 6546 474
E-Mail <orderdept@wkap.nl>

 Electronic Services <http://www.wkap.nl>

Library of Congress Cataloging-in-Publication Data

Molecular cardiology in clinical practice/edited by Michael R. Sanders, John B. Kostis.
  P. Cm. -- (Basic science for the cardiologist : 2)
Includes index.
ISBN 0-7923-8602-7
1. Heart--Diseases-Molecular aspects. I. Sanders, Michael, 1943-   . II. Kostis, John B. III. Series.
[DNLM: 1. Cardiovascular Diseases--physiopathology.   2. Cardiovascular Diseases--genetics. WG 120 M7177 1999] RC682.9.M645 1999
616.1'207--dc21
DNLM/DLC
for Library of Congress   99-37334
                                                           CIP

TABLE OF CONTENTS

LIST OF CONTRIBUTORS

Michael R. Sanders, M.D.
Clinical Professor of Medicine
Director of Molecular Medicine
Department of Medicine
University of Medicine and Dentistry of New Jersey
Robert Wood Johnson Medical School
New Brunswick, N.J. 08903

John B. Kostis, M.D.
John G. Detwiler Professor of Cardiology
Professor of Medicine and Pharmacology
Chairman, Department of Medicine
University of Medicine and Dentistry of New Jersey
Robert Wood Johnson Medical School
New Brunswick, N.J. 08903

Wilson S. Colucci, M.D.
Chief, Cardiovascular Medicine
Professor of Medicine and Physiology
Boston University School of Medicine
Boston, Massachusetts 02118

Jeffrey S.Borer, M.D.
Chief, Division of Cardiovascular Pathophysiology
New York Presbyterian Hospital-Weill Cornell University Medical College
Gladys and Roland Harriman Professor of Cardiovascular Medicine
Professor of Cardiovascular Medicine in Radiology and Cardiothoracic Surgery
Weill Medical College of Cornell University
New York, N.Y. 10021

Edmund McM. Herrold, M.D., Ph.D.
Director, Section of Biomechanics and Biophysics
Division of Cardiovascular Pathophysiology
New York Presbyterian Hospital-Weill Cornell University Medical College
Associate Professor of Medicine and Cardiovascular Medicine in Cardiothoracic
Surgery
Weill Medical College of Cornell University
New York, N.Y. 10021

Clare A. Hochreiter, M.D.
Director, Section of Clinical Epidemiology and Clinical Trials
Division of Cardiovascular Pathophysiology
New York Presbyterian Hospital-Weill Cornell University Medical College
Associate Professor of Medicine and Cardiovascular Medicine in Cardiothoracic
Surgery
Weill Medical College of Cornell University
New York, N.Y. 10021

Sharada L. Truter, Ph.D.
Division of Cardiovascular Pathophysiology
New York Hospital-Weill Cornell University Medical College
Assistant Professor of Cell Biology in Medicine and Cell Biology and Anatomy
Well Medical College of Cornell University
New Yrok, N.Y. 10021

John N. Carter, Ph.D.
Division of Cardiovascular Pathophysiology
Research Associate in Cardiovascular Surgery
Weill Medical College of Cornell University
Adjunct Assistant Professor of Chemical Engineering
Cornell University
Ithaca, N.Y. 14850

Steven M. Goldfine, Ph.D.
Senior Scientist, Department of Physiology and Biophysics
Health Sciences Center at SUNY Stony Brook
Stony Brook, N.Y. 11794

Avi Fischer, M.D.
Fellow in Cardiology
Zena and Michael A. Weiner Cardiovascular Institute
Mt. Sinai Medical Center
New York, N.Y. 10029

David E. Gutstein, M.D.
Fellow in Cardiology
Zena and Michael A. Weiner Cardiovascular Institute
Mt. Sinai Medical Center
New York, N.Y. 10029

Zahi A. Fayad, Ph.D.
Director, Cardiovascular Imaging Physics and Research
Assistant Professor
Zena and Michael A. Weiner Cardiovascular Institute and Department of Radiology
Mt. Sinai Medical Center
New York, N.Y. 10029

Valentin Fuster, M.D., Ph.D.
Director, The Zena and Michael A. Weiner Cardiovascular Institute
Richard Gorlin, MD / Heart Research Foundation Professor of Cardiology
Dean of Academic Affairs
Mount Sinai Medical Center
New York, N.Y. 10029

Robert A. Vogel, M.D.
Herbert Berger Professor of Medicine
Head, Division of Cardiology
University of Maryland School of Medicine
Baltimore, Maryland 21201

Richard E. Pratt, Ph.D.
Associate Professor of Medicine
Harvard Medical School
Director, Laboratory of Genetic Physiology
Brigham and Women's Hospital
Boston, Massachusetts 02115

Kenneth Walsh, Ph.D.
Associate Professor of Medicine
Tufts University School of Medicine
Boston, Massachusetts 02111

Masataka Sata, M.D.
Senior Physician
Department of Cardiovascular Medicine
Graduate School of Medicine
University of Tokyo
Tokyo, Japan

A.Koneti Rao, M.D.
Professor of Medicine and Thrombosis Research
Director, Thromboembolic Diseases
Temple University School of Medicine
Philadelphia, Pennsylvania 19140

Michael R. Rosen, M.D.
Gustavus A. Pfeiffer Professor of Pharmacology
Professor of Pediatrics
College of Physicians and Surgeons of Columbia University
New York, N.Y. 10032

Stephen Bakir, M.D.
Associate in Cardiology
Department of Medicine
University of Alabama at Birmingham
Birmingham, Alabama 35294

Suzanne Oparil, M.D.
Director, Vascular Biology and Hypertension of the Division of
Cardiovascular Diseases
Professor of Medicine
University of Alabama at Birmingham
Birmingham, Alabama 35294

FOREWORD

It had been several years since I had attended a national meeting of the American Heart Association Scientific Sessions. While the sessions on clinical cardiology had the same feel and tone I was long accustomed to, I was struck by the immense changes which had occurred within the basic scientific sessions. Not only were the topics foreign to what I had come to expect, but its very essence had undergone a profound metamorphosis; I found myself inside a molecular biologist's world! Instead of force-velocity curves or action potentials, the projection screen flourished Northern blots, PCR gels and supershift assays. Sarcomeres were replaced by phosphorylation cascades and contractility by apoptosis. Even the style and demeanor of the speakers had altered, exemplified by the custom of recognizing laboratory co-workers at the end of each presentation. I supposed that I should not have been surprised since I had recently noticed the changing format of some standard cardiology publications to make them look more like basic science journals.

It was true; cardiology had entered the world of molecular biology on a large scale. But it was also true that the practicing cardiologists and internists at this meeting seemed essentially unaware or disinterested in what appeared to me as a major shift in the emphasis of cardiologic science. There were, in essence, two parallel populations of attendees at the Scientific Sessions: the clinical and the scientific. On further reflection, however, it became clear to me that it was not the lack of awareness or interest that separated the practicing physicians from the new science. Rather, it was the lack of feeling of connectedness, which in turn, I realized, issued from the rapidly expanding field of "molecular cardiology" distancing itself by the sheer speed of its growth. But deeper, at the core of the problem, was the change in the very foundation of the *basic science* that today's previously trained physicians had been trained in.

While molecular biology is not a new field, it has not until relatively recently become an essential part of the standard medical school curriculum, an integral part of physician thinking. It was 1961 when Jacob and Monod proposed the molecular genetic basis for cellular adaptation, but Claude Bernard's 19th century model of homeostasis, rather than altered gene expression, has remained the mainstay of standard medical understanding to most of today's practicing clinicians.

Even "Molecular Medicine" might not be claimed a recent innovation, recalling Garrod's description of inborn errors of metabolism in 1909, or Pauling's explanation of the molecular basis of sickle cell disease in 1949. Nevertheless, the subject "molecular medicine" is not found in a literature search until the 1980's when a few scant references first appear. It is not until the mid and late 1990's that this topic becomes significantly represented by a corpulent body of research publications.

In truth, however, the term "molecular medicine", has taken on a modern meaning, different from just the biochemical explanation of pathophysiology.

On first consideration, "molecular medicine" might be taken as: the application of the principles of molecular biology to those issues which have been traditionally of interest in the *practice* and *science* of medicine. However, experience in post-graduate education of both medical practitioners and medical scientists has led me to the realization that these are such diverse, although intersecting worlds, that even their concept of "medicine" is different. Again this duality! Its background, indeed, inhabits the very history of medicine.

The practice of medicine is the ancient tradition, based on custom and folklore, in which a sufferer of a subjective feeling of being "unwell" or "sick" (a symptom) seeks aid in alleviating his distress. A medical practitioner applies some intervention which he has reason to believe may help. Only recently has medical science become *one* of those many different kinds of reasons to believe in the effectiveness of a medical intervention. Empiricism, that is observation or trial and error, played only a minor role until the scientific revolution, as seen in the early contributions of Morgagni, blossoming with eighteenth and nineteenth century science, as embodied by Jenner, Pasteur, Koch and Virchow.

Medical science, on the other hand, is a recent tradition in which an individual's symptoms are believed to be caused by a knowable disease process which has altered normal biologic (biochemical and physiological) mechanisms, and is therefore understandable in terms of those mechanisms. Medical practice treats persons who feel unwell, whereas medical science deals with individuals who are unhealthy. In this sense, a person may feel well but be unhealthy or feel unwell (sick), yet be entirely healthy. The medical practitioner may seek to have his patient feel "normal" again – that is, the way he normally feels or feels most of the time. Medical science seeks to return the patient to "normal" as objectively compared to other people who are believed or known to be without the disease causing his symptoms.

Medical science, then, has become a corpus of knowledge about the nature of the human body and its constituent parts in health and disease, based upon discoverable laws of nature; and known through proof by observation and experimentation, imitating the models of the physical sciences. This body of knowledge in which biological function (physiology) is explained in terms of observable structure has grown enormously during the past century, as technology has allowed the size of observable structures to become increasingly smaller: from organs to tissues to cells and finally to the molecular constituents of those cells. Medical science has evolved into the science of biochemical physiology, and most recently has absorbed the principles of molecular biology: hence, "Molecular Medicine".

Then what are these principles of molecular biology?

The eleventh century monk Gregor Mendle's observations on the inheritance of traits posed two important questions: (1) How are traits passed on from parent to offspring? and (2) How do these traits come to be expressed in individuals?

In response, profound discoveries over the first six decades of our century have revealed that: (1) All traits of all living beings, from bacteria to man, from microscopic mold to giant redwoods, are encoded within the DNA molecules of each cell's chromosomes; and that this DNA is faithfully copied each time a cell divides in order to pass on the encoded blueprints for all of those traits that go to make up that kind of being. (2) Equally as faithfully, genes (the DNA encoding specific traits) are selectively translated into those chemicals that are responsible for the expression of every particular trait of every different cell.

The mechanisms underlying these two basic principles have become the foundation of the science of molecular biology, opening the door for the complete chemical explanation of life processes. In our introductory chapter, these principles are reviewed, to help prepare the classically trained physician to participate in the exciting and illuminating discussions of molecular cardiology in the chapters that follow.

Cardiology is an area of great recent triumphs in pharmacological and surgical treatment. Yet cardiovascular disease remains the leading cause of death and disability in the industrialized world: *coronary disease, heart failure, stroke and sudden arrhythmic cardiac death* grimily challenge medical practitioners and scientists both.

With the dawning of the new "molecular" era, there is awakened hope that a more fundamental understanding of biologic processes may eventually lead to new progress in the prevention and treatment of these persistent and seemingly intransigent problems.

This book brings together an outstanding panel of experts in cardiovascular disease who have been at the forefront of the application of molecular medicine to cardiology. Its intent is to help bridge the gap between modern medical practice and modern science, in the belief that an understanding of basic principles can lead to new insight into the problems of cardiac patients who are cared for and about.

Michael R. Sanders, M.D.
New Brunswick, N.J.

PREFACE

Since ancient times cardiologists and their physician predecessors have applied the science of the day to the solution of clinical problems. In the year 490 B.C. Pheidippides ran 42 kilometers from Marathon to Athens, announced the victory of the Greeks over the Persians and immediately dropped dead. At that time, little was known about the anatomy and physiology of the cardiovascular system and the pathophysiology of sudden death. Logic was the science of the day, and the lesson learned was to do "everything in moderation". Many years later in the 16th century, gross anatomy was the science of the day. This led to the first correct description of the circulation of the blood by William Harvey in his famous *Exercitatio anatomica de motu cordis et sanguinis in animalibus*. In the beginning of the 18th century, William Cooper applied his knowledge of anatomy to the explication of the symptoms of aortic regurgitation. Development of a new science, physics, in the 18th century allowed Stephen Hales to measure the arterial pressure of the horse, the sheep and the dog by cannulating the carotid artery and observing the height of the blood column in a glass tube. Development of pathologic anatomy allowed clinicopathologic correlations such as those of Morgagni on correlation of clinical findings with post mortem pathology of mitral stenosis, aortic aneurysm, heart block, etc. The science of pathology combined with astute clinical observation resulted in the description of angina and its relationship to the coronary arteries by William Heberden and Everard Home. In the early 19th century emphasis on acoustics allowed Laennec to develop the stethoscope, and Dominic John Corrigan, Paul Louis Duroziez and Austin Flight to describe aortic regurgitation in more detail. William Withering described the use of digitalis. Developments in the field of electricity and magnetism allowed Willem Einthoven to register the human electrocardiogram. Based on that, Sir James Mackenzie described atrial fibrillation. Further development of physics resulted in the discovery of x-rays that gave a high impetus to cardiovascular diagnosis. In 1929 Werner Forssmann performed the first cardiac catheterization (on himself), walked to an X-ray room and took a film showing the catheter in his right heart. In this century, development of biochemistry resulted in elucidation of cardiac metabolism, understanding of receptors and intracellular signaling pathways and development of effective pharmacotherapies for many conditions. The new science of the 20th century is molecular biology. This book is dedicated to this new science and its relationship to clinical cardiology.

John B. Kostis, M.D.
New Brunswick, N.J.

1 INTRODUCTION TO MOLECULAR MEDICINE: A CONTEMPORARY VIEW OF HEART FAILURE

Michael R. Sanders, M.D.
University of Medicine and Dentistry of N.J.
Robert Wood Johnson School of Medicine

INTRODUCTION

Molecular medicine is the application of the principles of *molecular biology* to the theory and practice of medicine. Although it is most modern, its evolution can be viewed in the larger context of the development of *scientific medicine* and its quest for the fundamental explanation of disease.

THE INTERSECTION OF STRUCTURE AND FUNCTION

The beginnings of scientific medicine can be traced to ancient Greece, where Hippocrates, in the fourth century BC, is credited with developing the concept that illness is caused by factors inside the body, rather than supernatural external forces. This idea, successfully promulgated by Galen five hundred years later in Rome, survived the superstitions of the Middle Ages and reemerged during the Renaissance as the two parallel lines of scientific inquiry into human biology: *structure* and *function*. Andreas Vesalius established the careful observation and recording of human anatomy, while William Harvey was able to experimentally demonstrate the essential nature of circulatory physiology. By the eighteenth century, accurate post-mortem examination allowed Giovanni Morgagni to recognize that specific diseases could be correlated with the pathologic changes of certain organs. Likewise, the subsequent development of dependable microscopy permitted Rudolf Virchow, in the nineteenth century, to describe the cellular basis of disease.   At the same time, methodological advances in physiologic experimentation by Claude Bernard and others, allowed the formulation and resolution of certain questions concerning the relationship of normal and abnormal structure to function in human biology. Disease had come to be recognized as the consequence of abnormal function, which could be explained, by some level of abnormal structure (system, organ, or cell), and *scientific medicine* has sought to discover the most fundamental form of this relationship. The technologies of our current century allow the continuation of this search into the subcellular level, even beyond the resolution of light.

CONGESTIVE HEART FAILURE

We have chosen to illustrate the principles of molecular medicine by tracing the development of one example of an important medical issue, the search for the cause of congestive heart failure, as it evolved into our present day scientific understanding.   Please note that this illustration is not intended as a thorough exposition of the complex pathophysiology of this disease; rather it traces only one of its many aspects.

William Harvey had shown in 1628 that the contraction of the heart was responsible for the circulation of the blood.   By the eighteenth century, the constellation of symptoms of swollen ankles, easy fatigability and shortness of breath were known to be associated with enlargement and pathological changes of the heart.   In 1832, James Hope had suggested that in such patients, a weakened heart with failure of the ventricles to prevent the backing up of blood, led to congestion in the body and lungs, causing these symptoms; and James MacKenzie, in 1913, posited that the weakened heart was symptomatically failing to deliver an adequate supply of blood to the vital organs of the body.

Early understanding into the pathophysiology of this syndrome of *congestive heart failure* derived from Theodor Schwann's discovery in 1835, that stretching skeletal muscle increases the strength with which it contracts.   In 1895, Otto Frank extended this observation to the intact frog heart, showing that the strength of cardiac contraction could be augmented by increased filling of the ventricle. Ernest Starling, in 1914, confirmed that the output of the heart depends upon the length to which its fibers are stretched just prior to contraction. He also noted that beyond a certain limit, further lengthening actually decreased its strength.

In 1954, A.F.Huxley and H.E.Huxley attempted to explain "Starling's Law of the Heart" by the *sliding filament hypothesis* [1,2]. Cardiac muscle cells, or cardiomyocytes, are made up of extended fibers of individual contractile units, *sarcomeres*, each composed of interdigitating thick and thin filaments (Figure 1). The dark and light banding design, which had long been recognized microscopically as the hallmark of striated muscle, is due to the overlapping pattern of these filaments. Cardiac contraction occurs when sarcomeres shorten; however, the length of the filaments remains unchanged, as they slide past each other, altering only their banding pattern.

Starling had originally posited that "the mechanical energy set free on passage from the resting state to the contracted state depends on the area of chemically active surfaces, that is, on the length of the muscle fibers"[3].   In the sliding filament hypothesis, this "area" is represented by the degree of thin/thick overlap, which in turn reflects the actual number of thin/thick contact points, or cross-links. By stretching muscle fibers prior to contraction, the amount of overlap is increased, thereby increasing the strength of contraction, as predicted by Starling. Also, as predicted, there is a limit beyond which further lengthening reduces overlap, and thereby, cardiac strength.   Therefore, increasing ventricular dimensions, or fiber length, can improve cardiac performance, up to a limit, to compensate for demands put upon the heart by normal (exercise) or abnormal (valvular regurgitation) conditions. But further increases may cause the heart to "decompensate",   with   decreasing   performance   accompanying   increasing dimensions. Cardiac decompensation is seen clinically as congestive heart failure.

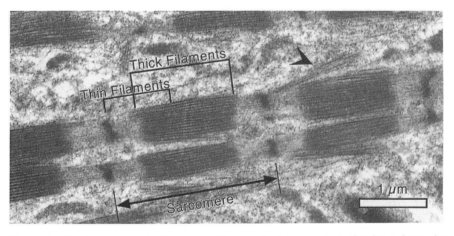

Figure 1.   Electron micrograph of myocyte.   The myofibril is comprised of series o f repeating sarcomeres. The broad, dark bands are the areas of thin/thick filament overlap. The sarcomeres contract as the thin filaments are drawn into this region of the thick filaments. See text for details. Arrowhead points to a new myofibril being added in parallel; see *Pressure Hypertophy* in text. (Courtesy of Dr. Donald Winkelmann)

BIOCHEMICAL PHYSIOLOGY

The sliding filament model was proposed as a *structural* explanation for the *functional* behavior of the normal and abnormal heart; i.e., cellular anatomy explaining cardiac cellular physiology and pathophysiology.

However, the association of any pathologic structure (e.g., over-stretched muscle fibers) with an abnormal function (decreased contractile work) does not necessarily explain how one causes the other, or how either causes disease. Realization that the underlying structural units of all living cells are the chemical constituents of which they are composed, and viewing biochemical reactions as the most basic biologic function, biochemistry has been proposed to promise the most fundamental kind of explanation. Indeed, in 1949, Linus Pauling was able to offer a successful chemical explanation of the pathophysiology of sickle cell anemia [4]. Biochemistry, with its reactants and reactions, ought to be able to give the most fundamental relationship between biologic structure and function; i.e., a *biochemical physiology*. Looking at biology in this way should satisfy the reductionism of scientific medicine by defining the most basic abnormalities underlying human disease.

How might heart failure be explained chemically? Cardiac contraction results in mechanical work; using glucose as its substrate, heart muscle is able to convert, or *transduce*, the chemical energy stored within the sugar molecule into the mechanical energy used during sarcomere shortening. The only chemical energy usable by the contractile machinery of the cell, however, is in the form of adenosine triphosphate (ATP). In the presence of adequate oxygen, for every mole of glucose consumed, 30-32 moles of ATP are produced by oxidative phosphorylation. But in the absence of oxygen, anaerobic ATP production is limited to the two moles released during the conversion of glucose to pyruvate. Might hypoxia due to inadequate blood flow, or *ischemia,* be "the" underlying cause of congestive heart failure, perhaps on the basis of disturbed myocardial microcirculation? Or, as in chronic pressure overloading due to hypertension or aortic valve stenosis, does compensatory thickening of the left ventricular muscle mass without the concomitant addition of new blood vessels result in an inadequate capillary density and an increased vulnerability to ischemia? [5]

While this kind of biochemical explanation has been advanced, it does not address the fundamental problem of how the actual process of contraction is affected. What does the shortfall of ATP have to do with the Starling mechanism? How does it affect the sliding filament model? This kind of purely biochemical description of disease is unsuccessful at providing an understanding of the basic mechanisms underlying the disease process. If the chemical constituents of the cell represent its fundamental structure, and their reactions correspond to their fundamental processes, or function, then to become rigorously effective in the explanation of disease, biochemical physiology has to be taken to the molecular level: i.e., where the structure of the chemical molecules themselves are used to explain the chemical reaction - a *molecular* biology.

CHEMICAL FOUNDATIONS OF MOLECULAR BIOLOGY

The chemical reactions, which take place within living cells, are the intra- and inter-molecular rearrangements of its chemical constituents. *Intra-molecular* refers to the association of atoms within the molecule, and *inter-molecular* refers to the association between different molecules.

In stable molecules, atoms are held together by the sharing of electrons in strong, or *covalent* bonds, which require larger amounts of energy to alter than the normal intracellular environment will allow. In order to perform the multitude of covalent reactions upon which life depends, the facilitation of catalysts, or *enzymes* is required. These reactions include the making, breaking or reconfiguration of existing bonds. For example, the first step in the metabolism of glucose, the addition of a phosphate atom (glucose + ATP → glucose-6-phosphate + ADP) requires the enzyme, hexokinase.

Many reactions between different molecules, especially the large molecular structures we will be discussing, result from the formation of weak, or *noncovalent* bonds, caused by the attractant or repellant electrochemical forces between each others' atoms or groups of atoms (hydrogen bonds, ionic bonds, van der Waals bonds and hydrophobic bonds). Since these are inherently weak, stability of intermolecular associations depends upon the co-ordination of large numbers of such interactions. These attractant and repellant chemically active sites are distributed over the molecule's external surface, so that its exact shape, or topology, determines the ability of one molecule to associate with another; this property is referred to as *complementarity*. The essential nature of noncovalent interactions is that they are weak in the sense that they can exert influence only over very small distances.

The chemical reactions which form and dissolve both covalent and noncovalent bonds are driven by the concentrations of the reactants, and are constrained by the intracellular environment as well as the universal thermodynamic forces of stabilization.

MOLECULAR BIOLOGY OF PROTEINS

Myocardial thick and thin filaments can be chemically separated and shown to be composed of the biologic chemicals myosin and actin respectively. In 1942, Szent-Gyorgyi isolated *myosin* and actin from skeletal muscle, and demonstrated that *in vitro* they combine to form actomyosin. In addition, while myosin was known to also act as an enzyme, catalyzing the hydrolysis of ATP (ATPase activity), he determined that a myosin-ATP complex, rather than free myosin, bound with actin to form actomysoin. Most importantly, however, during this reaction, the energy released by the splitting of ATP into ADP and inorganic phosphate was used to produce an actual mechanical shortening of the actomyosin molecule. This seminal observation suggested a molecular basis for muscle contraction

A biochemical explanation of the way in which the sliding filament model utilizes this reaction needs to be elucidated from an understanding of the molecular structure of its cellular chemical constituents.

Actin and myosin are both proteins. Although proteins ordinarily make up about twenty percent of most animal tissue, actin and myosin alone comprise about fifty percent of cardiac contractile cells. As is the case for all biologic molecules, protein function is dependent upon the physical chemistry of their surface: its topology and distribution of chemically active sites. The complementarity between proteins or between proteins and other chemical species (nucleic acids, carbohydrates, lipids) allows molecules to recognize and react with one another, thus determining the complex network of chemical reactions which constitute the biochemistry of living cells. This principle underlies the specificity of all protein-protein interactions, as between antibody and antigen, ligand and receptor, as well as subunit or monomer association into functional complexes. It allows enzymes to correctly recognize and bind their substrates.

An understanding of protein chemistry began with Emil Fischer's postulation in 1906 that proteins were polymers of amino acid subunits. However, it was not until 1946 that the exact proportions of specific amino acid residues, or their stoichiometry, was able to be measured; and not until 1953 that the actual chemical formula of a protein was successfully shown to be its amino acid sequence, or its *primary structure,* with Sanger's description of the insulin molecule.

Primary structure, the linear order of constituent amino acids, defines every protein as a unique chemical species. Although there are only twenty naturally occurring amino acids, they combine to form the hundreds of thousands of proteins found in nature. Each of the twenty amino acids is also unique, despite their identical format. A single carbon atom is covalently bonded to one amino group ($NH2$), one carboxyl group (COOH), one hydrogen atom (H), and one uniquely configured side group (R). The carboxyl group of the first, or *amino terminal* (N-terminal) residue is covalently linked to its immediate neighbor's amino group in a peptide bond (CO—NH); each subsequent amino acid is joined in a similar fashion until the last, or *carboxy terminal* (C-terminal) residue, forming a polypeptide chain. It is the unique configuration and particular electrochemical nature of the protruding side group R, whether it is hydrophilic (polar) or hydrophobic (nonpolar), positively, negatively or uncharged, which give each amino acid its specific abilities to participate in chemical associations. A polypeptide's primary structure or amino acid sequence, in turn, is the determinant of its chemical behavior.

Considering that active side groups will react with one another, as well as with the polypeptide backbone, protein chains should develop some higher order of structure. On the basis of interatomic distances, bond angles and "other configurational parameters" of crystallized protein, Pauling in 1951, was able to accurately predict that polypeptides must form intra-chain noncovalent bonds, causing them to automatically fold into two specific kinds of helical *secondary structures, α-helices* and *β-pleated sheets* [6,7].

In 1971, Anfinsen was able to show that secondarily folded proteins themselves folded into specific three dimensional *tertiary structures,* again "determined by the totality of the interatomic interactions, and hence by the amino acid sequence [8]." Since most proteins need to exist in an aqueous environment, hydrophobic forces cause the mostly nonpolar portions of the peptide chain to be sequestered in its interior *core,* while stretches of mainly polar residues remain exposed on its surface.

Although polypeptide chains may be many hundreds of residues long, a specifically folded tertiary structure usually averages about one hundred and twenty amino acids. These constrained structures, or *domains,* are connected together into complex three-dimensional superstructures constituting the entire protein in its natural state.

Structural proteins often require rigidity; a common motif is the intertwining of two or more α-helices into a "coiled-coil", as a *rod-like domain.* As we shall see, both thick and thin muscle filaments are essentially dimeric coiled-coils. Many functional proteins, however, are folded into ball-like, or *globular domains*, with their active sites on the surface. Globular domains are comprised of short α-helices and/or β-sheets connected by coils and sharp reverse turns, packed tightly together into complex folding patterns, where they are stabilized by noncovalent forces. An important effect of this tight polypeptide chain packing is to create internal active sites by bringing together a constellation of otherwise distant residues into close proximity; this also sets up the possibility for inter-atomic reactions which can determine protein function by causing intra-molecular *conformational change*. Cardiac contraction, as will be explained, depends upon such intra-molecular alterations within the globular myosin domain.

We shall require this concept of conformational change in our later discussion. Coils of secondary structure are folded together tightly inside globular protein domains. Although noncovalent forces are only able to act between immediately contiguous groups of atoms, the closeness of various residues to each other in this crowded micro-environment allows atomic changes at one point, in charge or position, to have an effect on all of the other atoms within range. Since it is the constellation of these weak forces that determines tertiary structure of a molecule, a small change introduced at any one site may be amplified by the consequent chain-reaction of noncovalent rearrangements, into new local folding patterns that can significantly alter that structure. This results in two important consequences. (1) A chemical reaction at one molecular site may have an effect at apparently distant sites; and (2) even small chemical changes may result in large molecular configurational alterations in which whole secondary structures move in relation to one another.

The result of these complex folding patterns is to endow each protein with its unique physical chemistry according to the topology of its exposed active sites and internal folding arrangement. It is the totality of shape and chemistry, or *stereochemistry*, which determines the recognition and interaction between molecules within the biologic milieu. In other words, a molecule's function can be explained in terms of its structure.

MYOSIN AND MUSCLE CONTRACTION

We are seeking an explanation for congestive heart failure based upon an abnormality in the structure, and thereby in the function, of the molecular constituents of the sliding filament unit, the cardiac sarcomere (Figure 1). It is the force generated by the concerted, coordinated contraction of the thousands of cardiac sarcomeres (4000 per cm^2 of muscle) in the heart that results in its pumping function. While the biology of sarcomere shortening is complex, depending upon a large number of different proteins, most of these are regulatory and not directly involved in force development. For the purpose of simplicity, the focus of the remainder of this chapter, will be on the contractile proteins, actin and myosin, whose movement produces the actual "sliding" between the thin and thick filaments. Their molecular structure and function in congestive heart failure is the basis for our illustration of how molecular biology can be applied to the understanding of medical problems.

Deteriorating ability of sarcomeres to contract (contract-ability, or *contractility*) is the final common feature of all causes of congestive heart failure, both primary (*e.g.,* idiopathic dilated cardiomyopathy) or secondary (*e.g.,* hypertensive heart disease). While severe increases in work requirement from abnormal volume or pressure overloading may even temporarily result in congestive symptoms in the normal heart, usual compensatory mechanisms, if chronically applied, will eventually lead to the gradual diminution of cardiac contractility, as discussed later in this chapter. The complex pathobiology of this syndrome, including abnormalities of many of the regulatory proteins referred to in the last paragraph, has been well reviewed elsewhere and is not the subject of this chapter. 9-11

In 1942, Szent-Gyorgyi had shown that synthetic fibers made from actin and myosin contract in the presence of ATP; and in 1953, Taeschler and Bing demonstrated that actomyosin fibers chemically extracted from heart muscle exhibited the Frank-Starling stretch response [12]. However it was not until H.E. Huxley was able to convincingly demonstrate physical contacts, or cross-bridges, between thin actin and thick myosin filaments, suggesting the "chemical active surfaces" predicted by Starling, that the biochemical explanation for cardiac contraction was established.

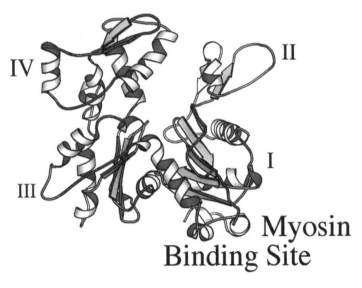

Figure 2. Tertiary structure of G-actin. Each molecule consists of 4 subdomains (I-IV), compacted into a globular monomer. Actin filaments (F actin) are formed by polymerization of these units end-to-end into linear chains, subdomains I and IV of one binding to the II and III of the next. Two such chains twist around each other to form a coiled-coil. α–helices represented by coils, β–sheets by arrows (Courtesy of Dr. Donald Winkelmann)

The protein actin was discovered by Straub in 1942. Its primary amino acid structure was determined in 1973, and its tertiary structure solved in 1990 [13] [14]. It consists of polymeric chains of globular subunits, G-actin, associated into stable filaments referred to as F-actin (Figure 2). Every sarcomere has two sets of thin actin filaments, one attached to either end, extending about 1.0 μm towards the center. They consist of two helical F-actin chains, coiled around each other (coiled-coils) and four regulatory proteins. Each G-actin monomer contains a series of four specific positively charged amino acids near its N-terminus, which we shall see later, can function as a myosin binding site. While its regulatory proteins serve as the on/off switch for each contraction, the thin filaments are otherwise passive, as they are pulled centripetally by surrounding thick filaments, about 0.2 μm (200 nanometers) every time the sarcomere is activated.

While myosin was first isolated by Kuhne in 1859, Szent-Gyorgyi in his chemical analysis of muscle fibers almost a century later, discovered that "...the thread-like very thin protein particles, out of which Nature has built contractile matter is, myosin [15]."

Over the past thirty years, a combination of biochemistry, electron microscopy and x-ray crytallography has been used to construct an accurate molecular picture of the functional structure of myosin. The myosin molecule has two distinct structural portions: a globular, egg-shaped "head" attached to a helical rod-like stalk, or *body*. In muscle, myosin molecules occur as pairs, or *dimers*, with the two helical rod domains twisted about each other into rigid coiled-coils. At the N-terminal end of the myosin dimer, the two helices uncouple to become short flexible necks for each one's globular head domain (Figure 3). The body, neck and head are respectively 130, 8.5 and 9 nm in length. Like actin, myosin is bound to several accessory proteins called *light chains*; the myosin molecule itself is therefore referred to as *myosin heavy chain (MHC)*.

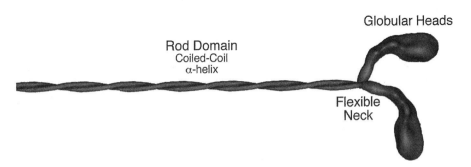

Globular Heads

Rod Domain
Coiled-Coil
α-helix

Flexible
Neck

Figure 3. Organization of the myosin filament. See text above. (Courtesy of Dr. Donald Winkelmann)

The thick myosin filaments are 1.6 μm long structures, centered at the middle of the sarcomere, and extending towards both ends (See Figure 1). Each filament is constituted as of a bundle of 300-400 myosin dimers, staggered spirally so that there is one exposed head unit protruding 90° every 14 nm. This allows multiple contact points with the surrounding parallel array of six thin filaments in the region of their overlap. The length of overlap determines the number of actin/myosin cross-bridges which can be formed, reflecting the Starling effect: stretching the sarcomere may increase the length of overlapping thin and thick filaments for a distance, but then decreases it. The optimal extent of overlap occurs at sarcomere lengths of 2.0-2.5 μm, which correlates with peak contractile performance [16].

During contraction, firmly cross-linked myosin heads flex about 45°, pulling their attached thin filament 10 nm centrally [17]. Since sarcomeres shorten about 200 nm during each episode of cardiac contraction, or *systole*, myosin must go through multiple attachment-flexion-detachment cycles per systole.

Knowledge of the stereochemistry of myosin has suggested a fundamental explanation for the molecular mechanisms of cardiac contraction [17-24]. The myosin head and neck are formed from a single 843 amino acid long polypeptide molecule which is attached at its C-terminal end to the coiled-coil myosin body (Figure 4). The N-terminal portion of this molecule is folded into an egg-shaped head comprised of complexly arranged, multiple short α-helices surrounding a seven stranded β-sheet structure; the C-terminal 8.5 nm of the polypeptide is the single chain α-helical neck.

The myosin head contains an actin binding site on one face (opposing its neighboring thin filament) and an ATP binding pocket directly behind it on the opposite face. The head is split by a deep cleft, dividing the actin binding site into two "jaw" regions. These jaws are hinged in their apex at the base of the cleft, Figure which is in direct contiguity with the bottom of the ATP binding pocket. The lower jaw is able to rotate about 10° as it opens and closes. When the cleft is closed, the actin binding site presents a sequence of negatively charged amino acids, which can form tight ionic bonds with the positively charged residues on its opposing actin molecule described above. When the lower jaw now rotates, the complementarity of the residues on the surfaces of the upper and lower jaws, which allows them to contact is lost; and the cleft opens. Before each flexion cycle begins, the closed position of the cleft also prevents its apex from allowing the entry of ATP into the contiguous binding pocket directly behind it. Therefore, at this point, when actin and myosin are bound, the myosin cleft is closed and the ATP pocket is empty.

ATP is an elongated molecule, with a nucleoside at one end and three phosphate atoms aligned at the other. As the phosphate end of an ATP molecule now enters the binding pocket and reaches its docking site at the apex of the cleft, noncovalent forces rearrange the internal myosin tertiary structure to allow its entry. This *conformational change* (see above) also causes the lower jaw region to begin to rotate and open by about 1 nm, disrupting the actin-myosin connection.

The usable energy of ATP resides in its terminal phosphate bond. As the conformational change, which occurs during the opening of the cleft, binds the phosphate atom more tightly, it also puts stress on this high-energy bond. Further change in the orientation of the terminal phosphate moves it close enough to a nearby water molecule for its bond to be completely ruptured by hydrolysis.

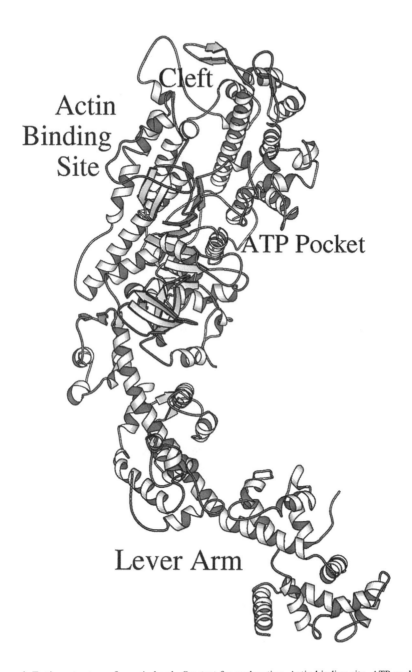

Figure 4. Tertiary structure of myosin head. See text for explanation. Actin binding site, ATP pocket, cleft are demonstrated. C-terminal helix, or lever arm, is extended by two associated proteins. (Courtesy of Dr. Donald Winkelmann)

Separation of the phosphate atom at the apex of the cleft is now accompanied by a reorientation of the lower jaw, which allows cleft closure to begin again. During this process, however, the myosin head has bent to face a new actin binding partner.

In the actin-bound state prior to the beginning of the flexion cycle, the myosin ATP binding pocket had been empty. These new conformational changes in myosin tertiary structure which have occurred as a consequence of ATP hydrolysis, now (1) re-establish actin contact, while at the same time (2) preventing the hydrolysis products from leaving as the jaws close. These changes have also rearranged the internal structure of the myosin head in such a way as to prepare it for its powerful flexion, once actin binding has been completed. Lower jaw closure now translates its rotation internally to the C-terminal helix, which acts as a *lever arm*, flexing the myosin head 45°, thereby "sliding" the attached actin thin filament about 10 nm toward the center of the sarcomere. As this happens, the ATP hydrolysis products, ADP and inorganic phosphate, are ejected; and myosin structure returns to its original "pre-flexion cycle" configuration. The chemical energy of ATP has been converted into mechanical motion.

We now have an explanation for the physiologic process of cardiac muscle contraction, in terms of both molecular function and structure. For the exact details of myosin tertiary structure and conformational change underlying sarcomere shortening, the reader is referred to Fisher, 1995 #17, Gulick, 1997 #10, and Dominguez, 1998 #161. The following sections will deal only with abnormalities of contractile protein structure in the explanation of congestive heart failure.

PROTEIN SYNTHESIS

For the purpose of our illustration in molecular medicine, we are considering congestive heart failure to be the manifestation of a disease of the heart muscle, or *cardiomyopathy*, which results from a derangement in the normal physiologic process of sarcomere shortening. We have described this process in terms of the normal structure and function of its contractile proteins, and now seek to explain impaired contractility as a corresponding protein abnormality. Abnormal protein function follows from its stereochemistry, which in turn depends upon it amino acid sequence, or its primary structure.

But what determines proteins' primary structure? They are part of the complete composite of an individual organism's molecular constituents that go to make up its particular physical structure, or *phenotype*. The information for this composite is transmitted from parent to offspring, from cell to cell, as a chemical "blueprint" for its total complement of proteins. This information is encoded within the ordered structure of the organism's deoxyribonucleic acid (DNA) *genes,* one gene specifying one protein [25].

An organism's genes are arranged on chromosomes, linear polymeric molecules of DNA, composed of subunits, much like the proteins they encode. However, instead of twenty amino acid subunits, DNA is constructed from only four *nucleotides,* each derived from one of the four purine or pyrimidine bases, adenine (A), thymine (T), cytosine (C) and guanine (G). Each base is covalently linked to an identical deoxyribose ring, with a phosphate group in its 5' position, and a hydroxyl group in its 3' position. DNA is polymerized into a chain by linking nucleotides serially together via their phosphate atoms in 5'-3' *phosphodiester* bonds, in similar fashion to the peptide bonds of protein.

In the gene for any protein, each of its constituent twenty amino acids is coded for by one or more unique nucleotide triplet sequences. The translation "script" from nucleotide triplets to amino acids is referred to as the *genetic code*. For example, the triplet CAG always codes for the amino acid glutamine, and CAU always codes for histidine. Therefore, a protein's unique amino acid sequence is determined exclusively by the nucleotide sequence, or DNA primary structure, of its corresponding gene. A change in one nucleotide (point mutation) can change the amino acid being specified; for example, if the final G of CAG were changed to U, histidine, rather than glutamine would then be specified.

Unlike polypeptide chains, which are single stranded, chromosomal DNA occurs in the form of double helices [26]. Each strand of the double helix is noncovalently linked to its partner by the stereospecific attachments, or *base-pairing*, between A and T nucleotides and C and G nucleotides. In this way, each strand is a base-pair inverse image, or *complement* of the other. Therefore during cell replication, DNA can be accurately duplicated by base-pair copying both strands at once. This is performed in the cell's nucleus by the enzyme *DNA-dependent DNA polymerase*, which catalyzes the formation of serial phosphodiester bonds utilizing an available pool of the four nucleoside triphosphates, ATP, TTP, CTP and GTP, making complementary base-pair copies of both strands simultaneously in their 5'→ 3' direction.

The DNA strand, which codes in a 5'→ 3' direction for proteins in their amino → carboxyl orientation is referred to the *coding strand.* Its complementary partner, the *template strand*, is used to transmit the coded information for eventual protein synthesis in a process called *transcription*. During this process, the DNA nucleotides are copied into a different form of nucleic acid, messenger ribonucleic acid (mRNA) by the enzyme *DNA-dependent RNA polymerase-II*. While similar in overall structure, RNA differs from DNA in several important ways. Ribose is used in its sugar backbone instead of deoxyribose and uracil (U) is used to base-pair with adenine instead of thymine. (2) mRNA occurs single-strandedly and is not limited to the nucleus. (3) mRNA's triplet coding sequences, or *codons*, are RNA copies of the original gene's DNA coding strand.

Transcription of a gene results in the production of a corresponding mRNA, which first needs to be chemically modified in the nucleus. Its structure is stabilized by covalent alterations at both ends. It is then edited by having non-coding sequences, or *introns*, excised. The remaining coding sequences, or *exons*, are spliced together, and the mature transcript moves to the cytoplasm for *translation* into protein.

mRNA transcipts are recognized by protein synthesizing *ribosomes*, large duplex structures composed of multiple small proteins as well as a second type of RNA, ribosomal RNA (rRNA). Ribosomes attach to mRNA and traverse the strand in a 5'→ 3' direction, sequentially polymerizing one amino acid after another into chains by the peptide-bond condensation reaction. In order for this process to occur, each amino acid must first be covalently linked to the stem end of a third type of RNA, a unique clover-leaf shaped molecule, *transfer RNA* (tRNA). The other end of each tRNA molecule contains the *anticodon* triplet, a base-pair complement of the corresponding mRNA codon specifying the amino acid which is attached to the stem.   Codon-anticodon matching allows the correctly ordered amino acids to be sequentially delivered to the ribosomal polymerization site as it reads along the mRNA strand.   tRNA's are detached, and the newly synthesized peptide chain is extruded from the ribosome.

Primary protein structure is therefore predetermined by the nucleotide sequence of its chromosomal gene. If variant forms of a certain proteins occur in an organism, they can be either (1) coded for by a different gene, (2) result from DNA mutation, (3) produced by variabilities in the splicing process, or (4) result from differences in chemical alteration following translation (*post-translational modification*).

VARIATION IN PROTEIN STRUCTURE

Abnormal contractile proteins may either result from an extrinsic insult (*secondary cardiomyopathy*), or an intrinsic flaw (*primary cardiomyopathy*). In the first case, the abnormal protein is a consequence of either direct cellular injury (e.g., toxic, ischemic, viral, immune), or as an indirect response to a chronic compensatory mechanism (e.g., pressure or volume overloading); this will be discussed later. We shall first turn our attention to primary cardiomyopathy, in which the abnormal protein is an inherent (inherited) characteristic of the individual in which is has been found [27].

Aberrant species of both myosin and actin have been found in different forms of human primary cardiomyopathy.

The first intrinsic contractile protein abnormality causing human disease was reported in the myosin heavy chain (MHC) molecule of patients with an unusual form of cardiomyopathy in which cardiac muscle is hypertrophied without any apparent cause, *idiopathic familial hypertrophic cardiomyopathy (FHC)*.   In these patients, a single amino acid alteration was discovered in the 403rd residue from the N-terminal end of the molecule.   This position, which is ordinarily occupied by a positively charged arginine residue, was found instead to be filled by an uncharged glutamine   This amino acid substitution results from a point mutation in the arginine 403 codon in the MHC gene on chromosome 14: CGA → CAA [28]. Subsequently, thirty-seven other MHC point mutations have been identified in patients with this condition [29].   Many of these mutations are in functionally important regions of the myosin polypeptide, including the actin and the ATP binding regions [30,31].   Accordingly, cardiac fibers containing these mutations demonstrate significant impairment in contractility. Decreased force generation leads to a compensatory hypertrophy of similarly impaired myocardial cells in an attempt at functional cardiac adaptation [Lankford, 1995 #62].   Eventually, however, heart failure may ensue as the disease process and its compensatory response progress. In addition, many of these mutations are strongly associated with premature death, especially when the amino acid substitution results in a differently charged residue [30]. Interestingly, point mutations at the ATPase site are not found, suggesting that certain functional changes in structure of essential proteins may be incompatible with life [30]. Over fifty mutations in MHC and six other sarcomeric proteins have also been associated with the FHC disease phenotype [29,32].

Two separate point mutations have been identified in patients in the gene for cardiac actin, which is located on chromosome 15. In one, arginine residue 312 is replaced by histidine, due to a $G \rightarrow A$ substitution, and in the other, an $A \rightarrow G$ change replaces glutamic acid 361 with a glycine. In both instances, congestive heart failure developed; but unlike the patients with myosin mutations, ventricular enlargement, rather than compensatory hypertrophy, occurred; and instead of cell overgrowth, there was cell death and interstitial fibrosis (*idiopathic dilated cardiomyopathy, IDC*). It is hypothesized that actin, rather than generating force like myosin, merely transmits force from the ends of the contracting sarcomeres to the surrounding intracellullar and extracellular architecture. Therefore, defective actin may not be able to support the transmission of force during sarcomere shortening, leading to damage of the contracting myocyte, and cell death rather than compensatory hypertrophy [33]. A similar mechanism has been proposed for the X-linked cardiomyopathy associated with another defective force-transmitting protein, dystrophin, and possibly with the extra-cellular matrix anchoring protein, merosin [34,35].

Since the causative factor in primary cardiomyopathy is a change in the patients' genetic information, these diseases are most often inherited within families. Most of our knowledge about the molecular biology of this condition has been obtained from studying members of afflicted families. However, point mutations of the involved genes may also occur *de novo* either by errors during DNA replication, or by biochemical alterations of germ line cells from such agents as chemical mutagens, ionizing radiation or oxygen free radicals. This is different, as we shall see, from direct toxic damage to somatic cells, the cardiac myocytes themselves, resulting in secondary forms of cardiomyopathy [36].

MYOSIN ISOENZYMES AND CONTRACTILITY

Using Starlings Law of the Heart, congestive heart failure might be construed simply as the result of decreased thin/thick overlap consequent to the cardiac fiber stretching occurring *pari passu* with compensatory ventricular dilatation. However, it was soon found that the force or tension exerted during muscle contraction is not solely a function of initial length. Indeed, many factors known to experimentally alter cardiac performance were found to change this basic length-tension relationship. An explanation for this discordance was sought in A.V. Hill's earlier studies on skeletal muscle energetics demonstrating the fundamental direct relationship between the force of contraction and its velocity [37,38]. If contractility were a function of the speed of sarcomeral shortening, then it should be traceable to the velocity of its underlying biochemical reactions.

Earlier, we described how enzymes can facilitate intracellular chemical reactions by alteration of their kinetics; enzyme action can, in fact, be described by the velocity of the reaction it catalyzes. Since the transduction of chemical to mechanical energy pivots about the hydrolysis of ATP, the velocity of this reaction might translate into the velocity of actin-myosin based contraction. The hydrolysis of ATP's high-energy terminal phosphate bond is catalyzed by the ATPase activity of the myosin molecule as described in a preceding section. This molecular function, as with others, is determined by the protein's stereochemical structure, which in turn derives from its primary amino acid sequence. If diminished contractility is a hallmark of congestive heart failure, then myosin ATPase activity should be considered in searching for its cause [39].

Barany, in 1967, reported his analysis of the speed of shortening of muscle obtained from fourteen different animal species. In all cases, the speed of shortening was proportional its myosin ATPase activity [40]. Even within the same species, cardiac myosins with different catalytic velocities have been found during different stages of life [41]. Such variants of the same enzyme are referred to as *isoenzymes,* or protein *isoforms.*

The isoenzymes we are considering are variants of the 843 amino acid polypeptide myosin heavy chain, MHC, which contain slight differences in primary structure in the vicinity of the ATP catalytic site. The residues at or near the terminal phosphate-binding loop are responsible for the multi-step hydrolytic cleavage described above, including its rate. The rest of the isoenzymes' tertiary structure must be similar enough to allow its other functions to operate.

In mammalian heart muscle, two isoforms of myosin heavy chain have been found: fast (α-MHC) and a slow (β-MHC). They are the protein products of two separate genes, both found on human chromosome 14 [42]. The ATPase activity of α-MHC is three to four times faster than the β isoform . In the human heart, α-MHC is preferentially expressed in atrial muscle, but is downregulated by pressure overloading [43]. The cardiac β-MHC isoenzyme is expressed primarily in ventricular myocardium, where it normally comprises about two thirds of myosin heavy chain. The remaining third of mysoin molecules contain the fast α-MHC isoform, as suggested by relative mRNA levels. In patients with chronic congestive heart failure, however, the expression of α-MHC falls to less than 5% of total $\alpha + \beta$ isoenzymes [44].

The down-regulation of fast α-MHC appears to be an adaptive response to myocardial injury or stress. It may be an attempt to preserve the vital integrity of the heart and ensure its survival by improving its metabolic energetics through the use of the slower, but more efficient β-isoform of myosin. The ATPase activity of α-MHC is more rapid, and therefore results in faster sarcomere shortening and greater contractility than the β-isoform. However, this occurs at the cost of a larger proportion of energy being lost in heat production. The more efficient β-MHC operates at a lower energy (ATP) cost, but necessarily results in decreased contractility.

We have spoken earlier of congestive heart failure as the failure of the heart to perform the work of propelling blood throughout the circulation; this mechanical work is accomplished by the ventricles exerting force upon the blood passing through their cavities. The amount of work done can be expressed as the volume of blood ejected per contraction (stroke volume) or per unit of time (cardiac output). The stroke volume is the difference between the volume of blood in the ventricular chamber before and after each contraction. Therefore, cardiac work can be increased in two ways: (1) increasing pre-ejection (end diastolic) volume or (2) decreasing post-ejection (end-systolic) volume. The first is an expression of the Starling relationship, and the second is manifestation of contractility, or contraction velocity.

When faced with stress or injury which diminishes sarcomere contractility, the heart can compensate temporarily by increasing pre-ejection volume (fiber length) or contractility. However, there is an upper limit to either. The Starling mechanism is limited by a fixed reserve of thin/thick overlap, and contractility is limited by the increased energy cost (reduced efficiency) of rapid ATPase activity. Eventually, successful chronic compensation requires the addition of new sarcomeres either in series to increase fiber length or in parallel to increase effective contractile force. In the first case, myocardial hypertrophy is associated with cardiac chamber enlargement, and in the second case, with increased ventricular wall thickness. Unfortunately, both forms of hypertrophic compensation eventually lead to further deterioration in myocardial function, resulting in the inexorably progressive nature of congestive heart failure [45].

HOMEOSTASIS

In the previous section, we have been speaking as if the heart "knows" it has been injured or is under stress and "knows" how to compensate. In fact, how does any biologic system know what is happening to it and how it should respond? The nineteenth century French physiologist, Claude Bernard, proposed an intrinsic self-regulating function whereby the internal environment of an organism, or *milieu interieur*, is held constant by sensing abnormalities and activating an interconnected network of adaptive physiologic processes to correct them. For example, if an animal becomes dehydrated, the increased serum osmolarity and decreased intravascular volume and pressure are sensed, and the kidney, intestine, lung and skin decrease water excretion while the neuroendocrine system promotes thirst and water seeking behavior.

Homeostasis also functions at the cellular level to maintain certain biological, chemical and physical parameters within those limits needed to sustain life : e.g., pH, charge, temperature, osmolarity, redox potential, ionic gradients, energy substrate supply, and the concentration of thousands of necessary biologic molecules. The levels of these parameters are controlled within the cell by a complex network of functional proteins such as we have been discussing. The questions of homeostasis can be reformulated into questions about the regulation of these controlling functional proteins. *The central issue of molecular medicine may well be the selective regulation of protein synthesis in health and disease.*

A succussful explanation for molecular homeostasis was proposed by Francois Jacob and Jacque Monod in 1961 from their discovery of how bacteria correctly adapt to the availability of certain sugar substrates by the controlled production of the appropriate metabolic enzymes [46]. How do bacteria "know" when to turn on the correct gene encoding the desired enzyme ? From Jacob and Monod's deductions, we now know that there are three different DNA sequences involved in this response. First, there is the sequence encoding the protein itself, the *structural gene*. Second, there is a nearby (*cis*) DNA sequence at the 5' end (upstream) of the structural gene, which turns its expression on or off, the *operator*. Third, there is a distant (*trans*) sequence coding for a separate diffusible protein which binds to and activates or inactivates the operator (*trans-activating factor*). Finally, there needs to be the chemical signal which is being sensed, and to which the cell is responding, the *inducer*.

For most human genes, unmodified trans-activating factors cannot attach to their operator, or *promoter*. The inducer molecule, or *signal*, is recognized and bound in the cytoplasm by the trans-activating protein which undergoes a conformational change, allowing it to move to the cell's nucleus, where it attaches to a stereochamically complementary DNA element in the gene's promoter region. These activated promoters, in turn, produce an increase in the frequency of *transcription* events for that gene, resulting in higher levels of mRNA, and thereby, increased targeted protein synthesis. Accordingly, trans-activating proteins are often referred to as *transription factors*.

We also now recognize that all communication between cells, cells and their environment and within cells is chemical. Even physical forces must be first transduced into chemical signals to affect a cellular adaptive response ; chemical signaling is the common language of molecular homeostasis. Chemical signals may enter cells directly, or may induce receptive molecules in the cell membrane (*receptors*) either enter the cell themselves, or produce a second chemical signaling event. This signal (*second messanger*) may pass directly to the nucleus as a trans-activating factor or may induce a multiplex cascade of downstream cytoplasmic or nuclear reactions which ultimately produce a functional transcription factor binding to an appropriate gene promoter. Therefore, *the cell senses and responds to incoming information by a change in gene expression.*

Cells, however, often reply to even simple signals by complex responses; that is, by the co-ordinated expression of many different genes together as a preset *program*. The ability to respond to different stimuli with specific gene-expression programs is part of an individual cell's phenotype. For example, an hepatocyte might respond to a given stimulus by a liver-specific gene program for that particular signal, whereas a cardiomyocyte might respond with a partially or entirely different panel of heart-specific genes to the same stimulus. Even different cells within the same organ might have differing responses, for example, atrial and ventricular cardiomyocytes.

How do cells, especially closely related cell types, "know " how to respond in their cell-type specific way to incoming chemical information ? The expression of a gene is under the control of its promoter, a contiguous region of upstream regulatory DNA, of about 200 nucleotides in length. This region contains multiple short DNA recognition sequences which bind specific trans-activating proteins. For example, the frequently encountered promoter sequence GGGCG binds a specific trans-activating protein, Sp-1. In addition, there may be similarly construcuted regulatory regions farther upstream from the gene, referred to as *enhancers*. The strength of a gene's response depends upon both the total number and type of regulatory sequences bound by the transcription factors which have been activated by the stimulus. The nucleotide sequeneces of the promotor regions of genes can be determined in much the same way as for the strucutural genes themselves. For example, the entire sequence of the human β-MHC gene on chromosome 14, along with its promoter region have been determined [42]. A specific cell's specific transcriptional response, therefore, is a function of both the pattern of its gene's regulatory sequences and the pattern of trans-activating factors produced by the incoming signal. This combinatorial arrangement allows both specificity of individual cell-type responses as well as preset programs of co-ordinated homeostatic responses in which multiple genes are expressed that share common recognition squences, or *response elements*, such as TGACTCA, which binds the trans-activating protein AP-1.

GENE EXPRESSION IN HEART FAILURE

A criticism often leveled at scientific medicine is paradoxically founded in its greatest strength; by looking too deeply into the nature of the parts, the whole is forgotten. Indeed, Hippocrates, the progenitor of scientific medicine, had stressed the importance of understanding the whole patient. Throughout much of this discussion, we have treated sarcomeres as though they exist in a vacuum and their contractility and force development as if they were ends in themselves. We have examined the operations of cardiac cellular and molecular homeostasis, but have not addressed their role in the homeostasis of the body's physiology.

We have dissected the structure and function of normal contractile proteins and have seen the seen how their aberrancy can lead to primary forms of cardiomyopathy. We need now to address the larger question of cardiomyopathies in general in order to complete our illustration of the molecular approach to congestive heart failure.

The heart plays an integral role in the maintenance the body's *internal environment* by satisfying all of the various local tissues' diverse metabolic requirements for oxygen delivery through modulating cardiac output. As a component in the homeostatic network, the heart senses moment-to-moment changes in circulatory pressure and volume, and responds contemporaneously using fiber length and contractility as discussed earlier. If needed, this it followed and augmented by a neuroendocrine-mediated expansion or contraction of the circulating blood volume. In the case of hemodynamically significant heart disease however, these temporary mechanisms cannot suffice to compensate for a severe or chronic inability of cardiac output to match the body's metabolic needs. We need to address role of molecular homeostasis in chronic cardiac compensation / decompensation within the greater context of whole body homeostasis.

In this regard, the heart must (1) sense the physiologic derangement as a change at the cellular level and (2) link it to a compensatory response in gene expression which will result in an appropriate physiologic resolution. Regardless of the cause of cardiac inadequacy, individual cardiomyocytes responds to the changes in tension that occur within the muscular wall of the challenged cardiac chamber (*intramural tension*), and transduce them into chemical messages which traverse the intracellular signaling pathways, emerging as activated transcription factors within the cell's nucleus.

In primary cardiomyopathy due to genetically abnormal sarcomeral proteins, or in secondary cardiomyopathy due to toxic, infectious, ischemic or inflammatory myocyte injury, there is contractile failure to generate adequate ventricular force to overcome the normal levels of circulatory resistance. In patients with arterial hypertension or valvular aortic stenosis, there is inadequate force developed to overcome persistently elevated outflow impedance. In either case, engagement of the normal Starling and contractile responses are required to maintain adequate blood flow, but in doing so, raises the amount of *intramural tension* experienced during systolic ejection. Alternatively, elevated levels of diastolic wall tension due chronic volume overload can be caused by aortic or mitral valvular regurgitation. A variety of compensatory programs of altered gene expression will be deployed in order deal with each particular type of hemodynamic stress [9]. Unfortunately, these responses will eventually fail, as can be seen in five-year patient survivals of less than fifty percent, once congestive heart failure has developed [45].

There are three patterns of altered gene expression encountered in the heart's attempt at a homeostatic response to these various forms hemodynamic stress: (1) myocyte hypertrophy, (2) apoptosis and (3) fetal gene re-expression. They may occur separately or in combination, depending upon the underlying pathophysiolgy of the heart failure [9,47].

Myocyte Hypertrophy. In the case of increased systolic resistance, there is inadequate contractile force being generated. Since cardiomyocytes are terminally differentiated cells which cannot duplicate, the most appropriate long-term compensatory mechanism available is hypertrophy – that is, the addition of new contractile units, sarcomeres, within the existing cells. Greater force can then be generated per cross-sectional area of ventricular wall muscle by the addition of more sarcomeres *in parallel* with the existing ones. This results in wider myocytes and concentric thickening of the chamber wall without any unnecessary lumenal enlargement [5].

However, while parallel sarcomere addition and concentric hypertrophy normalizes wall tension, this effect is inherently dysfunctional, and its benefit does not last. Firstly, the myocyte growth is not accompanied by a commensurate increase in either new capillaries or in new mitochondria, so there is increasing ischemia and impaired energetics [48]. Secondly, the gene programs which generate this hypertrophic response, also stimulate the synthesis of soluble growth factors for autocrine and paracrine amplification. Being somewhat non-specific, they also induce hyperplasia of local fibroblasts, resulting in increased interstitial fibrosis which interferes with the contractile performance of the myocardium. Thirdly, the relative proportion of fast (α) to slow (β) MHC decreases, resulting in *reduced* sarcomere contractility [44,49]. And fourthly, myocardial hypertrophy as a response to increased systolic wall stress is accompanied by an important loss of functioning myocytes (apoptosis) as an essential part of ventricular remodeling [50,51].

While the exact molecular mechanism responsible for the conversion of increased systolic wall tension into intracellular chemical signals is not fully understood, one of the most important signaling pathways to the nucleus begins with binding of the circulating peptide hormone *angiotensin-II* to its receptor in the cardiomyocyte cell-membrane. Occupancy of this GTP-coupled seven-pass transmembrane protein operates via the Ras / MAPK (mitogen-activated protein kinase) pathway to eventuate in the activation of AP-1, a transcription factor involved in cell growth [47,52,53]. However, it is clear that there are other non-angiotensin, non-MAP kinase repertoires with which to respond to increased tension [54].

When increased intramural tension is instead experienced during diastole, as occurs in volume overload, a different pattern of myocyte hypertrophy occurs as the expression of an alternate gene response program, resulting in the addition of new sarcomeres *in series*, rather than parallel. This produces an equivalent increase in chamber mass, but with a different morphology as the cardiomyocytes lengthen rather than thicken: chamber enlargement occurs, rather than concentric wall hypertrophy [5]. The pathways responsible for the differences in gene expression appears to operates through a different signaling system, beginning with activation of an interleukin-6-type cytokine receptor by the peptide *cardiotrophin-1*, and traveling to the nucleus via a JAK / STAT relay system [55,56]. In this program, β-MHC is not up-regulated, there is not as much interstitial fibrosis, and apoptosis is not an important factor [57]. Clinically, volume induced (diastolic) hypertrophy is tolerated for a much longer period of time than a comparable degree of pressure (systolic) induced hypertrophy.

While both angiotensin and cardiotrophin-1 are expressed in other tissues, the heart is capable of synthesizing these regulatory proteins itself, and participates in its own homeostatic response to systemic hemodynamic disequilibrium. This raises the question of how these proteins are themselves induced. The cardiotrophin gene, for example, contains an AP-1 recognition sequence in its promoter [58], suggesting that autocrine loops are important components, linking molecular and physiologic homeostasis.

Apoptosis.   We have already seen that apoptosis may be part of the heart's response to increased wall tension due to pressure overload. However, programmed cell death is most important as a mechanism in the wide variety of congestive heart failure due to diseases of the heart muscle, the dilated cardiomyopathies [59].

In those forms of primary dilated cardiomyopathy associated with failure of force- transmission, rather than force-generation, such as actin, dystrophin or merosin dysfunction, a dilated, poorly contractile, non-hypertrophied heart is seen as the consequence. These conditions are marked by too much stress for the natively aberrant proteins to support. Contractile force can be lessened by removing some of the contractile cells, the cardiomyocytes, through apoptosis. However, this only results in further Starling dependence, fiber overstetching and a progressive downward spiral of cardiac function.

More commonly, dilated cardiomyopathies are caused by toxic, infectious, ischemic or immune damage [27,60]. In these cases, the apoptosis program is often engaged as an adaptive response. For example, the anti-cancer drug, doxorubicin, is frequently associated with a secondary cardiomyopathy, presumably related to oxidative damage from reactive oxygen species [Singal, 1998 #68]. Irreversibly damaged cells would ordinarily die and lyse during the process of necrosis; the need for removal of the biologically active necrotic debris stimulate an inflammatory response in which a wave of invading leukocytes results in further oxidative stress. This additional injury can be pre-empted by engaging the apoptotic pathway for removing severely injured cells. The ordinarily pro-inflammatory intracellular contents are protectively degraded into non-inflammatory components, which can then be harmlessly removed by tissue macrophages. Biochemical evidence of apoptosis is commonly found in patients with end-stage decompensated heart failure[61] . An alternative explanation for the occurrence of apoptosis in heart failure has been suggested. Terminally differentiated cells, such as cardiomyocytes, may be unable to successfully respond to the genetic demands of hypertrophy and fetal gene expression (see below). Failure to complete these programs may result in abortive cell-cycle stimulation leading to irreversible lethal changes and a fall-back to the apoptotic response [9].

The overlapping of the hypertrophic and apoptotic programs may also be seen in the heart's response to infective injury, as occurs in Chagastic cardiomyopathy, where an acute inflammatory reaction is followed by an actual dilated ventricular hypertrophy. This phenomenon has been explained by the similarity between the receptors for the inflammatory cytokine interleukin-6 and for the cardiotrophin-1 peptide [62]. Chagastic pathology stands in contrast to other infectious cardiomyopathies, such as associated with HIV, in which destructive inflammatory histology predominates in the absence of significant hypertrophy [63].

Fetal Gene Re-expression.   Many of the proteins which are synthesized during the adaptive responses to cardiac stress we have been discussing are in fact the products of genes which had originally been expressed during fetal life, but not normally thereafter. For example, there are two separate genes on two separate chromosomes which encode the two different isoforms of α-actin found in skeletal and cardiac muscle. Their protein products differ by only four amino acid residues, and   there is no significant functional difference recognizable between them. During fetal life, cardiac tissue expresses both; but after birth, the heart's α-actin is limited to the cardiac isoform [64,65]. However, during the hypertrophic response to pressure (but not volume) stress, skeletal muscle α-actin is re-expressed in ventricular muscle [57]. This might be explained by the terminally differentiated adult cardiomyocyte not having the sufficient protein synthetic capacity to produce enough cardiac α-actin needed for new sarcomeres; it may therefore re-express the gene for the skeletal muscle isoform in order to be able to compensate [66].

However, a similar theory would not explain the re-expression of atrial naturetic peptide (ANP) in the ventricles of patient with end stage heart failure. ANP is found in fetal atrial and ventricular tissue, but normally only in adult atria [67]. ANP is released from the atrium in response to the stimulation of atrial stretch receptors which occurs during circulatory expansion, in order to reestablish volumetric homeostasis. During the early stages of volume overload, the Starling response, aided by competent tricuspid and mitral valves, maintain forward flow and prevent dilatation of the atria. However, as the ventricles begin to fail, atrial stretch occurs, and ANP is secreted to help control circulatory volume.

Nevertheless, the body's normal homeostatic response to decreasing cardiac output is to *increase* blood volume by secreting the anti-diuretic peptides aldosterone and vasopressin. Re-expression of ANP in the overloaded ventricle might be an adaptive attempt to help reduce wall stress by reducing circulatory volume, since there is an AP-1 recognition site in the ANP gene promoter [68].

Fetal hearts also contain a higher ratio of the fast (but less efficient) α-MHC to the slower β-MHC isoenzyme. Patients with severe congestive heart failure produce an increased expression of the α-MHC gene and decreased expression of β [44]. Therapy resulting in improvement of heart failure reverses this phenomenon [Bristow, 1997 #119]. These changes are mirrored by the switch of hypertrophic myocardial substrate utilization from the normal reliance on fatty acids to the fetal usage of glucose [69].

It is clear from this discussion, that the re-expression of specific genes which are normally restricted to fetal life, represents individual adaptive molecular responses to the specific types of homeostatic needs dictated by specific pathophysiologies, rather than a generic pattern of gene expression [47,70].

What are the mechanisms for these pathophysiology-specific patterns of gene expression in the same population of cells, the cardiomyocyte?

REGULATION OF GENE EXPRESSION

It may be clear now why we earlier stated that the control of gene expression was a central issue in molecular medicine. Cell behavior during health and disease is a manifestation of the genes expressed by each cellular phenotype, according not only to its cellular lineage, but also to the *specific* type of stress to which it is responding.

In discussing gene promoters earlier, it was pointed out that their ultimate activity was due to a combination of the number and kind of its transcription factor binding sites, as well as the number and kind of transcription factors activated by incoming signals. It is the modular nature of gene promoters and enhancers which allows for this kind of variability, in both specificity and intensity of transcriptional control, resulting in unique disease phenotypes.

On one level, there are certain nucleotide sequences which are found in the promoters from many proteins of all striated myocytes (muscle specific sequences), such as the CarG Box [CC(A/T$_6$)GG], the E Box (CACGTG) and M-CAT (CATTCCT) [71-73]. On a second level, there are promoter sequences which activate stress responses in many different cell types, such as AP-I (TGACTCA) and serum response element (CCATATTAGG) [53,68]. And thirdly, there are promoter sequences which act in concert with the first two categories to express unique phenotypes, such as GATA, which can act together with an M-CAT element in the β-MHC gene promoter to promote increased production in response to pressure stress, or can act with the DNA element which binds the transcription factor NF-AT3 resulting in either hypertrophic or dilated cardiomyopathy [73,74]. And finally, there are those ubiquitous sequences which appear to generally increase the rate of transcription, such as the SP-1 responsive GC box (GGGCGG) [69,75].

The modular nature of these elements allows cardiac myocytes to respond to a wide range of stimuli, such as pressure or volume stress, hypoxemia and reperfusion with a multiplex combination of patterns, such as hypertrophy, apoptosis and possibly de-differentiation. In different gene response patterns, the temporal and spatial expressions of specific cardiac proteins including α and β HCM, α cardiac and skeletal actin, and ANP are found to vary independently, according to the distribution of their promoter elements, resulting in the various particular homeostatic phenotypes we have been discussing 47,53,57,67,70,72,76,77.

SUMMARY

Molecular medicine is the innovative incorporation of molecular biology into the evolving science of medicine. We have seen how interactions between biologic molecules derive from their physical chemistry, which in turn derives from the information contained within chromosomal DNA. Disease processes are recognized as manifestations of abnormal physiology, or function, and are now potentially explicable in terms of the three-dimensional structures of these biologic molecules.

We have offered a paradigm for molecular medicine in one example of how the understanding of molecular structure and function can be used to explain the pathophysiology of one selected topic, congestive heart failure. The regulation of gene expression controlling molecular homeostasis is presented as the basis for the extraordinarily variable repertoire of cellular adaptive behaviors in health and disease.

REFERENCES

1. Huxley AF NR. Structural changes in muscle during contraction. *Nature*. 1954:971-973.
2. Huxley HE HJ. Changes in the cross-striations of muscle during contraction and stretch and their functional interpretation. *Nature*. 1954;173:973-976.
3. Patterson SW PH, Starling HE. The regulation of the heart beat. *J Physiol*. 1914;48:465-513.
4. Pauling L. Sickle ell anemia, a molecular disease. *Science*. 1949;110:543-548.
5. Anversa P, Ricci R, Olivetti G. Quantitative structural analysis of the myocardium during physiologic growth and induced cardiac hypertrophy: a review. *J Am Coll Cardiol*. 1986;7:1140-9.
6. Pauling L CR, Branson HR. The structure of proteins: two hydrogen-bonded helical configurations of the polypeptide chain. *Proc Nat Acad Sci USA*. 1951;37:205-211.
7. Pauling L CR. Configuration of polypeptide chains with favored orientations around single bonds: two new pleated sheets. *Proc Nat Acad Sci USA*. 1951;37:729-740.
8. Anfinsen CB. Principles that govern the folding of protein chains. *Science*. 1973;181:223-30.
9. Colucci WS. Molecular and cellular mechanisms of myocardial failure. *Am J Cardiol*. 1997;80:15L-25L.
10. Mittmann C ET, Scholz H. Cellular and molecular aspects of contractile dysfunction in heart failure. *Cardiovascular Research*. 1998;39:267-275.
11. Bristow M. Why does the myocardium fail? Insights from basic science. *Lancet*. 1998;352:8-14.
12. Taeschler M BR. Some properties of contractile protein of the heart as studied on the extracted heart muscle preparation. *Circulation Res*. 1953;1:129-134.
13. Elzinga M, Collins JH, Kuehl WM, Adelstein RS. Complete amino-acid sequence of actin of rabbit skeletal muscle. *Proc Natl Acad Sci U S A*. 1973;70:2687-91.

14. Holmes KC, Popp D, Gebhard W, Kabsch W. Atomic model of the actin filament [see comments]. *Nature*. 1990;347:44-9.

15. Svent-Gyorgyi A. Contraction in the heart muscle fibre. *Bull NY Acad Med*. 1952;28:3-10.

16. Gordon AM HA, Julian FT. The variations in isometric tension with sarcomere length in vertebrate muscle fibers. *J Physiol*. 1966;184:170-192.

17. Dominguez R, Freyzon Y, Trybus KM, Cohen C. Crystal structure of a vertebrate smooth muscle myosin motor domain and its complex with the essential light chain: visualization of the pre- power stroke state. *Cell*. 1998;94:559-71.

18. Winkelmann DA, Mekeel H, Rayment I. Packing analysis of crystalline myosin subfragment-1. Implications for the size and shape of the myosin head. *J Mol Biol*. 1985;181:487-501.

19. Tokunaga M, Sutoh K, Toyoshima C, Wakabayashi T. Location of the ATPase site of myosin determined by three-dimensional electron microscopy [published erratum appears in Nature 1987 Nov 26- Dec 2;330(6146):404]. *Nature*. 1987;329:635-8.

20. Yamamoto K. Binding manner of actin to the lysine-rich sequence of myosin subfragment 1 in the presence and absence of ATP. *Biochemistry*. 1989;28:5573-7.

21. Botts J, Thomason JF, Morales MF. On the origin and transmission of force in actomyosin subfragment 1. *Proc Natl Acad Sci U S A*. 1989;86:2204-8.

22. Gulick AM, Rayment I. Structural studies on myosin II: communication between distant protein domains. *Bioessays*. 1997;19:561-9.

23. Fisher AJ, Smith CA, Thoden J, Smith R, Sutoh K, Holden HM, Rayment I. Structural studies of myosin:nucleotide complexes: a revised model for the molecular basis of muscle contraction. *Biophys J*. 1995;68:19S-26S; discussion 27S-28S.

24. Rayment I, Holden HM, Whittaker M, Yohn CB, Lorenz M, Holmes KC, Milligan RA. Structure of the actin-myosin complex and its implications for muscle contraction [see comments]. *Science*. 1993;261:58-65.

25. Beadle GW, Tatum, E.L. Genetic control of biochemical reactions in Neurospora. *Proc Natl Acad Sci*. 1941;27:499-506.

26. Watson JD, Crick, F.H.C. A structure for deoxyribonucleic acid. *Nature*. 1953;171:737-738.

27. Towbin JA. Molecular genetic aspects of cardiomyopathy. *Biochemical Medicine and Metabolic Biology*. 1993;49:285-320.

28. Geisterfer-Lowrance AA, Kass S, Tanigawa G, Vosberg HP, McKenna W, Seidman CE, Seidman JG. A molecular basis for familial hypertrophic cardiomyopathy: a beta cardiac myosin heavy chain gene missense mutation. *Cell*. 1990;62:999-1006.

29. Vikstrom KL, Leinwand LA. Contractile protein mutations and heart disease. *Curr Opin Cell Biol*. 1996;8:97-105.

30. Watkins H, Rosenzweig A, Hwang DS, Levi T, McKenna W, Seidman CE, Seidman JG. Characteristics and prognostic implications of myosin missense mutations in familial hypertrophic cardiomyopathy [see comments]. *N Engl J Med*. 1992;326:1108-14.

31. Rayment I, Holden HM, Sellers JR, Fananapazir L, Epstein ND. Structural interpretation of the mutations in the beta-cardiac myosin that have been implicated in familial hypertrophic cardiomyopathy. *Proc Natl Acad Sci U S A*. 1995;92:3864-8.

32. McKenna WJ, Coccolo F, Elliott PM. Genes and disease expression in hypertrophic cardiomyopathy [In Process Citation]. *Lancet*. 1998;352:1162-3.

33. Olson TM, Michels VV, Thibodeau SN, Tai YS, Keating MT. Actin mutations in dilated cardiomyopathy, a heritable form of heart failure. *Science*. 1998;280:750-2.

34. Ortiz-Lopez R, Li H, Su J, Goytia V, Towbin JA. Evidence for a dystrophin missense mutation as a cause of X-linked dilated cardiomyopathy [see comments]. *Circulation*. 1997;95:2434-40.

35. Spyrou N, Philpot J, Foale R, Camici PG, Muntoni F. Evidence of left ventricular dysfunction in children with merosin- deficient congenital muscular dystrophy. *Am Heart J*. 1998;136:474-6.

36. Singal PK, Iliskovic N. Doxorubicin-induced cardiomyopathy. *N Engl J Med*. 1998;339:900-5.

37. Abbott BC, Wilke, D.R. The relation between velocity of shortening and the tension-length curve of skeletal muscle. *J Physiol*. 1953;120:214-223.

38. Abbott BC, Mommaerts, W.F.H.M. A study of inotropic mechanisms in the papillary muscle preparation. *J Gen Physiol*. 1959;42:533-551.

39. Alpert NR, Mulieri LA, Litten RZ. Functional significance of altered myosin adenosine triphosphatase activity in enlarged hearts. *Am J Cardiol*. 1979;44:946-53.

40. Barany M, Conover TE, Schliselfeld LH, Gaetjens E, Goffart M. Relation of properties of isolated myosin to those of intact muscles of the cat and sloth. *Eur J Biochem*. 1967;2:156-64.

41. Nadal-Ginard B, Mahdavi V. Molecular basis of cardiac performance. Plasticity of the myocardium generated through protein isoform switches. *J Clin Invest*. 1989;84:1693-700.

42. Saez LJ, Gianola KM, McNally EM, Feghali R, Eddy R, Shows TB, Leinwand LA. Human cardiac myosin heavy chain genes and their linkage in the genome. *Nucleic Acids Res.* 1987;15:5443-59.
43. Kurabayashi M, Tsuchimochi H, Komuro I, Takaku F, Yazaki Y. Molecular cloning and characterization of human cardiac alpha- and beta- form myosin heavy chain complementary DNA clones. Regulation of expression during development and pressure overload in human atrium. *J Clin Invest.* 1988;82:524-31.
44. Nakao K, Minobe W, Roden R, Bristow MR, Leinwand LA. Myosin heavy chain gene expression in human heart failure. *J Clin Invest.* 1997;100:2362-70.
45. Katz AM. Cardiomyopathy of overload. A major determinant of prognosis in congestive heart failure [see comments]. *N Engl J Med.* 1990;322:100-10.
46. Jacob F, Monod, J. Genetic regulatory mechanisms in the synthesis of proteins. *J Mol Biol.* 1961;3:318-356.
47. Hefti MA, Harder BA, Eppenberger HM, Schaub MC. Signaling pathways in cardiac myocyte hypertrophy. *J Mol Cell Cardiol.* 1997;29:2873-92.
48. Anversa P, Olivetti G, Melissari M, Loud AV. Stereological measurement of cellular and subcellular hypertrophy and hyperplasia in the papillary muscle of adult rat. *J Mol Cell Cardiol.* 1980;12:781-95.
49. Bristow MR, Gilbert, E.M., Lowes, B.D.,, Minobe WA, Shakar, S.F., Quaife, R.A., Abraham, W.T. Changes in gene expression asociated with b-blocker-related improvements in ventricular systolic function. *Circulation.* 1997;96:I - 92.
50. Cheng W, Li B, Kajstura J, Li P, Wolin MS, Sonnenblick EH, Hintze TH, Olivetti G, Anversa P. Stretch-induced programmed myocyte cell death. *J Clin Invest.* 1995;96:2247-59.
51. Teiger E, Than VD, Richard L, Wisnewsky C, Tea BS, Gaboury L, Tremblay J, Schwartz K, Hamet P. Apoptosis in pressure overload-induced heart hypertrophy in the rat. *J Clin Invest.* 1996;97:2891-7.
52. Glennon PE, Kaddoura S, Sale EM, Sale GJ, Fuller SJ, Sugden PH. Depletion of mitogen-activated protein kinase using an antisense oligodeoxynucleotide approach downregulates the phenylephrine-induced hypertrophic response in rat cardiac myocytes. *Circ Res.* 1996;78:954-61.
53. Sadoshima J, Jahn L, Takahashi T, Kulik TJ, Izumo S. Molecular characterization of the stretch-induced adaptation of cultured cardiac cells. An in vitro model of load-induced cardiac hypertrophy. *J Biol Chem.* 1992;267:10551-60.
54. Kudoh S, Komuro I, Hiroi Y, Zou Y, Harada K, Sugaya T, Takekoshi N, Murakami K, Kadowaki T, Yazaki Y. Mechanical stretch induces hypertrophic responses in cardiac myocytes of angiotensin II type 1a receptor knockout mice. *J Biol Chem.* 1998;273:24037-43.
55. Wollert KC, Taga T, Saito M, Narazaki M, Kishimoto T, Glembotski CC, Vernallis AB, Heath JK, Pennica D, Wood WI, Chien KR. Cardiotrophin-1 activates a distinct form of cardiac muscle cell hypertrophy. Assembly of sarcomeric units in series VIA gp130/leukemia inhibitory factor receptor-dependent pathways. *J Biol Chem.* 1996;271:9535-45.
56. Heinrich PC, Behrmann I, G Ml-N, Schaper F, Graeve L. Interleukin-6-type cytokine signalling through the gp130/Jak/STAT pathway1. *Biochem J.* 1998;334:297-314.
57. Calderone A, Takahashi N, Izzo NJ, Jr., Thaik CM, Colucci WS. Pressure- and volume-induced left ventricular hypertrophies are associated with distinct myocyte phenotypes and differential induction of peptide growth factor mRNAs. *Circulation.* 1995;92:2385-90.
58. Erdmann J, Hassfeld S, Kallisch H, Fleck E, Regitz-Zagrosek V. Cloning and characterization of the 5'-flanking region of the human cardiotrophin-1 gene. *Biochem Biophys Res Commun.* 1998;244:494-7.
59 .Narula J, Haider N, Virmani R, DiSalvo TG, Kolodgie FD, Hajjar RJ, Schmidt U, Semigran MJ, Dec GW, Khaw BA. Apoptosis in myocytes in end-stage heart failure [see comments]. *N Engl J Med.* 1996;335:1182-9.
60. Dec GW, Fuster V. Idiopathic dilated cardiomyopathy [see comments]. *N Engl J Med.* 1994;331:1564-75.
61. Olivetti G, Abbi R, Quaini F, Kajstura J, Cheng W, Nitahara JA, Quaini E, Di Loreto C, Beltrami CA, Krajewski S, Reed JC, Anversa P. Apoptosis in the failing human heart. *N Engl J Med.* 1997;336:1131-41.
62. Chandrasekar B, Melby PC, Pennica D, Freeman GL. Overexpression of cardiotrophin-1 and gp130 during experimental acute Chagasic cardiomyopathy. *Immunol Lett.* 1998;61:89-95.
63. Barbaro G, Di Lorenzo G, Grisorio B, Barbarini G. Incidence of Dilated Cardiomyopathy and Detection of HIV in Myocardial Cells of HIV-Positive Patients. *N Engl J Med.* 1998;339:1093-1099.
64. Garner I, Sassoon D, Vandekerckhove J, Alonso S, Buckingham ME. A developmental study of the abnormal expression of alpha-cardiac and alpha-skeletal actins in the striated muscle of a mutant mouse. *Dev Biol.* 1989;134:236-45.
65. Buckingham ME. Actin and myosin multigene families: their expression during the formation of skeletal muscle. *Essays Biochem.* 1985;20:77-109.

66. Katz AM. The cardiomyopathy of overload: an unnatural growth response in the hypertrophied heart. *Ann Intern Med.* 1994;121:363-71.

67. Takahashi T, Allen PD, Izumo S. Expression of A-, B-, and C-type natriuretic peptide genes in failing and developing human ventricles. Correlation with expression of the Ca(2+)-ATPase gene. *Circ Res.* 1992;71:9-17.

68. Cornelius T, Holmer SR, Muller FU, Riegger GA, Schunkert H. Regulation of the rat atrial natriuretic peptide gene after acute imposition of left ventricular pressure overload. *Hypertension.* 1997;30:1348-55.

69. Sack MN, Disch DL, Rockman HA, Kelly DP. A role for Sp and nuclear receptor transcription factors in a cardiac hypertrophic growth program. *Proc Natl Acad Sci U S A.* 1997;94:6438-43.

70. Yue P, Long CS, Austin R, Chang KC, Simpson PC, Massie BM. Post-infarction heart failure in the rat is associated with distinct alterations in cardiac myocyte molecular phenotype [In Process Citation]. *J Mol Cell Cardiol.* 1998;30:1615-30.

71. Boxer LM, Miwa T, Gustafson TA, Kedes L. Identification and characterization of a factor that binds to two human sarcomeric actin promoters. *J Biol Chem.* 1989;264:1284-92.

72. Navankasattusas S, Sawadogo M, van Bilsen M, Dang CV, Chien KR. The basic helix-loop-helix protein upstream stimulating factor regulates the cardiac ventricular myosin light-chain 2 gene via independent cis regulatory elements. *Mol Cell Biol.* 1994;14:7331-9.

73. Hasegawa K, Lee SJ, Jobe SM, Markham BE, Kitsis RN. cis-Acting sequences that mediate induction of beta-myosin heavy chain gene expression during left ventricular hypertrophy due to aortic constriction [see comments]. *Circulation.* 1997;96:3943-53.

74. Molkentin JD, Lu JR, Antos CL, Markham B, Richardson J, Robbins J, Grant SR, Olson EN. A calcineurin-dependent transcriptional pathway for cardiac hypertrophy. *Cell.* 1998;93:215-28.

75. Zilberman A, Dave V, Miano J, Olson EN, Periasamy M. Evolutionarily conserved promoter region containing CArG*-like elements is crucial for smooth muscle myosin heavy chain gene expression. *Circ Res.* 1998;82:566-75.

76. Schiaffino S, Samuel JL, Sassoon D, Lompre AM, Garner I, Marotte F, Buckingham M, Rappaport L, Schwartz K. Nonsynchronous accumulation of alpha-skeletal actin and beta-myosin heavy chain mRNAs during early stages of pressure-overload--induced cardiac hypertrophy demonstrated by in situ hybridization. *Circ Res.* 1989;64:937-48.

77. Xiao Q, Ojamaa K. Regulation of cardiac alpha-myosin heavy chain gene transcription by a contractile-responsive E-box binding protein. *J Mol Cell Cardiol.* 1998;30:87-95.

2 MOLECULAR MECHANISMS OF MYOCARDIAL REMODELING

Wilson S. Colucci, M.D.
Boston University School of Medicine

INTRODUCTION

Myocardial dysfunction is a progressive condition. Early after an insult to the myocardium (e.g., myocardial infarction) there may be little or no immediate reduction in overall pump function, particularly if the damage has been mild. However, with time there is a relentless deterioration in both the structure and function of the ventricle by a process referred to as "remodeling" (1). The specific features of the remodeling process depend, to a large extent, on the nature of the underlying stimulus.

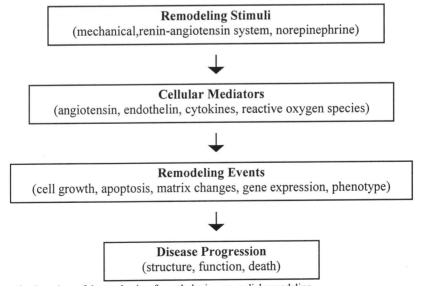

Figure 1. Overview of the mechanism for pathologic myocardial remodeling.

Although myocardial remodeling is a normal feature during maturation, and may be a useful adaptation to increased demands (e.g., with athletic training) in the adult, when it is the result of a pathologic stimulus (e.g., increased wall stress), the result is usually maladaptive and often eventuates in further myocardial dysfunction (2). The mechanism that mediates myocardial remodeling involves a variety of molecular and cellular alterations including hypertrophy of individual myocytes, altered gene expression, changes in the extracellular matrix, and possibly, the death of cardiac myocytes by apoptosis (Figure 1). Observations in vitro systems, and more recently, in transgenic mice, have led to the thesis that myocardial remodeling is mediated by a variety of signaling systems which are activated in response to pathologic stimuli known to be present in patients with myocardial dysfunction. (Figure 1). In this review we will first describe the major cellular events that appear to be important in myocardial remodeling. We will then consider the possible role of several stimuli and mediators for these events.

CELLULAR EVENTS IN MYOCARDIAL REMODELING

Myocyte hypertrophy. Hemodynamic overload typically results in an increase in myocardial mass that is associated with a change in the shape of the ventricle. Grossly, the type of shape change is related to the nature of the stimulus (3). When the stimulus is primarily systolic in nature (e.g., with aortic constriction), there is an increase in systolic wall stress that is associated with the parallel addition of sarcomeres and widening of cardiac myocytes. This form of hypertrophy has been referred to as "concentric" hypertrophy. If the hemodynamic stimulus is primarily due to an increase in ventricular diastolic volume (e.g., with arteriovenous fistula or mitral regurgitation), sarcomeres are added in series and there is lengthening of cardiac myocytes. This form of hypertrophy has been referred to as "eccentric" hypertrophy. In the clinical setting it is common for the two types of stimulus to coexist, and thus, there may be features of both eccentric and concentric hypertrophy.

The increase in myocardial mass is due mainly to hypertrophy of individual myocytes. As discussed subsequently, cardiac myocytes cultured from neonatal or adult rat hearts have proven to be a valuable tool for studying the mechanisms of myocyte hypertrophy under highly controlled conditions *in vitro*. Using this approach it has been shown that several stimuli can cause an increase in myocyte size due to increased protein synthesis in the absence of cell division. These include norepinephrine (4,5), angiotensin (6), endothelin (7), inflammatory cytokines (8), and mechanical stretch (9).

Myocyte apoptosis. The increase in myocyte size may be counter-balanced by the chronic loss of myocytes by the process of apoptosis. Apoptosis (also referred to as "programmed cell death"), is a normal feature of tissue development in the fetus and is common in rapidly dividing adult tissues such as the thymus. In distinction to necrosis, apoptosis is a genetically-regulated process that is energy-dependent and involves a series of molecular and biochemical events culminating in the engulfment of targeted cells by neighboring cells in the absence of inflammation. Apoptosis is characterized by condensation of nuclear chromatin within an intact nuclear membrane, condensation of the cytosol and shrinkage of the cell. DNA undergoes double-stranded breaks resulting in nucleosome-sized fragments of 180-200 base pairs, that can be seen as a characteristic "ladder" of small DNA fragments in multiples of 180 - 200 base pairs on agarose gel electrophoresis. Double-stranded DNA breaks can also be visualized by histologic staining with the terminal deoxynucleotidyl transferase-mediated dUTP nick end-labeling (TUNEL) technique.

Narula et al. (10) and Olivetti et al. (11) have provided the first evidence that apoptosis may occur in failing human myocardium. These observations were at first surprising because apoptosis is generally associated with cells that are undergoing mitosis, and not in terminally-differentiated adult cells such as cardiac myocytes. However, increasing evidence from several *in vitro* systems and animal models has supported the thesis that cardiac myocytes can undergo apoptosis, and have implicated a variety or insults that can stimulate the process, including ischemia-reperfusion (12), myocardial infarction (13,14), rapid ventricular pacing (15), mechanical stretch (16), and pressure overload due to aortic constriction (17). Despite the persuasive evidence that apoptosis can occur in the myocardium, it is not known if apoptosis actually contributes to myocardial failure. Indeed, the percentage of apoptotic cells observed in failing human myocardium is very low, on the order of than 0.2 % (11). Although this appears to be an insignificant number of cells to affect cardiac function, it should be noted that apoptosis is a transient event, lasting only hours. Therefore, the observation that 0.2% of cells are involved at any given time, when summated over months or years, could account for the loss of a large fraction of the total myocyte pool (18). The demonstration of apoptosis in failing human hearts has led to the thesis that continuing loss of viable myocytes is a mechanism for progressive myocardial failure.

Altered interstitial matrix. The interstitial matrix of the heart plays an important role in determining the structural characteristics of the myocardium. The extracellular matrix consists of a large number of components including several types of collagen, proteoglycans, glycoproteins, peptide growth factors, proteases and protease inhibitors. Changes in the nature and quantity of the extracellular matrix may play a role in determining the response of the myocardium to pathologic stimuli (19). For example, a reduction in the quantity or quality of collagen might reduce the integrity of the extracellular skeleton leading to chamber dilation. Alternatively, increased expression of interstitial matrix proteins may result in interstitial fibrosis that can impair relaxation of the myocardium(20) and/or limit the delivery of nutrients to myocytes. The biology of the interstitial matrix is affected by several substances that may be present or increased in the failing heart such as norepinephrine, which can act on β-adrenergic receptors on fibroblasts to stimulate DNA and protein synthesis (21), and endothelin-1, which can affect both the synthesis and degradation of collagen in the myocardium (22)

Components of the extracellular matrix (e.g., collagen, fibronectin, osteopontin) can also serve as ligands for cell membrane integrins that interact with adhesion molecules (e.g., ICAM, VCAM) that may be expressed on the surface of myocytes and other cells in the myocardium under various conditions (23-25). Although little is known about integrin signaling in the myocardium, it is likely that such interactions play an important role in directing biologic events such as cell growth and apoptosis that are involved in myocardial remodeling.

Fetal phenotype.   A characteristic of remodeled myocardium is the re-induction of fetal genes that are normally not expressed in adult myocardium. Atrial natriuretic peptide (ANP) and brain natriuretic peptide (BNP) are normally expressed in fetal cardiac tissue but not normal adult ventricular tissue. However, both are re-expressed in left ventricular myocardium from patients with heart failure (26). The re-expression of fetal genes is often associated with a reciprocal decrease in the expression of certain adult, muscle-specific genes such as sarcoplasmic reticulum Ca^{++}-ATPase (SERCA2). SERCA, a protein which is important for excitation-contraction coupling, is normally expressed in abundance in normal adult myocardium, but is reduced in ventricular myocardium from patients with heart failure (27).

There is evidence that different types of remodeling may be associated with distinct patterns of gene expression reflecting different molecular phenotypes (21). We found that in rats with pressure overload caused by aortic constriction there was induction of mRNAs for α-skeletal actin and β-myosin heavy chain, whereas with volume overload due to aorto-caval fistula neither was induced. Likewise, there is heterogeneity in the expression of peptide growth factors (e.g., transforming growth factor-β, fibroblast growth factor) which might exert important effects on the growth and phenotype of myocardial cells , and thus may be involved in orchestrating specific form phenotypes (21).   In support of this thesis, cardiotrophin-1 (CT-1), a cytokine related to the interleukin-6 family, can induce myocyte hypertrophy that is characterized by an increase in cell length (but not width), suggesting that CT-1 is a stimulus-specific determinant of myocyte phenotype of the type observed with volume overload (28). The expression of a fetal phenotype may occur in distinct stages during the development of heart failure (29,30). For example, in rats with pressure overload due to aortic banding, the expression of SERCA2 mRNA is normal at 10 weeks when myocardial hypertrophy is well established, but is decreased at 20 weeks when heart failure has developed (29).

Impaired calcium handling.   Calcium homeostasis is abnormal in failing myocardium.   In ventricular myocytes isolated from patients with severe dilated cardiomyopathy, there is prolongation of both the action potential and the intracellular calcium transient (31).   In these cells, the intracellular calcium transient does not rise normally after stimulation and remains elevated for a prolonged time. This perturbation in calcium handling is associated with abnormal levels of the mRNAs for several important calcium-handling proteins such as the voltage-dependent Ca^{++} channels (VDCC), SERCA2 and phospholamban, all of which are depressed in myocardium from patients with dilated cardiomyopathy (27,32,33). The mRNA for the calcium release channel (CRC), which mediates the release of calcium by the sarcoplasmic reticulum, is reduced in myocardium obtained from patients with ischemic, but not idiopathic cardiomyopathy (34). There may also be functional abnormalities in some of these proteins (35). These observations have led to the thesis that one or more of these alterations in the expression or function of excitation-contraction coupling proteins contributes to myocardial dysfunction.

Contractile proteins. The proteins responsible for generating contractile force in the myocardium include actin, myosin, and a complex of regulatory proteins (tropomyosin, troponin C, troponin I and troponin T). There are 3 isoenzymes of myosin designated V_1, V_2 and V_3. Of these, V_2 and V_3 have reduced ATPase activity and a slower velocity of shortening. It has long been known that chronic pressure overload in rodent models is associated with increased expression of the fetal isoforms, V_2 and V_3, and conversely, chronic endurance-type exercise (e.g., swimming) was associated with a decrease in the V_2 and V_3 isoforms and an increase in ATPase activity and shortening velocity. These observations led to the suggestion that a shift to fetal myosin isoforms could contribute to myocardial dysfunction. For many years it was believed that the slow V_3 isoform already predominated in human myocardium, and that no further shift toward a fetal phenotype occurred with hypertrophy or failure.

This situation was changed dramatically by the recent demonstration by Lowes et al. (36) that there is in fact a significant shift toward fetal myosin isoforms in failing human myocardium associated with reduced contractile function. Many of the stimuli that cause myocyte hypertrophy (e.g., norepinephrine, endothelin, angiotensin) can induce a shift in myosin isoforms, and thus may contribute to dysfunction of hypertrophied cells. Other members of the contractile apparatus regulatory proteins may also be altered in remodeling. Troponin T regulates the interaction of actin and myosin. In normal myocardium, there is a single isoform, referred to as troponin T_1. However, in failing human myocardium a second, fetal isoform (troponin T_2) is increased (37). It is not known if this isoform shift has functional significance.

Apoptosis as a fetal response. Why does apoptosis occur in remodeling myocardium? One possibility is that that apoptosis reflects an aborted growth response to pathologic stimuli that cause re-expression of a fetal growth program in cells that are no longer capable of undergoing mitosis. By analogy to its role in normal fetal tissue development, apoptosis may be part of a fetal response to growth stimuli in adult myocardium exposed to abnormal stresses. In support of the view, several factors that can cause hypertrophy in cardiac myocytes *in vitro,* including catecholamines, angiotensin, inflammatory cytokines, reactive oxygen species and mechanical stress, have been shown to cause apoptosis. Of note, most of these factors have also been implicated as being present in remodeling myocardium.

STIMULI AND MEDIATORS FOR MYOCARDIAL REMODELING

In vitro studies have shown that several stimuli and molecules can mimic features of myocardial remodeling (e.g., myocyte hypertrophy, fetal gene induction, apoptosis) (Figure 1). These observations are of interest because many of factors (e.g., mechanical stress, catecholamines, angiotensin, endothelin, inflammatory cytokines, and reactive oxygen species) appear to be present in remodeling myocardium. Taken together, these findings have led to an intense interest in the stimuli for myocardial remodeling.

Mechanical strain.   Hemodynamic overload is a frequently studied stimulus for myocardial remodeling. *In vitro* it can be shown that an increase in mechanical stresses on the cardiac myocyte can be a direct stimulus for growth and altered gene expression. In cardiac myocytes grown on a silastic membrane, stretching in length by 20% increases cellular protein content by approximately 30% (38). This effect is associated with the activation of multiple second messenger pathways including calcium influx, inositol phosphate generation, activation of protein kinase-C and mitogen-activated protein kinase, and the induction of early response (e.g., c-*fos*) and fetal genes (e.g., prepro-ANF). Only myocytes are present in this experiment, and therefore these findings suggest that mechanical deformation of the myocyte, per se, can stimulate growth and gene expression in the myocyte. Myocyte stretch may also cause the release of peptides such TGF-β (39), angiotensin (9) and endothelin (40). Chang et al. (16) have shown that mechanical stretching of the myocardium can cause apoptosis of cardiac myocytes, which, as discussed later, is associated with the generation of increased amounts of superoxide; and that the stretch-induced apoptosis can be attenuated by a nitric oxide donor that may work by scavenging the superoxide.

Catecholamines.   Sympathetic innervation has been implicated as a major stimulus for myocardial remodeling. Much of the evidence for this thesis is based on the observation that *in vitro* norepinephrine stimulates myocyte hypertrophy (4,5,41), expression of fetal genes, down-regulation of calcium-regulating genes and the expression of TGF-β (42). In neonatal rat myocytes, this response to norepinephrine is mediated primarily by the α_1-adrenergic pathway, whereas both α_1- and β-adrenergic receptors appear to be coupled in adult rat myocytes (41).

In vitro studies by Mann et al. (42) showed that the exposure of cardiac myocytes to norepinephrine caused a concentration-dependent decrease in the number of viable cells. This effect was inhibited by a β-adrenergic antagonist indicating that it is mediated by β-adrenergic receptors. We examined whether this effect was due to apoptosis by exposing myocytes cultured from the adult rat hearts to norepinephrine for 24 hours (43). Under these conditions there was an approximately 4-fold increase in the number of apoptotic cells as assessed by the TUNEL method. As with the work of Mann et al. (42), this effect was inhibited by a β-adrenergic antagonist, but not an a-adrenergic antagonist, indicating that it is mediated by the β-adrenergic pathway. Norepinephrine has effects on other cardiac cell types including fibroblasts, in which it stimulates DNA and protein synthesis, also via activation of β-adrenergic receptors (44).

Transgenic mice that over-express the G_s-protein α-subunit develop left ventricular dilation, reduced systolic contraction, and increased mortality (45). Of note, an increased rate of myocyte apoptosis has been observed in the hearts of these mice, supporting the thesis that tonic activation of the β-adrenergic pathway could contribute to myocardial failure by causing myocyte apoptosis (45). Taken together with the *in vitro* studies, this later observation suggests that norepinephrine may play an important role in pathologic myocardial remodeling.

Angiotensin.   Like norepinephrine, angiotensin can stimulate protein synthesis in cardiac myocytes and DNA synthesis in cardiac fibroblasts *in vitro* (6). Angiotensin has also been shown to cause apoptosis in cardiac myocytes in culture (46), and both the hypertrophic and apoptotic effects are blocked by an AT_1-selective antagonist. These observations indicate that angiotensin has the potential to act directly on cardiac cells, independent of its vascular and metabolic actions.

All of the components of the renin-angiotensin system are present in the myocardium. Interestingly, several components of the myocardial renin-angiotensin system, including angiotensin converting enzyme activity, angiotensinogen and angiotensin-II receptors (47-49) are up-regulated in hypertrophied or failing myocardium. It has further been shown that angiotensin is present in cardiac myocytes (9), and that stretch of the myocyte can cause release of the angiotensin that appears to mediate the effects of stretch on myocyte growth, gene expression, and apoptosis (9). Thus, the tissue-based production of angiotensin could play a central role in pathologic myocardial remodeling in response to hemodynamic overload.

Endothelin and other peptides.   Like angiotensin, endothelin-1 (ET-1) is a potent vasoconstrictor peptide with important effects on cardiac myocyte growth and phenotype. *In vitro* exposure to endothelin for 24 hours stimulates cellular hypertrophy in neonatal rat cardiac myocytes (7). Also like angiotensin, ET-1 can be synthesized within the myocardium, and both the synthesis of ET-1 and its receptors are increased in hypertrophied myocardium (50). Inhibition of the ET_A subtype receptor with the non-peptide antagonist BQ-123 increased survival in rats following myocardial infarction (51), suggesting that ET-1 may play a role similar to that of angiotensin as an autocrine/paracrine mediator of myocardial remodeling in response to hemodynamic overload (52).

In vitro, several other peptides have been shown to affect the growth and phenotype of cardiac myocytes or fibroblasts, including acidic fibroblast growth factor, basic fibroblast growth factor, transforming growth factor-$β_1$ and platelet-derived growth factor (53). A role for these peptide growth factors in myocardial remodeling is suggested by the demonstration that their expression is regulated *in vitro* by remodeling stimuli such as norepinephrine (39) and stretch, and that their level of expression is increased in myocardium following myocardial infarction (54) or with hemodynamic overload (21).

Inflammatory cytokines.   Plasma levels of the inflammatory cytokines tumor necrosis factor-α (TNF-α) and interleukin-6 (IL-6) are elevated in patients with heart failure (55,56). The levels of TNF-α and IL-6 correlate with each other, but not with neurohormones such as plasma norepinephrine, renin, vasopressin or atrial natriuretic peptide. The pathophysiologic role of inflammatory cytokines remains to be determined. However, there is evidence that plasma TNF-α is a better predictor of survival than norepinephrine. The failing myocardium may be a source of inflammatory cytokines which might thus be present in high local concentrations (57).

Inflammatory cytokines might influence myocardial remodeling by several mechanisms. The cytokines might directly stimulate myocyte and fibroblast receptors. *In vitro*, interleukin-1β (IL-1β) stimulates hypertrophy of cardiac myocytes and re-expression of a fetal gene program (8). At least one cytokine, TNF-α has been shown to cause apoptosis in cultured cardiac myocytes (58), whereas other cytokines (e.g., IL-6) can induce the expression of adhesion molecules such as intercellular adhesion molecule-1 (ICAM-1) (59,60). Inflammatory cytokines might also act through the induction of reactive oxygen species including superoxide and nitric oxide (NO).

Reactive oxygen species and NO.   Exposure to high levels of free radicals appears to play a central role in causing injury to the myocardium during hypoxia and reperfusion. There is growing evidence that reactive oxygen species may also mediate myocardial remodeling over longer periods of time. The stretching of rat papillary muscle for 3 hours causes increased generation of superoxide, induction of the Fas protein and apoptosis of myocytes and fibroblasts (16). The addition of a NO-releasing agent attenuated both the generation of reactive oxygen species and apoptosis, perhaps by scavenging superoxide. These findings led to the suggestion that increased generation of reactive oxygen species due to mechanical strain may be a cause of myocardial apoptosis. It has also been shown that inflammatory cytokines such as TNF-α can stimulate superoxide generation (61).

We have found that chronic exposure to a modest increase in superoxide can stimulate apoptosis in cardiac myocytes in culture (62).   Reactive oxygen species have also been shown to induce the expression of immediate early genes (63), and to stimulate fibroblast proliferation (64). Prior work suggested that oxidative stress is increased in the myocardium during the transition from compensated hypertrophy to failure (65,66). For example, in guinea pigs with chronic pressure overload due to banding of the aorta, endogenous antioxidant activity is increased at 10 weeks, at a time when the hearts have compensated hypertrophy (65). However, by 20 weeks, at a time when there is myocardial dysfunction as evidenced by a decrease in left ventricular developed pressure and an increase in left ventricular end-diastolic pressure, endogenous antioxidant pathways are depleted as reflected by a decreased ratio of reduced to oxidized glutathione and increased lipid peroxidation. Of note, administration vitamin-E, an endogenous antioxidant, prevented the development of hemodynamic failure at 20 weeks (66). These observations raise the possibility that increased oxidative stress in the myocardium contributes to myocardial failure, and therefore, that antioxidants may be of value in the prevention of myocardial failure.

The human myocardium expresses at least two isoforms of the enzyme nitric oxide synthase NOS, termed NOS2 and NOS3 (67,68). The inducible isoform of NOS (NOS2) is not normally expressed in the myocardium, but is synthesized *de novo* in response to inflammatory cytokines thereby causing high levels of NO production within the myocardium (69,70). It appears that the expression and activity of NOS2 are increased in myocardium obtained from patients with severe heart failure (67,68).

There a several ways that NO might affect the myocardium (71). It has been shown that NO mediates the inhibitory effect of inflammatory cytokines on the contractile response to β-adrenergic stimulation in cardiac myocytes and myocardium by the induction of NOS2 (72,73). We have used the intracoronary infusion of the NOS inhibitor N^G-monomethyl-L-arginine (L-NMMA) to demonstrate the relevance of these observations to patients with LV dysfunction. Under these conditions, inhibition of NOS potentiated the positive inotropic response to β-adrenergic receptor stimulation in patients with heart failure, but not those with normal LV function (74,75). Similar observations were made *in vitro* in isolated cardiac myocytes obtained from dogs with pacing-induced heart failure (76). Thus, it appears that increased NO production in the myocardium contributes to impaired adrenergic responsiveness of the myocardium in patients with heart failure.

Beyond these functional effects, NO may contribute to the death of cardiac myocytes due to direct toxicity (77). For example, in vascular smooth muscle cells it has been shown that exposure to high levels of NO induces apoptosis (78). The mechanism of this toxic action is not known, but might involve NO's ability to form reactive oxygen species such as peroxynitrite. Alternatively, there is evidence from *in vitro* experiments that atrial natriuretic peptide can cause apoptosis of neonatal rat cardiac myocytes (79). Since ANP, like NO, increases cGMP production, this observation suggests that cGMP could also mediate the toxic effect of NO.

SUMMARY

Myocardial remodeling is a central mechanism in the development of myocardial failure. Myocardial remodeling consists of changes in the structure and function of the myocardium associated with myocyte hypertrophy and apoptosis, a shift in the molecular phenotype with re-expression of a fetal gene program, and changes in the extracellular matrix. Activation of the sympathetic nervous and the renin-angiotensin systems appear to be causes of remodeling due to direct effects on the biology of the myocardium. Recent recognition that myocardial failure is associated with myocardial expression of endothelin, inflammatory cytokines, and reactive oxygen species such as superoxide and NO, raises the possibility that these factors may also be involved in myocardial remodeling. Understanding the basic mechanisms that stimulate and mediate myocardial remodeling may lead to novel strategies to slow the process of myocardial remodeling and the development of clinical heart failure.

REFERENCES

1. Cohn JN. Structural basis for heart failure. Ventricular remodeling and pharmacological inhibition. Circulation 1995; 91: 2504-2507.

2. Katz AM. The cardiomyopathy of overload: an unnatural growth response in the hypertrophied heart. Annals of Internal Medicine 1994; 121:363-371.

3. Anversa P, Ricci R & Olivetti G. Quantitative structural analysis of the myocardium during growth and induced cardiac hypertrophy: A review. Journal of the American College of Cardiology 1986; 7:1140-1149.

4. Simpson P & McGrath A . Norepinephrine-stimulated hypertrophy of cultured rat myocardial cells is an alpha$_1$ adrenergic response. Journal of Clinical Investigation 1983; 72:732-738.

5. Knowlton KU, Michel MC, Itani M, Shubeita HE, Ishihara K, Brown JH & Chien KR. The α_{1A} adrenergic receptor subtype mediates biochemical, molecular, and morphologic features of cultured myocardial cell hypertrophy. Journal of Biological Chemistry 1993; 268: 15374-15380.

6. Sadoshima J-i & Izumo S. Molecular characterization of angiotensin II-induced hypertrophy of cardiac myocytes and hyperplasia of cardiac fibroblasts. Critical role of the AT$_1$ receptor subtype. Circulation Research 1993; 73:413-423.

7. Shubeita HE, McDonough PM, Harris AN, Knowlton KU, Glembotski CC, Brown JH & Chien KR. Endothelin induction of inositol phospholipid hydrolysis, sarcomere assembly, and cardiac gene expression in ventricular myocytes. A paracrine mechanism for myocardial cell hypertrophy. Journal of Biological Chemistry 1990; 265:20555-20562.

8. Thaik CM, Calderone A, Takahashi N & Colucci WS. Interleukin-1B modulates the growth and phenotype of neonatal rat cardiac myocytes. Journal of Clinical Investigation 1995; 96:1093-1099.

9. Sadoshima J-i, Xu Y, Slayter HS & Izumo S. Autocrine release of angiotensin II mediates stretch-induced hypertrophy of cardiac myocytes in vitro. Cell 1993; 75:977-984.

10. Narula J, Haider N, Virmani R, DiSalvo TG, Kolodgie FD, Hajjar RJ, Schmidt U, Semigran MJ, Dec GW, Khaw B-A. Programmed myocyte death in end-stage heart failure. N Eng J Med 1996; 335: 1182-1189.

11. Olivetti G, Abbi R, Quaini F, Kajstura J, Cheng W, Nitahara JA, Quaini E, DeLoreto C, Beltrami CA, Krajewski S, Reed JC & Anversa P. Apoptosis in the failing human heart. New England Journal of Medicine 1997; 336:1131-1141.

12. Gottlieb RA, Burleson KO, Kloner RA, Babior BM, Engler RL. Reperfusion injury induces apoptosis in rabbit cardiomyocytes. J Clin Invest 1994;94:1621-1628.

13. Kajstura J, ChengW, Reiss K, Clark WA, Sonnenblick EH, Krajewski S, Reed JC, Olivetrti G, Anversa P. Apoptotic and necrotic myocyte cell death are independent contributing variables of infarct size in rats. Lab Invest 1996; 74: 86-107.

14. Saraste A, Pulkki K, Kallajoki M, Henriksen K, Parvinen M, Voipio-Pulkki L-M. Apoptosis in human acute myocardial infarction. Circulation 1997;95:320-323.

15. Liu Y, Cigola E, Cheng W, Kajstura J, Olivetti G, Hintze TH, Anversa P. Myocyte nuclear mitotic division and programmed myocyte death characterize the cardiac myopathy induced by rapid ventricular pacing in dogs. Lab Invest. 1995; 73 771-787.

16. Cheng W, Li B, Kajstura J, Li P, Wolin MS, Sonnenblick EH, Hintze TH, Olivetti G, Anversa P. Stretch-induced programmed myocyte cell death. J Clin Invest 1995; 96: 2247-2259.

17. Teiger E, Dam T-V, Richard L, Wisnewsky C, Tea B-S, Gaboury L, Tremblay J, Schwartz K, Hamet P. Apoptosis in pressure overload-induced heart hypertrophy in the rat. J Clin Invest 1996; 97:2891-2897.

18. Colucci WS. Apoptosis in the heart. N Eng J Med 1996; 335: 1224-1226.

19. Weber KT & Brilla CG. Pathological hypertrophy and cardiac interstitium. Fibrosis and renin-angiotensin-aldosterone system. Circulation 1991; 83:1849-1865.

20. Conrad CH, Brooks WW, Hayes JA, Sen S, Robinson KG, Bing OHL. Myocardial fibrosis and stiffness with hypertrophy and heart failure in the spontaneously hyertensive rat. Circulation 1995; 91: 161- 170.

21. Calderone A, Takahashi N, Izzo NJ, Thaik CM & Colucci WS. Pressure- and volume-induced left ventricular hypertrophies are associated with distinct myocyte phenotypes and differential induction of peptide growth factor mRNAs. Circulation 1995; 92; 2385-2390.

22. Guarda E, Katwa LC, Myers PR, Tyagi SC, Weber KT. Effects of endothelins on collagen turnover in cardiac fibroblasts. Cardiovasc Res 1993;27:2130-2134.

23. Terracio L, Rubin K, Gullberg D, Balog E, Carver W, Jyring R, Borg TK. Expression of collagen binding integrins during cardiac development and hypertrophy. Circ Res 1991;68:734-744.

24. Burgess ML, Carver WE, Terracio L, Wilson SP, Wilson MA, Borg TK. Integrin-mediated collagen gel contraction by cardiac fibroblasts. Circ Res 1994;74:291-298.

25. Ikeda U, Ikeda M, Kano S, Shimada K. Neutrophil adherence to rat cardiac myocyte by proinflammatory cytokines. J Cardiovasc Pharmacol 1994;23:647-652.

26. Takahashi T, Allen PD & Izumo S. Expression of A-, B-, and C-type natriuretic peptide genes in failing and developing human ventricles. Circulation Research 1992; 71:9-17.

27. Arai M, Alpert NR, MacLennan DH, Barton P & Periasamy M. Alterations in sarcoplasmic reticulum gene expression in human heart failure. 1993; Circulation Research 72:463-469.

28. Wollert KC, Taga T, Saito M, Narazaki M, Kishimoto T, Glembotski CC, Vernallis AB, Heath JK, Pennica D, Wood WI & Chien KR. Cardiotrophin-1 activates a distinct form of cardiac muscle cell hypertrophy. Assembly of sarcomeric units in series VIA gp130/leukemia inhibitory factor receptor-dependent pathways. J Biol Chem 1996; 271(16):9535-45.

29. Feldman AM, Weinberg EO, Ray PE and Lorell BH. Selective changes in cardiac gene expression during compensated hypertrophy and the transition to cardiac decompensation in rats with chronic aortic banding. Circulation Research 1993; 73:184-192.

30. Boluyt MO, O'Neill L, Meredith AL, Bing OHL, Brooks WW, Conrad CH, Crow MT, Lakatta EG. Alterations in cardiac gene expression during the transition from stable hypertrophy to heart failure. Circ Res 1994;75:23-32.

31. Beuckelmann DJ, Nabauer M & Erdmann E. Intracellular calcium handling in isolated ventricular myocytes from patients with terminal heart failure. Circulation 1992; 85:1046-1055.

32. Takahashi T, Allen PD, Lacro RV, Marks AR, Dennis AR, Schoen FJ, Grossman W, Marsh JD & Izumo S. Expression of dihydropyridine receptor (Ca^{2+} channel) and calsequestrin genes in the myocardium of patients with end-stage heart failure. Journal of Clinical Investigation 1992; 90:927-935.

33. Feldman AM, Ray PE, Silan CM, Mercer JA, Minobe W & Bristow MR. Selective gene expression in failing human heart. Quantification of steady-state levels of messenger RNA in endomyocardial biopsies using the polymerase chain reaction. Circulation 1991; 83:1866-1872.

34. Brillantes A-M, Allen P, Takahashi T, Izumo S & Marks AR. Differences in cardiac calcium release channel (ryanodine receptor) expression in myocardium from patients with end-stage heart failure caused by ischemic versus dilated cardiomyopathy. Circulation Research 1992; 71:18-26.

35. Gómez AM, Valdivia HH, Cheng H, Lederer MR, Santana LF, Cannell MB, McCune SA, Altschuld RA, Lederer WJ. Defective excitation-contraction coupling in experimental cardiac hypertrophy and heart failure. Science 1997;276:800-806.

36. Lowes BD, Minobe W, Abraham WT, Rizeq MN, Bohlmeyer TJ, Quaife RA, Roden RL, Dutcher DL, Robertson AD, Voelkel NF, Badesch DB, Groves BM, Gilbert EM, Bristow. Changes in gene expression in the intact human heart. Downregulation of alpha-myosin heavy chain in hypertrophied, failing ventricular myocardium. J Clin Invest. 1997;100:2315-24.

37. Anderson PAW, Malouf NN, Oakeley AE, Pagani ED & Allen PD. Troponin T isoform expression in the normal and failing human left ventricle: a correlation with myofibrillar ATPase activity. Basic Research in Cardiology 1992; 87:117-127.

38. Sadoshima J-i, Jahn L, Takahashi T, Kulik TJ & Izumo S. Molecular characterizations of the stretch-induced adaptation of cultured cardiac cells. An in vitro model of load-induced cardiac hypertrophy. Journal of Biological Chemistry 1992; 267:10551-10560.

39. Takahashi N, Calderone A, Izzo NJ Jr, Maki TM, Marsh JD & Colucci WS. Hypertrophic stimuli-induced transforming growth factor-β_1 expression in rat ventricular myocytes. Journal of Clinical Investigation 1994; 94:1470-1483.

40. Yamazaki T, Komuro I, Kudoh S, Zou Y, Shiojima I, Hiroi Y, Mizuno T, Maemura K, Kurihara H, Aikawa R, Takano H & Yazaki Y. Endothelin-1 is involved in mechanical stress-induced cardiomyocyte hypertrophy. Journal of Biological Chemistry 1996; 271:3221-3227.

41. Clark WA, Rudnick SJ, LaPres JJ, Andersen LC & LaPointe MC. Regulation of hypertrophy and atrophy in cultured adult heart cells. Circulation Research 1993; 73:1163-1176.

42. Mann DL, Kent RL, Parsons B & Cooper G. Adrenergic effects on the biology of the adult mammalian cardiocyte. Circulation 85;790-804.

43. Communal C, Singh K, Pimentel D, Colucci WS. Norepinephrine stimulates apoptosis in adult rat ventricular myocytes by activation of the β-adrenergic pathway. Circulation 1998;98: 1329-1334.

44. Calderone A, Thaik CM, Takahashi N, Colucci WS. Norepinephrine-stimulated DNA and protein synthesis in cardiac fibroblasts are inhibited by nitric oxide and atrial natriuretic factor. Circulation 1995; 92(Suppl I):I-384.

45. Geng YJ, Ishikawa Y, Vatner DE, Wagner TE, Bishop SP, Vatner SF, Homcy CJ. Overexpression of Gsα accelerates programmed cell death (apoptosis) of cardiomyocytes in transgenic mice. Circulation 1996; 94 (Suppl. 1): 1640 (abstr).

46. Kajstura J, Cigola E, Malhotra A, Li P, Cheng W, Meggs L & Anversa P. Angiotensin II induces apoptosis of adult ventricular myocytes in vitro. J Cell Cardiol 1997; 29:859-870.

47. Hirsch AT, Talsness CE, Schunkert H, Paul M & Dzau VJ. Tissue-specific activation of cardiac angiotensin converting enzyme in experimental heart failure. Circulation Research 1991; 69:475-482.

48. Lindpaintner K, Lu W, Niedermajer N, Schieffer B, Just H, Ganten D & Drexler H. Selective activation of cardiac angiotensinogen gene expression in post-infarction ventricular remodeling in the rat. Journal of Molecular and Cellular Cardiology 1993; 5:133-143.

49. Meggs LG, Coupet J, Huang H, Cheng W, Li P, Capasso JM, Homcy CJ & Anversa P (1993) Regulation of angiotensin II receptors on ventricular myocytes after myocardial infarction in rats. Circulation Research 72:1149-1162.

50. Sakai S, Miyauchi T, Sakurai T, Kasuya Y, Ihara M, yamaguchi I, Goto K, Sugishita Y. Endogenous endothelin-1 participates in the maintenance of cardiac function in rats with

congestive heart failure: marked increase in endothelin-1 production in the failig heart. Circulation 1996; 93:1214-1222.

51.   Sakai S, Miyauchi T, Kobayashi M, Yamaguchi I, Goto K & Sugishita Y. Inhibition of myocardial endothelin pathway improves long-term survival in heart failure. Letters to Nature 1996; 384:353-355.

52.   Colucci WS. Myocardial Endothelin. Does it play a role in myocardial failure?   1996; Circulation 93:1069-1072.49.Parker TG, Packer SE & Schneider MD. Peptide growth factors can provoke "fetal" contractile protein gene expression in rat cardiac myocytes. Journal of Clinical Investigation 1990; 85:507-514.

53.   Parker TG, Packer SE & Schneider MD. Peptide growth factors can provoke "fetal" contractile protein gene expression in rat cardiac myocytes. Journal of Clinical Investigation 1990; 85:507-514.

54.   Casscells W, Bazoberry F, Speir E, Thompson N, Flanders K, Kondaiah P, Ferrans VJ, Epstein SE & Sporn M. Transforming growth factor- 1 in normal heart and in   myocardial   infarction. Annals of the New York Academy of Science 1990; 593:148-160.

55.   Levine B, Kalman J, Mayer L, Fillit HM, Packer M. Elevated circulating levels of tumor necrosis factor in severe chronic heart failure. N Engl J Med 1990;223:236-241.

56.   Torre-Amione G, Kapadia S, Benedict C, Oral H, Young JB, Mann D. Proinflammatory cytokine levels in patients with depressed left ventricular ejection fraction: A report from the studies of left ventricular dysfunction (SOLVD). J Am Coll Cardiol 1996;27:1201-1206.

57.   Torre-Amione G, Kapadia S, Lee J, Durand JB, Bies RD, Young JB, Mann DL. Tumor necrosis factor-α and tumor necrosis factor receptors in the failing human heart. Circulation 1996;93:704-711.

58.   Krown KA, Page MT, Nguyen C, Zechner D, Gutierrez V, Comstock KL, Glembotski CC, Quintana PJE & Sabbadini RA. Tumor necrosis factor alpha-induced apoptosis in cardiac myocytes. Involvement of the sphingolipid signaling cascade in cardiac cell death. Journal of Clinical Investigation 1996; 98:2854-2865.

59.   Youker K, Smith CW, Anderson DC, Miller D, Michael LH, Rossen RD & Entman ML. Neutrophil adherence to isolated adult cardiac myocytes. Journal of Clinical Investigation 1992; 89:602-609.

60.   Ikeda U, Ikeda M, Kano S, Shimada K. Neutrophil adherence to rat cardiac myocyte by proinflamatory cytokines. J Cardiovasc Pharmacol 1994; 23: 47-652.

61.   Meier B, Radeke HH, Selle S, Younes M, Sies H, Resch, K & Habermehl GG. Human fibroblasts release reactive oxygen species in response to interleukin-1 or tumour necrosis factor-alpha. Biochem J 1989; 263:539-545.

62.   Tzortzis JD, Siwik DA, Chang DL-F, Singh K, Commuanal C, Pagano P, Colucci WS. Chronic oxidative stress induces a hypertrophic phenotype and apoptosis in neonatal rat cardiac myocytes. Circulation 1997; 96 (suppl. I): I-605.

63.   Webster KA, Discher DJ, Bishopric NH. Regulation of *fos* and *jun* immediate-early genes by redox or metabolic stress in cardiac myocytes. Circ Res 1994;74:679-686.

64.   Murrell A C, Francis M & Bromley L. Modulation of fibroblast proliferation by oxygen free radicals. Biochem J 1990; 265:659-665.

65.   Dhalla AK & Singal PK. Antioxidant changes in hypertrophied and failing guinea pig hearts. American Physiological Society 1994; H1280-H1285.

66.   Dhalla AK, Hill MF & Singal PK. Role of oxidative stress in transition of hypertrophy to heart failure. J Am Coll Cardiol 1996; 28:506-514.

67. DeBelder AJ, Radomski MW, Why JF, Richardson PJ, Martin JF. Myocardial calcium-independent nitric oxide synthase activity is present in dilated cardiomyopathy, myocarditis, and postpartum cardiomyopathy but not in ischaemic or valvar heart disease. Br Heart J 1995;74:426-430.

68. Haywood GA, Tsao PS, von der Leyen HE, Mann MJ, Keeling PJ, Trindade PT, Lewis NP, Byrne CD, Rickenbacher PR, Bishopric NH, Cooke JP, McKenna WJ, Fowler MB. Expression of inducible nitric oxide synthase in human heart failure.Circulation 1996;931087-1094.

69. Schulz R, Nava E, Moncada S. Induction and potential biological relevance of a Ca^{2+}-independent nitric oxide synthase in the myocardium. Br J Pharmacol 1992;105:575-580.

70. Balligand J-L, Ungureanu-Longrois D, Simmons WW, Pimental D, Malinski TA, Kapturczak M, Taha Z, Lowenstein C, Davidoff AJ, Kelly RA, Smith TW, Michel T. Cytokine-inducible nitric oxide synthase (iNOS) expression in cardiac myocytes: Characterization and regulation of iNOS expression and detection of iNOS activity in single cardiac myocytes in vitro. J Biol Chem 1994;269:27580-27588.

71. Hare JM, Colucci WS. Role of nitric oxide in the regulation of myocardial function. Prog Cardiovasc Dis 1995;38:155-166.

72. Balligand J-L, Ungureanu D, Kelly RA, Kobzik L, Pimental D, Michel T, Smith TW. Abnormal contractile function due to induction of nitric oxide synthesis in rat cardiac myocytes follows exposure to activated macrophage-conditioned medium. J Clin Invest 1993;91:2314-2319.

73. Brady AJB, Poole-Wilson PA, Harding SE, Warren JB. Nitric oxide production within cardiac myocytes reduces their contractility in endotoxemia. Am J Physiol 1992;263:H1963-H1966.

74. Hare JM, Loh E, Creager MA, Colucci WS. Nitric oxide inhibits the contractile response to β-adrenergic stimulation in humans with left ventricular dysfunction. Circulation   1995;92:2198-2203.

75. Hare JM, Givertz MM, Creager MA, Colucci WS. Increased sensitivity to nitric oxide inhibition in patients with heart failure: Potentiation of β-adrenergic inotropic responsiveness. Circulation 1998; 97: 161-166.

76. Yamamoto S, Tsusui H, Tagawa H, Saito K, Takahashi M, Tada H, Yamamoto M, Katoh M, Egashira K & Takeshita A. Role of myocyte nitric oxide in β-adrenergic hyporesponsiveness in heart failure. Circulation 1997; 95:1111-1114.

77. Pinsky DJ, Cai B, Yang X, Rodriguez C, Sciacca RR, Cannon PJ. The lethal effects of cytokine-induced nitric oxide on cardiac myocytes are blocked by nitric oxide synthase antagonism or transforming growth factor beta. J Clin Invest 1995;95:677-685.

78. Fukuo K, Hata T, Suhara T, Nakahashi T, Shinto Y, Tsujimoto Y, Morimoto S, Ogihara T. Nitric oxide induces upregulation of Fas and apoptosis in vascular smooth muscle. Hypertension 1996;27:823-826.

79. Wu C-F, Bishopric, Pratt RE. Atrial natriuretic peptide induce apoptosis in neonatal rat cardiac myocytes. J Biol Chem 1997; 272: 1460-14866.

3 PATHOPHYSIOLOGY OF HEART FAILURE IN REGURGITANT VALVULAR DISEASES: RELATION TO VENTRICULAR DYSFUNCTION AND CLINICAL DEBILITY

Jeffrey S. Borer, M.D.
Edmund M. Herrold, M.D., Ph.D.
Clare A. Hochreiter, M.D.
Sharada L. Truter, Ph.D.
John N. Carter, Ph.D.
Steven M. Goldfine, Ph.D.
Cornell Univeristy Medical College

INTRODUCTION

Regurgitant valvular heart diseases and, most particularly, insufficiency of the aortic and/or mitral valves (AR, MR), are among the more common, and most predictable, causes of congestive heart failure. Current data suggest that these conditions also confer a proclivity for sudden death, even among asymptomatic or minimally symptomatic patients (1,2,3).

Most often, regurgitant valvular conditions are chronic and, even when hemodynamically severe, usually are not associated with debilitating clinical sequelae until the regurgitant lesion has been established for many years. Consequently, longitudinal study of these diseases is difficult: evaluation requires prolonged serial assessment of many patients using both clinical and objective methods. In an era of increasing cost-consciousness and decreasing support for clinical research, the resources required to support such study seldom are available. Animal models suitable for study of the fundamental pathophysiology of these diseases do not exist in nature and, in part because of the prolonged natural course of the diseases, are relatively difficult to create and maintain.

During the past 20 years, the availability of clinically applicable non-invasive imaging modalities has enabled collection of considerable data defining the natural history of cardiac function associated with these diseases and enabling prognostication for clinical outcomes. This information has been employed to generate hypotheses concerning cellular and molecular variations that may account for clinical phenomena and envisioning potentially beneficial pharmacological interventions. In parallel, investigators have overcome some of the problems associated with creating useful animal models (4,5) and, in addition, have begun to harness the increasing technical facility for cellular and molecular studies in small tissue samples to interrogate both animal specimens and human biopsies in search of answers to fundamental questions. As a result, knowledge of the pathobiology of regurgitant valvular diseases has increased considerably, holding hope for development of new and increasingly effective management strategies and treatment modalities.

This essay will review the clinical data which have driven recent cellular and molecular studies, the whole animal studies which have modeled the clinical disease, and a selection of the recent cellular and molecular experiments and observations which are adding importantly to our understanding of the fundamental basis of cardiac dysfunction and clinical debility in patients with regurgitant valvular diseases.

Relatively few investigators focus specifically on the basic pathobiology of valvular diseases and, thus, this review will be heavily skewed toward work performed in our own laboratories during the past 15 years. In addition, while much effort in the general area of heart failure has focused on the importance of biological variations of cardiac myocytes, our work with regurgitant valvular diseases, like that of others studying stenotic lesions (6), has highlighted the potential pathogenic importance of disease-induced variations of the cardiac fibroblast (7). Therefore, though this chapter will provide some corollary background data concerning abnormalities associated with cardiomyocytes, the primary focus of our review of basic science studies will be the cardiac fibroblast. Since some of our data, and particularly those involving molecular techniques, are preliminary and/or not yet published in peer-reviewed literature, many of the more recent observations will be presented summarily. The chapter will end with a discussion of the therapeutic implications of these findings. It is hoped that this review will provide a focused overview of current knowledge and, of equal importance, will elucidate the many major gaps in our knowledge that require additional investigation.

THE SCOPE OF THE PROBLEM

The true incidence and prevalence of regurgitant valvular diseases are not well defined, but all available evidence suggests that these abnormalities are far more common than generally is appreciated. For example, in a recent echocardiographic survey of 4000 patients younger than age 35, ≥1+ aortic regurgitation was present in 2% of the population while $\geq$2+ mitral regurgitation was present in 1½% (8). This is a minimal estimate: today, most common causes of valvular regurgitation involve inborn variations in connective tissue structures (mitral valve prolapse, idiopathic aortic root dilatation, etc.) for which the association with valve dysfunction (and the severity of such dysfunction) increases with age. Thus, several million Americans have regurgitant valvular abnormalities, and a large subset has hemodynamically severe and potentially clinically important disease. However, at any one time, most of these people are not clinically ill. "Decompensation" (i.e., cardiac functional and symptomatic debility) results when the mechanical loads on the left ventricle (LV) and, in the case of MR, the right ventricle (RV), exceed the capacity of the ventricles to pump blood in sufficient quantity to meet systemic demands; this situation usually is associated with, and preceded by, development of subnormal myocardial contractility ("systolic function") and compromised chamber compliance and/or active relaxation ("diastolic dysfunction"). Regurgitation can result from sudden loss of valve integrity (cordal rupture, leaflet avulsion) but, more commonly, regurgitation increases slowly, associated with ventricular geometric remodeling and myocardial growth which initially retard the occurrence of decompensation but which ultimately may potentiate organ dysfunction.

From the development of hemodynamically severe valvular regurgitation, many years typically intervene before objective evidence of cardiac dysfunction can be detected by any but the most sophisticated testing methods and before heart failure (CHF) becomes clinically apparent or sudden death occurs. Finally, the prevalence of these lesions, while not on a par with coronary artery disease or hypertension as a cause of CHF, nonetheless is sufficient to render valvular regurgitation a true public health concern.

NATURAL HISTORY AND PROGNOSTICATION

As noted above, even when valvular regurgitation is severe, progression to clinical debility typically is slow. From epidemiological studies in patients with pure, isolated severe AR who are first evaluated when they are asymptomatic or minimally symptomatic, rate of progression to CHF, subnormal LV ejection fraction at rest or sudden death varies from 4% to 6.2% (1,9,10,11). In the absence of confounding intercurrent processes, precipitous deterioration in LV function does not occur among asymptomatic patients. Nonetheless, though uncommon, sudden death can occur even in the asymptomatic patient with normal LV ejection fraction at rest. This problem has been recognized only recently, with the publication of the longest and largest of the epidemiological studies, in which 4% of patients died suddenly, generally before manifesting clinical deterioration (1). (Once congestive symptoms develop, progression to death is considerably faster.) Thus, there is great need for recognition of fundamental processes which may enable therapies to retard cardiac dysfunction or, at the very least, which can be interrogated to help optimize timing of currently available management strategies, most particularly including surgical replacement or repair of the defective valve.

Currently, prognostication in AR is best achieved with reference to measures of LV performance or function (1,9,10,11,12). Recent data suggest that prognostication is most accurate when measures are obtained not only at rest but also during the interposition of the added stress of exercise (1). Our group has shown that markedly subnormal intrinsic LV contractility, measured as the change in LV ejection fraction from rest to exercise normalized to the change in LV end systolic wall stress from rest to exercise, can predict imminence of subnormal LV ejection fraction at rest (itself a very powerful prognosticator which appears only relatively late in the course of disease) and of congestive symptoms. The same measure can predict patients at risk of sudden death while still asymptomatic, though this risk is relatively small (1), and retains its prognostic power when made shortly before surgical aortic valve replacement to predict long-term post-operative outcome (13).

Thus, natural history among patients with AR is most closely related to intrinsic myocardial contractility, suggesting the fundamental importance of the biology of the myocyte-derived contractile elements in the pathophysiology of the disease. However, as discussed below, the function of the contractile apparatus depends importantly upon the interaction of the myocyte with the extracellular matrix. Data obtained from patients studied after valve replacement also support the pathophysiological importance of non-myocyte elements of the myocardium. Serial measurements of LV ejection fraction after valve replacement in our patients with AR revealed that maximal post-operative recovery of this parameter requires approximately 3 years (14). The duration of this process indicates the high likelihood that it depends either on neurovascular adaptation, myocardial extracellular matrix protein metabolism, or both, as discussed below.

Hemodynamically, the problem posed by MR is importantly different from that associated with AR. Like AR, MR imposes an abnormal volume load on the LV; unlike AR, MR involves a backflow of blood into the relatively low impedence left atrium, increasing outflow impedance to the RV. Ultimately, pressure overload of the RV can lead to dysfunction paralleling the LV dysfunction which occurs in consequence of volume loading. In addition, the dynamics of LV volume loading are different in AR and MR: the low impedance of the left atrium allows more rapid and complete systolic emptying of the LV in MR than is possible in AR, in which ejection occurs totally into the relatively high impedence aorta. These global hemodynamic differences suggest that the stresses applied directly to myocardial cells (myocytes and fibroblasts) in AR and MR also may differ, potentially altering the cellular and molecular responses to these diseases.

Outcome in patients with MR, as in AR, can be predicted from measures of LV performance (2,15,16). Subnormal LV ejection fraction long has been recognized as a harbinger of relatively poor survival even if valve replacement or repair is performed. However, because the LV ejects partially into the low impedance left atrium, LV ejection fraction in MR bears a different relation to intrinsic contractility than it does in patients with AR or without structural heart disease. As a result, several investigators have attempted empirically to define a LV ejection fraction cut-point which can be employed to predict poor outcome with and without operation. Recent data suggest that a cut point 10 ejection fraction units (10%) above the putative lower limit of normal may be most effective in identifying patients whose risk potentially can be mitigated with operation, even if they are totally asymptomatic (15).

Because both ventricles are target organs in MR, it is not surprising that additional prognostic value can be obtained by supplementing information about LV performance with parallel data for the RV. Thus, among totally asymptomatic patients with normal LV and RV ejection fractions at rest, the change in RV ejection fraction from rest to exercise has been the most powerful predictor of clinical deterioration to CHF (17). RV ejection fraction at rest has proven the most potent predictor of death among clinically stable patients with no symptoms or with symptoms acceptably compensated with pharmacological therapy (2).

While the pathologic hemodynamics of MR differ importantly from those of AR, the time course of recovery of LV ejection fraction after operation is remarkably similar in the 2 diseases. Preliminary data suggest that, as in AR, maximal LV ejection fraction after mitral valve surgery requires up to 3 years of remodeling (18).

PATHOPHYSIOLOGIC IMPLICATIONS OF PROGNOSTIC DESCRIPTORS

Several inferences can be drawn from the foregoing presentation of natural history and its predictors. First, as suggested above, the predominance of contractility as a predictor of outcome in AR strongly suggests that qualitative and/or quantitative abnormalities of myocyte-derived proteins are fundamental to the genesis of LV dysfunction and CHF in this disease. The lack of direct measurement of contractility in MR precludes firm parallel conclusions for this disease, but the concordance of LV ejection fraction data (and RV ejection fraction data, as both parameters are determined by contractility modified by loading factors) in MR are consistent with the importance of myocyte-derived protein metabolic abnormalities in the pathogenesis of clinical debility in this disease as well.

Second, for both diseases, the relatively long time course of LV ejection fraction recovery after operation suggests the involvement of processes other than those primarily associated with myocyte-derived protein metabolism. The half-life of contractile proteins is measured in days, not months or years (19). Thus, a process requiring 3 years to reach its conclusion suggests either peripheral neurovascular adaptation, known from experience with CHF to be relatively slow, or metabolism of proteins with longer half-lives than those derived from myocytes. The latter include some of the proteins of the extracellular matrix, a major myocardial component and an important determinant of both systolic and diastolic function.

The relation of the matrix to diastolic function has been clear for some time. Increase in extracellular matrix, and particularly in collagen, can be expected to increase chamber wall stiffness and to reduce ventricular compliance. These variations lead to abnormal ventricular diastolic pressures when normal forward blood flow impinges on the LV or RV. In the left heart, ventricular diastolic pressures are reflected backward into the pulmonary circulation, and can result in pulmonary vascular congestion and dyspnea.

The relation of matrix composition to systolic function has become evident as the interactions of the myocyte cytoskeleton and the extracellular matrix have been progressively clarified. It is now known that the external mechanical efficiency of myocyte contraction depends in large measure on appropriate tethering of the myocyte to the matrix. Indeed, genetically determined alteration of the dystrophins, structural elements formed within the myocytes and extending through the sarcolemma to mediate connection of the myocyte cytoskeleton to the matrix, results in systolic dysfunction and CHF (20). Though not yet described, it is clear that abnormalities of the matrix elements to which the dystrophins normally are anchored also can be expected to result in ventricular mechanical dysfunction.

In summary, clinical studies suggest that variations in myocyte-derived contractile proteins are importantly involved in the pathophysiology of CHF in regurgitant valvular diseases. However, additional observations, in concert with recent data derived in non-valvular cardiomyopathic states, suggest equal or perhaps even greater importance in causing cardiac mechanical/contractile dysfunction may be attributable to variations of non-contractile structural proteins of the myocyte, as well as of non-myocyte-derived matrix proteins. These inferences suggest the value of defining the biology not only of the cardiomyocyte, but also of the cell responsible for extracellular matrix proteins, the cardiac fibroblast, in seeking the basis for CHF in valvular diseases.

DISORDERS OF MYOCARDIAL CELL BIOLOGY

The inferences noted above, derived from clinical studies of natural history and its predictors, are confirmed by studies of the biology of myocytes and fibroblasts from hearts afflicted with regurgitant valvular diseases.

To evaluate these processes, we developed animal models of hemodynamically severe chronic AR and hemodynamically severe chronic MR which manifest geometrical, functional and myocardial mass variations which mimic those seen in humans afflicted with disease of similar severity (4,19,21,22,23).

The animal model we have employed is the New Zealand White rabbit in which AR or MR are induced via mechanical injury to the valve leaflets. To create AR, we introduce a bevel-tipped 4F catheter into the carotid artery and advance the instrument until, by echocardiography, the tip is immediately superior to the aortic valve. Then, with echocardiographic guidance, the catheter is passed through a valve leaflet repeatedly until the regurgitant jet is of the desired magnitude. Verification of regurgitation severity is obtained using Doppler echocardiography; geometric and functional variations in response to valvular regurgitation also are made with echocardiography, according to methods validated in our laboratory (23).

In early studies, mild to moderate AR was created (regurgitant fraction = 20% to 35%). As facility with the surgical techniques increased, animals routinely have been created with regurgitant fractions of 50% to 65% . These hemodynaimally severe abnormalities are sustained with excellent perioperative survival and relatively prolonged late post-operative survival (often extending 2 to 3 years prior to sacrifice), providing a model of chronic, pure, isolated severe AR.

To create MR, a bioptome is passed through the open aortic valve into the LV and is then directed toward a mitral valve leaflet, from which a portion is resected. Using this method, creation of MR with regurgitant fractions in the range of 35% to 50% regularly has been achieved, again with excellent perioperative and "late" post-operative survival.

These models have revealed, first, that, as expected, LV cardiomyocyte-derived contractile protein metabolism is abnormal in AR and MR. In a dynamic diseased state such as valvular regurgitation, complete assessment of contractile protein metabolism requires definition of the kinetics of contractile protein synthesis independently from those of contractile protein degradation. We achieved this with a novel method developed for this purpose (19). First, synthesis rates are defined from the kinetics of tritiated leucine incorporation into Langendorff preparations of normal and diseased NZW rabbit hearts. Myocardial mass increases expected during a suitable time interval then are calculated from the synthesis rates. Degradation rates are determined by subtraction of the actual echocardiographically determined LV mass change during the interval from that which would have been expected.

Like earlier investigators, we found that, early after AR induction, LV growth is rapid and is driven predominantly by an increase in contractile protein synthesis rates, a process which continues for approximately one week. When we evaluated animals in which AR had been maintained during longer periods (not previously studied), we found that LV growth proceeds at a slower but still supernormal rate during the succeeding 3 months. This later growth is driven not by abnormal protein synthesis (indeed, protein synthesis rates are subnormal during this interval) but, rather, by markedly subnormal degradation rates of myocyte derived contractile proteins (19). Among animals followed longer than 3 months, LV growth slows markedly, reaching a relative "plateau" featuring mass increments only slightly greater than those of age-matched controls. During this interval, animals which remain functionally/clinically compensated manifest global synthesis and degradation rates that are equal and are indistinguishable from normal. Further analysis reveals abnormal protein metabolic kinetics in individual myofibrillar proteins, the significance of which is not yet clear (24). More strikingly, however, in animals that develop LV dysfunction and are sacrificed, myocardial protein synthesis and degradation rates both are markedly subnormal (25). It is not yet clear whether this phenomenon precedes functional deterioration or results from hemodynamic changes; the pulmonary vascular congestion in the sacrificed animals was relatively modest, suggesting this process, alone, was not the mediate cause of the metabolic abnormalities, but further research is necessary to resolve this issue. Preliminary studies in experimental MR suggest qualitatively similar myocardial contractile protein metabolic kinetic changes as those seen in AR, despite differences in the causative hemodynamics (26).

The fundamental basis of these striking metabolic changes remains to be elucidated. However, histopathologic studies among animals with AR prepared similarly and simultaneously with those evaluated in metabolic assessments reveal important variations in other cellular elements which may affect the function of the cardiomyocyte. Most prominently, an exuberant proliferation of extracellular matrix, or fibrosis, invariably is present among those animals that develop CHF (7). Among animals that remain clinically and functionally compensated despite severe AR, fibrous tissue invariably is present in supernormal quantities, but the magnitude of fibrosis generally varies from very mild to moderately severe and seldom reaches the severity associated with CHF (7, 27). Studies in MR as yet are preliminary, but suggest a pattern of LV extracellular matrix proliferation qualitatively similar to that of AR.

These findings cannot be interpreted unequivocally. They may be affected by species-related peculiarities or by the specific temporal characteristics of the development of AR and LV volume overload. However, importantly, parallel findings have been reported in humans with AR at endomyocardial biopsy and at valve replacement (28,29). Moreover, our animal studies indicate that fibrosis is very modest at the "subacute" stage, one month after AR induction, and can be minimal in compensated animals more than 2 years after AR has been established. (The earliest evidence of severe fibrosis in our series has been observed after 7 months of AR in an animal that died spontaneously with severe CHF.) Also, it is known that fibroblasts from other tissues and organ systems typically proliferate and hyperproduce extracellular matrix when placed under physical stretch in culture, a maneuver that parallels some of the stresses believed to impinge on mural cellular elements in the setting of LV volume overload (30). (Study of the response of cultured cardiac fibroblasts to such exogenous stimuli now is being pursued actively in our laboratory.) Thus, it is reasonable to hypothesize that myocardial fibrosis in valvular regurgitation largely or exclusively is a primary process. Whether primary or secondary, the biology of this process is of interest because quantitative alteration of myocardial extracellular matrix and variation in its physical relation to cardiomyocytes can be expected to affect ventricular mechanical performance profoundly. Therefore, modulation of this process has potentially important therapeutic implications.

The fibrous tissue is distributed throughout the full thickness of the ventricular myocardium, though preliminary studies suggest a relative preponderance in the subendocardium (31). The pattern of distribution may reflect the distribution of physical stresses which impinge upon and, perhaps, stimulate the fibroblast to produce extracellular matrix. These stresses are relatively complex, vary among different regions of the ventricle, and are modulated by ventricular shape changes that typically accompany chamber remodeling in response to valvular regurgitation (32). These physical stresses also may cause myocyte injury, with inflammation and secondary fibrosis. Finally, fibrosis might be a response to ischemic injury to myocytes, perhaps resulting from abnormal diastolic pressure and subendocardial stresses which compromise subendocardial blood flow. To evaluate the latter possibility, we have measured regional myocardial blood flow in AR and have related this to regional LV wall stresses. Results suggest that global and subendocardial myocardial flows are relatively normal in most LV regions, with subnormal subendocardial flow found only at the apex (33). These findings suggest that ischemia is unlikely to be a primary determinant of fibrosis distribution, though it may modulate responses to other stimuli.

Precise determination of the biology of the fibrotic response is important because this information will affect interpretation of associated variations at the molecular level as well as potential management strategies based on modulating fibrosis. Several lines of evidence now suggest, but do not yet prove, that extracellular matrix proliferation is a primary response to volume loading. First, our experimental AR hearts demonstrating the most severe myocardial fibrosis invariably are devoid of inflammatory cellular response. Though myocyte necrosis is seen in association with fibrosis in these severely abnormal specimens, the lack of apparent inflammation raises the possibility of an apoptotic process rather than inflammation-induced fibrosis. No definitive evidence yet has been accumulated to support this possibility, but in parallel CHF settings in the absence of valvular diseases, several studies have suggested a role for apoptosis. Second, in animals which have not yet developed LV dysfunction or heart failure and in which fibrosis is modest to minimal, extracellular matrix is quantitatively abnormal in areas devoid of myocyte necrosis. Third, as noted previously, physical stresses which model those of ventricular volume overload, when applied to fibroblasts in non-myocardial tissues, result in cellular proliferation and enhancement of extracellular matrix production (30).

Irrespective of its genesis, abundant evidence now suggests that the extracellular matrix produced in regurgitant valvular diseases is abnormal in composition. In our first series of studies, we undertook to characterize the collagen content of the myocardium in AR. The results were surprising in that they differed considerably from those previously reported in the setting of experimental aortic stenosis. The latter disease is characterized by pure LV pressure overloading associated with marked and significant overproduction of myocardial collagen (6). In contrast, in animals with clinically and functionally compensated AR, in which fibrosis was visible but relatively modest by light microscopy and Masson trichrome staining, myocardial hydroxyproline content was indistinguishable from that among control animals (34). In animals with CHF and subnormal LV performance characteristics, Masson trichrome staining revealed exuberant fibrosis but hydroxyproline content tended to be *subnormal.* To confirm this unexpected finding, tissues were studied by staining with Picro-Sirius Red, an agent that binds specifically to collagen (a characteristic not shared by Masson trichrome stain). Though the latter procedure revealed dense and convoluted collagen bundles in the specimens of animals with LV dysfunction, total collagen content did not differ from control (34). (Preliminary assessment did not reveal qualitative change in myocardial collagen isoforms as compared with control, but this issue remains to be definitively resolved.)

Fibroblasts isolated and cultured from normal and AR rabbit hearts support the tissue findings. Preliminary data, obtained using hearts only from animals with compensated AR and not with CHF, indicate that tritiated proline uptake (a measure of collagen synthesis) is virtually identical in AR and control cells, whereas tritiated glucosamine uptake (a measure of synthesis of numerous non-collagen matrix elements) is markedly and significantly upregulated (35).

THE MOLECULAR BIOLOGY OF THE CARDIAC FIBROBLAST

Taken together, the results of histopathological evaluation, tissue content determination and cell culture studies all highlight variations in fibroblast biology in the pathogenesis of CHF in valvular regurgitation. Therefore, we undertook to elucidate the molecular mechanisms underlying the disordered biology of the cardiac fibroblast in AR.

The first step, reported preliminarily, was isolation of RNA from cultured fibroblasts from each of 3 non-CHF AR animals and 3 matched normal controls. Differential display of cDNA after amplification by polymerase chain reaction methodology indicated several clear and consistent differences in gene expression among normal and AR fibroblasts (36). Preliminary data also suggest that abnormal gene expression is related directly to the magnitude of AR. Importantly, these abnormalities were seen in fibroblasts taken from animals *without* evidence of LV dysfunction or CHF, suggesting (but not rigorously proving) that previously-noted extracellular matrix variations are involved in the pathogenesis of cardiac dysfunction and are not merely epiphenomena due to myocyte damage.

Specific aspects of the study design have raised important questions about the mechanism by which the alterations in gene expression are propagated. Differential display (and subsequent studies employing selective subtraction hybridization techniques) indicated that gene expression differed consistently between AR cells and normal cells as late as the sixth passage of fibroblasts in culture, though immunohistochemistry indicated that the cells maintained their fibroblast characteristics at this passage. This finding may be attributable to factors extrinsic to the fibroblast which somehow are transmitted through several passages. Alternatively, stereotyped somatic mutations may be induced by AR, perhaps enabled by an abnormal rate of fibroblast proliferation, increasing the opportunities for common mutations. Another attractive theoretical possibility is that stress responsive genomic elements in fibroblasts, like those shown to be expressed in endothelial cells placed under mechanical stress (37), may be activated by the stresses of volume loading in AR. In the endothelium, the stress responsive elements alter expression of other genes. The products of stress responsive elements may remain active even after the inciting mechanical stress is removed, thus maintaining abnormal expression of other genes in the affected cells.

Once differential display PCR established the existence of differential fibroblast gene expression, identification of the differentially expressed DNA was undertaken. Two approaches have been employed. The first has been the conventional approach, initially involving the cloning of differentially expressed gene fragments isolated from differential display PCR and from contemporaneous selective subtraction hybridization studies involving RNA from normal and AR cultured fibroblasts. After preliminary confirmation of differential expression by reverse Northern analysis, final confirmation is achieved by quantitative Northern analyses.

As yet, these studies are incomplete. However, preliminarily, 7 differentially expressed gene fragments have been confirmed by Northern analysis in at least one AR-normal cell line pair and have proven to be portions of unique genes upon sequencing and GENBANK comparison for homology with known genes (38). Of these 7 unique genes, 4 code for intracellular or cell surface components; one of these, though different from the calcium channel previously identified, also is involved in fibroblast calcium metabolism. One, which we have found to be down-regulated, codes for an enzyme believed to mediate fibroblast collagen production. Each of the other 3, all upregulated relatively markedly on preliminary assessment, codes for a different non-collagen extracellular matrix protein. Preliminarily, these proteins include fibronectin, thrombospondin and amyloid prescursor protein (38) . Thus, these preliminary results are fully consistent with, and may be responsible for, earlier evidence that AR causes hyperproduction of extracellular matrix and that this excessive matrix selectively comprises proteins other than collagen.

A second approach to identifying differentially expressed genes has involved quantification of expression of specific genes which are likely to be involved in a fibrotic response. Thus, because calcium is required for the fibroblast proliferation and motility, common features of fibrosis, Northern analyses were performed to assess expression of genes coding for portions of sarcolemmal calcium channels. Preliminary studies revealed that the alpha-2 subunit of the dihydropyridine receptor, part of the L-type calcium channel, is present in fibroblasts and is up-regulated in AR (39). The quantitative and pathophysiologic importance of this finding is not yet clear.

THERAPEUTIC IMPLICATIONS

As noted earlier, clinical studies of post-operative LV functional recovery in AR and MR suggest the importance of processes separate from contractile protein replacement and possibly involving matrix remodeling. Parallel whole animal experimental studies (consistent with the few published clinical tissue assessments) indicate the development of myocardial fibrosis prior to appearance of LV dysfunction or CHF; tissue analysis of this model reveals that the fibrous tissue predominantly comprises extracellular matrix elements other than collagen. Cultured fibroblasts from this model selectively produce abnormal amounts of non-collagen matrix proteins and preliminary molecular studies indicate abnormal expression of genes that code for such matrix proteins.

Taken together, these findings suggest that, to retard the development of heart failure and to reduce the necessity for surgical correction of regurgitant valvular lesions, interventions that modify the biology of the cardiac fibroblast may prove particularly useful. (As a corollary, procedures which identify emergence of specific abnormalities of fibroblast biology may be useful in optimizing the timing of currently available therapy.) Our studies suggest that such therapy is possible in practice.

Further studies have indicated the potential availability of this approach in practice. Thus, using vesnarinone as a pharmacological probe, we have demonstrated the capacity to suppress the survival of the cardiac fibroblast (40). Vesnarinone is a quinolone derivative with multiple actions in the cardiomyocyte. Clinically, the drug has been shown to reduce several manifestations of congestive heart failure, but the pharmacologic basis of these clinical effects have not been elucidated clearly. At the clinically employed doses, arrhythmogenesis is a potential problem, as well. At tissue bath doses which roughly parallel those employed clinically, vesnarinone also manifests diverse, occasionally deleterious, pharmacologic effects in selected lines of non-cardiac fibroblasts. Importantly, in these earlier studies, the magnitude of effects on fibroblasts has been directly related to drug dose. Building on these earlier findings, we employed vesnarinone in cultured fibroblasts aiming to suppress fibroblast metabolic activity, hypothesizing that this action can be expected to prevent myocardial fibrosis *in vivo*.

Our results indicated that, at tissue bath concentrations corresponding to doses more than an order of magnitude *lower* than those which have been employed clinically, vesnarinone reduces survival of normal cardiac fibroblasts by approximately 50%. Suppression of AR cardiac fibroblasts is even more dramatic: cell survival >50% lower than that observed in the untreated state is achieved by doses even lower than those effective in normal cells. Perhaps the most unusual result of these experiments was that the effect of vesnarinone on cardiac fibroblasts varied *inversely* with dose: as vesnarinone concentration was increased to levels corresponding to those normally employed clinically, the effect on fibroblast survival disappeared (40). This finding suggests that vesnarinone has multiple pharmacologic effects on cardiac fibroblasts and that the dose-response relations of these effects interact in a complex pattern. More importantly, these results illustrate the potential for therapy in AR based on pharmacologic modification of cardiac fibroblast biology.

Acknowledgments

Preparation of this chapter was supported by grants from The Howard Gilman Foundation, New York, N.Y., The Schiavone Family Foundation, Whitehouse Station, N.J., The Jean and Charles Brunie Foundation, Bronxville, N.Y., The Margolis Foundation, New York, N.Y., The Hansen Foundation, New York, N.Y., The Mary A. H. Rumsey Foundation, New York, N.Y., and by much appreciated gifts from Steven and Suzanne Weiss and Maryjane Voute Arrigoni and the late William Voute.

REFERENCES

1. Borer JS, Hochreiter C, Herrold EM, Supino P, Aschermann M, Wencker D, Devereux RB, Roman MJ, Szulc M, Kligfield P, Isom OW. Prediction of indications for valve replacement among asymptomatic or minimally symptomatic patients with chronic aortic regurgitation and normal left ventricular performance. Circulation 1998; 97:525-534.

2. Hochreiter C, Niles N, Devereux RB, Kligfield P, Borer JS. Mitral regurgitation: relationship of non-invasive descriptors of right and left ventricular performance to clinical and hemodynamic findings and to prognosis in medically and surgically treated patients. Circulation 1986;73:900-912.

3. Kligfield P, Hochreiter C, Niles N, Devereux RB, Borer JS. Relation of sudden death in pure mitral regurgitation, with and without mitral valve prolapse, to repetitive ventricular arrhythmias and right and left ventricular ejection fractions. American Journal of Cardiology 1987;60:397-399.

4. Magid NM, Young MS, Wallerson DC, Goldweit RS, Carter JN, Devereux RB, Borer JS. Hypertrophic and functional response to experimental chronic aortic regurgitation. Journal of Molecular and Cellular Cardiology 1988;20:239-246.

5. Yamazaki T, Uematsu T, Mizuno A, Takiguchi Y, Nakashima M. Alterations of cardiac adrenoceptors and calcium channels subsequent to production of aortic insufficiency in rats. Arch Int Pharmacodyn Ther 1989;299:155-168.

6. Weber KT, Brilla CG. Pathological hypertrophy and the cardiac interstitium. Fibrosis and the renin-angiotensin-aldosterone system. Circulation 1991; 83:1849-1865.

7. Liu S-K, Magid NM, Fox PR, Goldfine SM, Borer JS. Fibrosis, myocyte degeneration and heart failure in chronic experimental aortic regurgitation. Cardiology, 1998, in press.

8. Reid CL, Gardin JM, Yunis C, Kurosaki T, Flack JM, for the Coronary Artery Risk Development inYoung Adults Research Group.   Prevalence and clinical correlates of aortic and mitral regurgitation in young adult population: The Cardia Study.   Circulation 1994;90(Suppl I):I-282(Abs).

9. Siemienczuk D, Greenberg B, Morris C, Massie B, Wilson RA, Topic N, Bristow JD, Cheitlin M. Chronic aortic insuffiency: factors associated with progression to aortic valve replacement. Ann Intern Med. 1989;110-587-592.

10. Bonow RO, Rosing DR, McIntosh CL, Jones M, Maron BJ, Lan KKG, Lakatos E, Bacharach SL, Green MV, Epstein SE. The natural history of asymptomatic patients with aortic regurgitation and normal left ventricular function. Circulation. 1983;68:509-517.

11. Linsay J, Silverman A, Van Voorhees LB, Nolan NG. Prognostic implications of left ventricular function during exercise in asymptomatic patients with aortic regurgitation.   Angiology 1987;38:386-392.

12. Henry WL, Bonow RO, Borer JS, Ware JH, Kent KM, Redwood DR, McIntosh CL, Morrow AG, Epstein SE. Observations on the optimum time for operative intervention for aortic regurgitation, I: evaluation of the results of aortic valve replacement in symptomatic patients. Circulation 1980;61:471-483.

13. Borer JS, Hochreiter C, Herrold EM, Roman MJ, Kligfield P, Szulc M, Supino P, Isom OW, Krieger K, Kaufman JD. Prediction of outcome late after aortic valve replacement for aortic regurgitation utilizing pre-operative wall-stress-sdjusted change in ejection fraction from rest to exercise. Circulation 1998; in press (Abs).

14. Borer JS, Herrold EM, Hochreiter C, Roman M, Supino P, Devereux RB, Kligfield P, Nawaz H. Natural history of left ventricular performance at rest and during exercise after aortic valve replacement for aortic regurgitation. Circulation 1991;84 (Suppl III):III-133-III-139.

15. Enrique-Sarano M, Tajik AJ, Schaff HV, Orszulak TA, Bailey KR, Frye RL. Echocardiographic prediction of survival after surgical correction of organic mitral regurgitation. Circulation 1994;90:830-837.

16. Philips HR, Levine FH, Carter JE, Boucher C, Osbakken MD, Okada RD, Akins CW, Daggett WM, Buckley MJ, Pohost GM. Mitral valve replacement for isolated mitral regurgitation: analysis of clinical course and late postoperative left ventricular ejection fraction. American Journal of Cardiology 1981;48: 647-654.

17. Rosen S, Borer JS, Hochreiter C, Supino P, Roman M, Devereux RB, Kligfield P. Natural history of the asymptomatic/minimally symptomatic patient with normal right and left ventricular performance and severe mitral regurgitation due to mitral valve prolapse. American Journal of Cardiology 1994;74:374-380.

18. Borer JS, Wencker D, Hochreiter C. Management decisions in valvular heart disease: the role of radionuclide-based assessment of ventricular function and performance. Journal of Nuclear Cardiology 1996; 3:72-81.

19. Magid NM, Borer JS, Young MS, Wallerson DC, De Monteiro C. Suppression of protein degradation in progessive cardiac hypertrophy of chronic aortic regurgitation. Circulation 1993;871249-1257.

20. Leiden JM. The genetics of dilated cardiomyopathy-emerging clues to the puzzle. New England J Med 1997;337:1080-1081.

21. Magid NM, Opio G, Wallerson DC, Young MS, Borer JS. Heart failure due to chronic experimental aortic regurgitation. American J Physiology 1994;267:H556-562.

22. Magid NM, Wallerson DC, Bent SJ, Borer JS. Hypertrophy and heart failure in chronic experimental mitral regurgitation. J American College Cardiology 1994;23 (Special Issue) : 248A (Abs.).

23. Young MS, Magid NM, Wallerson DC, Goldweit RS, Devereux RB, Carter JN, Im J, Hall MA, Borer JS. Echocardiographic left ventricular mass measurement in small animals: anotomic validation in normal and aortic regurgitant rabbits. American Journal of Noninvasive Cardiology 1990;4:145-153.

24. King RK, Magid NM, Opio G, Borer JS. Protein turnover in compensated chronic aortic regurgitation. Cardiology 1997;88:518-525.

25. Magid NM, Opio G, Wallerson DC, Borer JS. Suppressed protein turnover in congestive heart failure due to severe chronic aortic regurgitation. Circulation 1992;86:I-540.

26. Carter JN, Borer JS, Jacobson MN, Herrold EM, Magid NM. Myofibrillar protein synthesis rates in mitral regurgitation. Circulation 1997;96(Suppl I): I-469 (Abs).

27. Herrold EM, Lu P, Zanzonic P, Goldfine SM, Szulc M, Magid NM, Borer JS. Antimyosin antibody-mediated detection of myocardial injury: relation to wall stress in chronic aortic regurgitation. Computers in Cardiology 1995; IEEE Publication #0276-6547/95: 59-62.

28. Oldershaw PJ, Brooksby IAB, Davies MJ, Coltart DJ, Jenkins BS, Webb-Peploe MM: Correlations of fibrosis in endomyocardial biopsies from patients with aortic valve disease. B Heart J 1980; 44:609-611.

29. Donaldson RM, Florio R, Rickards AF, et al: Irreversible morphological changes contributing to depressed cardiac function after surgery for chronic aortic regurgitation. B Heart J 1982;48:589-597.

30. Hannafin JA, personal communication.

31. Lu P, Zanzonico P, Goldfine SM, Hardoff R, Gentile R, Magid N, Herrold EM, Borer JS. Antimyosin antibody imaging in experimental aortic regurgitation. Journal of Nuclear Cardiology 1997;4:25-32.

32. Herrold EM, Carter JN, Borer JS. Volume-overload-related shape change limits mass increase with wall thickening but only minimally reduces wall stress. Computers in Cardiology, 1992; IEEE publication #0276-6547/92:287-290.

33. Herrold EM, Goldfine SM, Magid NM, Borer JS. Myocardial blood flow in aortic regurgitation: computer-based predictions from wall stress compared with fluorescent microsphere measurements. Computers in Cardiology 1994; IEEE Publications #0276-6547/94:729-732.

34. Goldfine SM, Pena M, Magid NM, Liu S-K, Borer JS. Myocardial collagen in cardiac hypertrophy resulting from chronic aortic regurgitation. American Journal of Therapeutics, in press, 1998.

35. Borer JS, Pena M, Falcone D, Truter S, Goldfine S. Chronic aortic regurgitation causes fibrosis featuring hyper-production of non-collogen, glucosamine-containing matrix elements. J American College of Cardiology (Abstract), submitted, action pending 1999.

36. Goldin D, Borer JS, Goldfine SM. Abnormal gene expression of cardiac fibroblasts in experimental aortic regurgitation. Circulation 1997; 96(Suppl I): I-205(Abs).

37. Gimbrone MA, Nagel T, Topper JN. Biomechanical activation: an emerging paradigm in endothelial adhesion biology. J Clin Invest 1997;99:1809-1813.

38. Truter S, Kolesar J, Dumlao T, Borer JS. Chronic aortic regurgitation causes abnormal cardiac fibroblast gene expression leading to myocardial fibrosis. J American College Cardiology (Abs.), submitted, action pending 1999.

39. Liu F, Truter SL, Magda P, Borer JS. Aortic regurgitation alters the expression of dihydropyridine-sensitive L-type calcium channels in cardiac fibroblasts. J American College of Cardiology 1998; 31 (Suppl A):424A (Abs.).

40. Ross JS, Goldfine SM, Herrold EM, Borer JS. Differential response to vesnarinone by cardiac fibroblasts isolated from normal and aortic regurgitation hearts. American Journal of Therapeutics 1998, in press.

4 CORONARY ATHEROTHROMBOSIS: PATHOPHYSIOLOGY AND CLINICAL IMPLICATIONS

Avi Fischer, M.D.
David E. Gutstein, M.D.
Zahi A. Fayad, PhD.
Valentin Fuster, M.D., PhD.
Mt. Sinai Medical Center

INTRODUCTION

The past two decades have witnessed a significant improvement in post-myocardial infarction (MI) survival in the United States [1-3]. Significant decreases in mortality have been noted in several other countries, as well [4-8]. The progressive improvement in survival after MI began prior to the introduction of thrombolytic therapy and appears to be related to a variety of improvements in the care of cardiac patients. Most recently, these advances in patient care have included improvements in post-MI medical therapy, revascularization techniques and risk reduction.

Important advances in our understanding of the underlying mechanisms of the acute coronary syndromes has led to a more targeted treatment approach for coronary disease. Much of this progress derives from advances made in basic science. Furthermore, a better understanding of the importance of different components in the atherosclerotic plaque has led to the search for imaging modalities able to identify vulnerable plaques before the appearance of clinical manifestations of coronary artery disease.

This chapter will discuss recent advances in our understanding, prevention, diagnosis and medical treatment of the acute coronary syndromes. First, we will review aspects of the biology of the developing atherosclerotic plaque. We will focus on factors which lead to plaque instability and discuss the clinical syndromes which result from plaque rupture. A review of diagnostic imaging, prevention and treatment of atherosclerotic disease then follows. This review is intended to summarize current thinking regarding the pathophysiology underlying the acute coronary syndroms.

CLASSIFICATION OF ATHEROSCLEROTIC LESIONS

The origin of the atherosclerotic lesion.   A lipid-rich region in the intima, the innermost layer of medium and large arteries, forms the atherosclerotic lesion. Segments of adaptive intimal thickening, particularly at bifurcations, are present from birth. Thickening occurs in areas of turbulent flow and is accelerated by diabetes mellitus, hypertension, hyperlipidemia and smoking. These thick areas of intima that contain lipid deposits represent early atherosclerotic lesions[9].

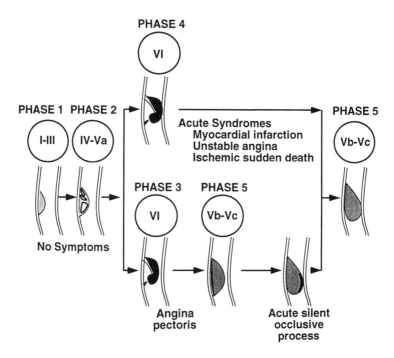

Figure 1. Schematic diagram illustrating the phases of progression of coronary atherosclerosis and the associated lesion morphology and clinical findings. See text for more details. Reproduced with permission[14].

Phases of the atherosclerotic lesion.   Atherosclerotic lesions can be classified into lesion types and grouped into phases, constituting a continuum of events evolving over time (Figure 1). Lesion types I and II, referred to as the "early lesions," are noted as early as childhood[9]. Type I lesions are characterized by lipid-laden macrophage or foam cell infiltration[10]. These lesions progress and mature into plaques where smooth muscle infiltration and lipid deposition predominate (the "fatty streak" or type II lesion). When extracellular connective tissue, fibrils and lipid deposits surround the smooth muscle cells, the lesion becomes known as type III. Lesion types I-III constitute phase 1 of atherosclerotic plaque progression and generally occurs in persons under age 30[10]. The arterial wall is not thickened appreciably and the arterial lumen is not narrowed by phase 1 lesions[9].

Phase 2 characterized by type IV and V lesions represents the progression of the atherosclerotic plaque to a more vulnerable state. Phase 2 is often asymptomatic but may be associated with stable angina[11]. Type IV lesions, the "atheroma" and first of the advanced lesions, are marked by disarrangement of intimal structure secondary to accumulation of extracellular lipid with intertwined fibrous tissue localized in the lipid core. These lesions when first appearing in younger persons are found in the same locations as adaptive intimal thickening and at least initially, are eccentric. In addition to the presence of macrophages and smooth muscle cells, lymphocytes and mast cells have been identified in the region between the lipid core and the endothelial surface. In these lesions, the tissue layer between the lipid core and the endothelial surface is the intima that preceded lesion development. Even though this lesion may not cause much lumenal narrowing, it may be susceptible to fissuring and rupture[9].

Type V lesions, the second variant of Phase 2 lesions, are characterized by prominent new fibrous connective tissue and intimal thickening. When a lipid core underlies the connective tissue formation, the lesion is referred to as Va or fibroatheroma. This lesion may be multilayered, with several lipid cores separated by thick layers of fibrous tissue above one another. A type V lesion with prominent calcification of the lipid core or other areas is referred to as type Vb, or calcific. In these lesions mineralization may replace the entire lipid core. The absence of a lipid core, with minimal lipid deposition in general, constitutes a Vc lesion, a fibrotic lesion[9]. Fibrotic lesions may represent organization of thrombi, extension of adjacent fibroatheroma or resorption of the lipid core. Type V lesions are more occlusive than type IV lesions but like type IV lesions, are prone to developing fissures, hematomas and thrombi[9].

Phase 3 is marked by the acute disruption of type IV and V lesions leading to mural thrombus formation within the vessel wall (the complex or type VI lesion). These events are often asymptomatic because thrombus formation in the vessel during phase 3 may not be flow limiting[10]. While phase 3 may not result in an acute clinical syndrome, the net result is a rapid progression of plaque size that may ultimately result in symptomatic stable angina[12, 13].

The acute coronary syndromes of unstable angina and myocardial infarction are associated with phase 4 plaque disruption and associated flow limiting thrombus (also type VI lesion) [10]. After a phase 3 or 4 event, the thrombus over the disrupted plaque often calcifies (type Vb) or fibroses (type Vc), forming a chronic stenotic lesion. This phase 5 lesion often underlies chronic stable angina. Frequently, the phase 5 lesion contains organizing thrombus from prior episodes of plaque rupture, ulceration, hemorrhage and organization. Severely stenotic phase 5 plaques may progress to complete occlusion from intravascular stasis rather than from acute plaque rupture[11].

DYNAMIC CHANGES IN THE EARLY ATHEROSCLEROTIC PLAQUE

Lipoprotein transport in plaque formation.   The accumulation of lipid within the atherosclerotic plaque represents a breakdown of defenses which normally prevents lipid deposition in the vessel wall (Figure 2). Most lipids deposited in atherosclerotic lesions are derived from plasma low-density lipoprotein (LDL), which enters the vessel wall through dysfunctional endothelium[14]. Endothelial injury due to shear forces from turbulent flow occurs and is enhanced by many other factors. Hypertension, diabetes mellitus, hypercholesterolemia, tobacco and vasoactive amines are several of the many factors affecting integrity of the vascular endothelium. As a result of the often-synergistic effects of these influences, chronic endothelial injury leads to accumulation of lipids, monocytes and macrophages[15, 16]. In addition to chronic endothelial damage and forces increasing the lipid influx into the plaque, a low serum high-density lipoprotein (HDL) level may decrease the efflux of lipid from the plaque. Additionally, by inhibiting oxidation of LDL, HDL may protect against excess lipid accumulation in the vessel wall. Disturbances in the protective effects of the endothelium and HDL result in an increase in the overall lipid content of the atherosclerotic plaque[14].

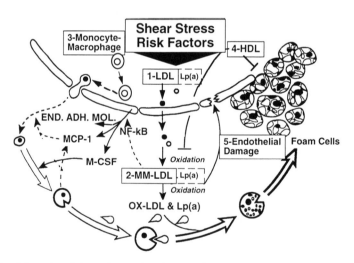

Figure 2. Schematic of the pathogenesis of progression of the atherosclerotic plaque. ENDO = endothelial; END.ADH.MOL. = endothelial adhesion molecule; HDL = high density lipoprotein; LDL = low density lipoprotein; Lp(a) = lipoprotein (a); MCP-1 = monocyte chemotactic protein -1; M-CSF = monocyte colony stimulating factor; MM = minimally modified; NF-KB = necrosis factor-KB; OX = oxidized. Reproduced with permission[17]

All major cell types in the vessel wall have the ability to oxidize LDL, but probably the most important cell at early stages is the endothelial cell[17, 18]. Through the elaboration of two adhesive cell-surface glycoproteins, intercellular adhesion molecule-1 (ICAM-1) and vascular cell adhesion molecule-1 (VCAM-1) monocyte recruitment occurs[19, 20]. Subsequent monocyte adhesion to the vessel wall surface begins a second cascade of events. Specific chemokines such as monocyte chemotactic protein-1 (MCP-1) and monocyte colony stimulating factor (M-CSF) attract monocytes causing their entrance into the vessel wall and their differentiation into macrophages. These differentiated macrophages scavenge oxidized LDL to become foam cells[14].

Factors in plaque instability and disruption.

External physical forces. Blood flow impacting on the plaque and vessel wall stress are key external factors affecting plaque stability[14]. These external forces may be influenced by systemic factors, such as environmental or pharmacologic stressors (Table 1).

Table 1. Thrombotic Complications of Plaque Disruption: Local and Systemic Thrombogenic Risk Factors

Local Factors
     Degree of plaque disruption (i.e., fissure, ulcer)
     Degree of stenosis (i.e., change in geometry)
     Tissue substrate (i.e., lipid-rich plaque)
     Surface of residual thrombus (i.e., recurrence)
   Vasoconstriction (i.e., platelets, thrombin)
 Systemic Factors
     Catecholamines (i.e., smoking, stress, cocaine)
     Renin-angiotensin (i.e., DD genotype)
     Cholesterol, lipoprotein (a)
     Metabolic states (i.e., homocystinemia, diabetes)
     Fibrinogen, impaired fibrinolysis (i.e., plasminogen activator inhibitor - 1)
     Activated platelets and clotting (i.e., Factor VII)
     Thrombin generation (fragment 1+2) or activity (fibrinopeptide A)

High Risk, presumably by the presence of several local or systemic thrombogenic risk factors at the time of plaque disruption, indicates acute occlusive labile thrombus versus fixed mural thrombus (unstable angina and non-Q wave and Q wave myocardial infarction).   **Low Risk,** presumably by the paucity of thrombogenic risk factors at the time of plaque disruption, indicates only mural thrombus (progressive atherogenesis)   Reproduced with permission [86].

Factors intrinsic to the plaque which make it particularly sensitive to external physical forces include the size, location and content of the lipid core, as well as the integrity of the fibrous cap. A weak point in the cap which is vulnerable to shear forces appears to be at its insertion into the vessel wall[10, 12]. Here, the fibrous cap thins and is often replete with lipid-packed macrophages (foam cells) as seen in Figure 3 [12, 21].

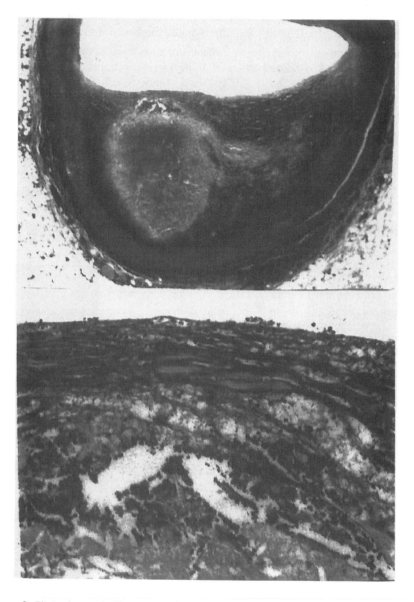

Figure 3. Photomicrograph of a coronary atheroma. A large lipid core and thin fibrous cap are evident at low magnification. At higher power, foam cell infiltration into the fibrous cap is noted. Erythrocytes are noted just below the fibrous cap , the result of cap disruption or plaque hemorrhage. Reproduced with permission[23].

Internal forces. Inflammatory cell activity in the atherosclerotic plaque appears to have an important impact on plaque stability [21, 22]. For instance, macrophages secrete metalloproteinases which have activity against the collagen component of the plaque and may act to weaken the fibrous cap[23-26]. Macrophage-derived foam cells have also been shown to activate matrix metalloproteinases by elaborating reactive oxygen species [27].

Macrophages in the atherosclerotic plaque derive from circulating monocytes, which adhere to the vessel wall in areas of turbulent flow. Monocytes are drawn into the vessel wall by chemotactic factors such as MCP-1, which also acts to induce tissue factor expression in monocytic and smooth muscle cell lines (see below) [28]. In addition to macrophages, T-lymphocytes are found in abundance in atheromatous plaques[29].   Systemic infections (e.g. C. pneumoniae, cytomegalovirus and H. pylori) have been linked to atherosclerotic disease, although a causal relationship is far from clear[30-34]. Infectious agents may affect endothelial function[35, 36], and activate monocytes and macrophages to secrete inflammatory cytokines[37]. These cytokines, in turn, stimulate the production of reactive oxygen species and proteolytic enzymes which may influence plaque stability. Oxidative stress and the anti-oxidant capacity of the arterial wall appear to play important roles in the progression of atherosclerotic disease, in addition to plaque rupture [38, 39].

Both T-lymphocytes and macrophages have been shown to undergo apoptosis in the advanced atherosclerotic plaque[29, 40]. Smooth muscle cells express Bax, a proapoptotic protein, in carotid plaques[41] and can be induced to undergo apoptosis in the presence of cytokines secreted by macrophages and T-lymphocytes[42]. Apoptotic cell death, particularly involving smooth muscle cells in the fibrous cap, may contribute to the destabilization of advanced atherosclerotic plaques[29, 43].

There is marked heterogeneity in the composition of the atherosclerotic plaque, even within the same individual, and the disruption of plaques exposes different vessel wall components to blood[10]. In a disrupted plaque with ulceration, several plaque components demonstrate marked thrombogenicity. Of these components, the lipid rich core, that is abundant in cholesteryl ester, has the greatest degree of thrombogenicity and tissue factor staining[10, 44] (Figure 4).

Tissue factor (TF), a glycoprotein elaborated by cells infiltrating the plaque, is believed to be a major regulator of coagulation, thrombosis and hemostasis[10]. TF forms a high - affinity complex with coagulation factors VII/VIIa; TF/VIIa complex activates factors IX and X, which generate thrombin[45]. TF is normally present in the arterial adventitia, but all of the major cell types found in the atherosclerotic plaque - smooth muscle cells, macrophages and endothelial cells, are able to express TF. Additional sites of TF are extracellular, in the lipid - rich core and fibrous matrix. As previously mentioned, the lipid - rich core, the most thrombogenic substrate, exhibits the most intense TF staining, suggesting that tissue factor is an important determinant of thrombogenicity after spontaneous or mechanical plaque disruption[10].

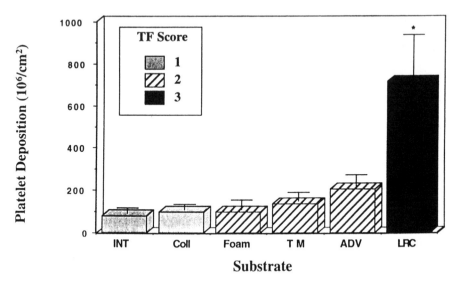

Figure 4. Tissue Factor Activity and Platelet deposition. Platelet deposition data are expressed as mean ±SEM ; TF staining intensity is expressed as the average of the independant observers. Note the positive correlation between platelet-thrombus formation and TF score on the exposed human substrates (p<0.01). INT = normal intima; COLL = collagen-rich matrix; FOAM = foam cell-rich matrix; TM = normal tunica media; ADV = adventitia; LCR = lipid-rich core (*p=0.0002); ANOVA. Reproduced with permission[121].

CLINICAL SEQUELLAE OF PLAQUE RUPTURE

From a clinical standpoint, a spectrum of acute coronary events may follow atherosclerotic plaque rupture. These events range from the asymptomatic, to those resulting in critical illness or sudden death. The pathophysiology underlying these clinical events involves a reduction in blood flow supporting myocardium distal to the site of acute plaque rupture. As reviewed above, blood flow is reduced by accumulated thrombus, as well as vasospasm over the ruptured plaque. The severity of the resulting coronary event appears to be related to the change in blood flow around the site of plaque disruption. In those cases where blood flow is essentially unaffected, plaque rupture may result only in asymptomatic progression of the atherosclerotic lesion. If blood flow is reduced, a change in the pattern of angina may result, producing unstable angina. If complete vessel occlusion follows plaque rupture acutely in the absence of sufficient collateral blood flow, acute MI results[15, 46].

The risk of adverse outcomes after acute coronary syndromes appears to be related to the type of event. Cumulative six-month mortality is highest in acute MI when compared with unstable and stable angina [47]. Clinical outcome data, including cumulative death or MI and cardiac event rates, are similar for non-Q and Q-wave MI [48, 49]. The risk of adverse outcome with unstable angina is highest in the post-MI setting, or with recent (<48 hours) onset of rest angina. The process of plaque rupture may play a major role in the pathogenesis of these entities. On the other hand, if external factors which trigger worsened angina (e.g., anemia, environmental stresses) can be identified and corrected, prognosis may be improved[50].

An important cause of mortality in the setting of intracoronary thrombosis is sudden death[51]. Up to one half of all cardiovascular deaths in the United States result from sudden arrhythmic death. Most sudden death, in turn, occurs in the setting of coronary artery disease[52]. Acute ischemia has been shown in experimental models to predispose to malignant arrhythmias[53, 54]. Several pathologic studies of patients that died suddenly implicate acute coronary thrombosis as a possible cause of sudden death, in addition to primary arrhythmias from a pre-existing ventricular scar[51, 55-58].

Acute coronary syndromes also play an important role in the progression of heart failure. It is estimated that the majority of cases of cardiomyopathy in the United States is ischemic in origin[59]. Furthermore, interventions which slow the progression of coronary artery disease (i.e., lipid lowering therapy) also appear to reduce the incidence of congestive heart failure[60].

IMAGING OF THE ATHEROSCLEROTIC LESION

Imaging alternatives to identify and characterize coronary atherosclerotic lesions have broadened considerably in the last several years. The driving forces behind the development of various alternatives to image the coronaries include the improvement of sensitivity and specificity for detection of disease, while limiting risk, cost and exposure to radiation. The modalities in use for the visualization of coronary atherosclerosis presently include angiography, angioscopy, intravascular ultrasound, electron beam computed tomography (CT) and magnetic resonance. While the use of these modalities varies significantly, each has demonstrated clinical usefulness in trials on human subjects. In contrast, B-mode ultrasound has not proven useful for the direct imaging of the coronaries, although correlative studies have demonstrated an increased risk of coronary events in patients with carotid atherosclerosis by duplex scanning [61, 62]. It is useful to note that several radiotracers capable of identifying components of the atherosclerotic lesion, such as LDL and monocytes, or intra-arterial thrombus, have shown promise in animal models of atherosclerosis, but are not yet available clinically [63].

Invasive Imaging Techniques. The most widely used technique for the visualization of coronary atherosclerosis remains angiography [64]. Although coronary angiography is an invasive procedure, it is safely performed on a routine basis at many centers and allows the option of percutaneous intervention upon diagnosis of significant atherosclerotic stenoses.   Angiography, however, only visualizes the lumen of the vessel, and can not provide reliable information regarding the content of the atherosclerotic lesion.   Furthermore, angiography is best at identifying advanced coronary lesions, but it is not a sensitive test for identifying the early atheroma.   Consequently, angiography can miss many vulnerable lesions.

The addition of angioscopy and intravascular ultrasound to angiography allows for a more complete characterization of the coronary artery. Angioscopy is particularly sensitive for the detection of intravascular thrombus in comparison to both angiography and intravascular ultrasound [65]. Intravascular ultrasound allows for a higher sensitivity in the detection of atherosclerotic disease.   In addition, intravascular ultrasound can distinguish between soft, fibrotic and calcified plaques based on differences in echogenicity within the atherosclerotic lesion.

Electron Beam CT.   Electron beam CT is a fast-growing modality for the detection of coronary calcification. It allows for the rapid acquisition of images of the coronary arteries at less cost and with less radioactivity exposure than angiography [66]. By detecting calcification of the coronaries, electron beam CT serves as a screening technique for the presence of atherosclerosis. The calcium score obtained with the electron beam CT appears to provide reliable diagnostic information regarding the extent of coronary disease [67, 68].   With adequate imaging, electron beam CT can be useful in the detection of high-grade coronary stenoses [69]. In addition, improvements in the calcium score obtained with electron beam CT have been noted with HMG-CoA reductase inhibitor treatment of hypercholesterolemia [70].While the sensitivity of electron beam CT is between 80 to 100 percent for the detection of obstructive coronary disease, some concern has been raised regarding the low specificity of the test (40-60%) [66, 71, 72]. As a result of the low specificity of electron beam CT, the American Heart Association is not supporting the use of electron beam CT for routine population-based screening for the presence of atherosclerosis [73].

Magnetic Resonance.   The use of MR for the visualization of coronary atherosclerotic lesions is still investigational. The cardiac and respiratory cycles cause motion artifacts and are the limiting factors in MR imaging.   Even so, the resolution of MR is accurate enough to allow for the visualization of aortic disease in transgenic mice [74].   Because of its resolving capability, MR holds the most promise of the available imaging techniques for the identification of the lesion at risk for rupture. On the basis of chemical composition, molecular motion, diffusion, physical state, or water content, MR is able to identify the components of the atherosclerotic lesion, such as the lipid core, fibrous cap, intraplaque hemorrhage and acute thrombus (Figure 5) [75-77]. MR angiography is routinely used for the detection of carotid, aortic and peripheral atherosclerosis, and is able to detect

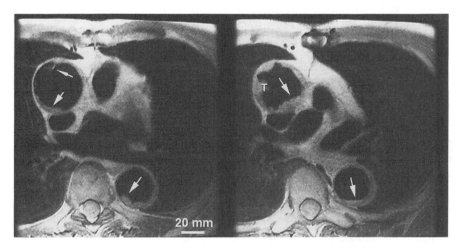

Figure 5. In-vivo aortic plaque magnetic resonance (MR) imaging of a patient with atherosclerotic plaques in both the descending and ascending aorta. T2-weighted (MR) images were acquired with a double inversion-recovery, fast spin-echo sequence. In the ascending aorta, we see a severely thrombotic plaque (AHA type VI) with a very irregular surface and increased wall thickness (right panel). A thrombus (T) in the arterial lumen is also shown (right panel). In the ascending aorta, the site of plaque rupture is seen (left panel, narrow arrow). In the descending aorta, a fibrotic plaque (AHA type Vc) with increased wall thickness (arrows, both panels) is present. Plaque characterization was based on the information obtained from T1-proton density and T2 weighted MR images.

coronary stenosis. At this time, it is unlikely that MR coronary angiography (MRCA) is going to replace conventional coronary angiography, but there are a variety of clinical applications for MRCA . Potential uses include the visualization of coronary artery anomalies, proximal coronary bypass graft patency and proximal coronary tree follow-up post coronary intervention [78].

Recently, we have reported in patients with aortic atherosclerotic plaques, an MR method for the direct assessment of aortic plaque thickness, extent and composition [79]. This method may lend itself to use as a screening tool for the prediction of future cardiovascular events and evaluation of therapeutic interventions. New methods are currently being developed for in-vivo coronary plaque characterization.

PREVENTION OF ACUTE CORONARY SYNDROMES

In addition to lifestyle modifications such as smoking cessation, weight loss and exercise, other risks for coronary artery disease must be controlled in order to prevent the occurrence of coronary events. The aggressive lowering of serum lipids by primary and secondary prevention is essential in prevention of acute coronary syndromes. In hypercholesterolemic patients without coronary artery disease and following acute coronary events, lipid lowering has been shown to significantly improve prognosis[80-82]. Despite the proven benefits of lipid lowering, there is no equivalent evidence of atherosclerotic plaque regression by angiography accounting for the reduction in coronary events [83, 84]. However, by stabilizing the atheromatous plaque and decreasing its lipid content, cholesterol lowering may make the plaque more resistant to disruption [85, 86].

Plaque stabilization may occur through several mechanisms. Reduction in serum lipid levels decreases lipid infiltration into the plaque. The result is a net efflux of lipid from the atherosclerotic plaque. The reduced lipid content in the plaque is associated with reduced macrophage infiltration and therefore reduced metalloproteinase, free radical and cytokine elaboration[87-89]. Additionally, the process of programmed cell death, known as apoptosis, which occurs in cells of the atherosclerotic plaque, seems to be reduced by lipid lowering, as is the expression of the proapoptotic protein Bax in the plaque[43].

Secondary prevention of the complications of coronary events may involve treatment with systemic anticoagulation. Anticoagulation is clearly indicated both acutely and long-term after MI in those at risk for systemic emboli (patients with atrial fibrillation, left ventricular thrombus, or a large MI). Anticoagulation is also indicated for 48 hours after thrombolysis with alteplase [90]. However, long-term anticoagulation with warfarin or a combination of low fixed doses of warfarin and ASA does not appear to be more effective than ASA alone[91, 92]. Given the excess bleeding sequellae and complicated dosing of warfarin, ASA appears preferable [93].

New risk factors of coronary artery disease are now emerging. Some of these factors, homocysteine and P-selectin, are associated with endothelial dysfunction[28]. Others, such as tissue factor, factor VII and fibrinogen, herald a thrombotic state. Estrogen deficiency states are associated with dyslipidemia and endothelial dysfunction [46]. These potential risk factors, their actions and putative therapies need better elucidation.

TREATMENT OF PLAQUE RUPTURE AND ITS COMPLICATIONS

As atherosclerotic plaque rupture represents an important aspect of the pathophysiology of the acute coronary syndromes, the clinical approach to these syndromes must address the potential complications of plaque rupture. Thus, antithrombotic therapy, designed to halt or reverse the accumulation of thrombus over the disrupted plaque, has become a mainstay of therapy in acute coronary syndromes. Antianginal therapy helps treat the coronary vasospasm associated with the ruptured plaque. In addition, antianginals reduce the metabolic needs of the heart and the propensity towards arrhythmia associated with the acute coronary syndromes[94]. Most importantly, prevention in coronary disease is geared towards increasing the stability of the atherosclerotic plaque, preventing its progression, and reducing systemic thrombogenic factors which may complicate plaque rupture.

Antithrombotic and anti-platelet therapies. Antithrombotic therapies, designed to reverse or halt the accumulation of thrombus over the disrupted plaque, have become a mainstay in acute coronary syndromes. While thrombolytic agents have been shown to improve outcome following acute MI [95, 96], to date there has been no evidence supporting their use in unstable angina and non-Q wave MI [97]. A proposed mechanism to explain this difference may relate to the importance of fibrin in addition to platelets in the pathogenesis of acute MI. In contrast, in unstable angina, platelets appear to predominate in the intracoronary thrombus [98].

The most widely used and least toxic antithrombotic agent, used in both acute and chronic coronary artery disease is aspirin. It is effective in unstable angina[99], acute myocardial infarction, during and after coronary revascularization as well as in the prevention of cerebrovascular events[14, 15]. Aspirin reduces the risk of fatal or nonfatal MI by 71% during the acute phase[100, 101], by 60% at 3 months[101, 102] and by 52% at 2 years[103]. The mechanism accounting for the beneficial effects is the irreversible inhibition of cyclooygenase pathways in platelets, blocking formation of thromboxane A2 and platelet aggregation. Drugs that inhibit thromboxane synthase, the thromboxane receptor, or both have not proven to be more advantageous than aspirin.

The thienopyridines, ticlopidine and clopidogrel, block platelet aggregation induced by ADP and the transformation of Glycoprotein IIb/IIIa into its high affinity state. Ticlopidine and clopidogrel are acceptable alternatives for secondary prevention in patients with poor tolerance to aspirin; however, their role in acute situations has not been evaluated[46]. In addition, the cost and potential side effects of these therapies are important considerations.

Heparin is recommended in the management of unstable angina based on documented efficacy in many trials and supported by meta-analyses[104, 105]. In the setting of acute MI, heparin is strongly indicated as an adjunct to the use of tissue plasminogen activator (tPA). Heparin is given as an intravenous bolus followed by infusion at levels titrated to activated partial thromboplastin time 1.5 - 2 times the upper limit of normal.

Low-molecular-weight heparins have shown promise in the treatment of acute coronary syndromes. These agents induce less platelet activation, can be given subcutaneously once or twice daily, do not need to be monitored, have better bioavailibility and produce more reproducible anticoagulation[46].

Direct thrombin inhibitors, hirudin and hirulog, which act by blocking the early stage of thrombin-related platelet activation and fibrin formation, have been widely investigated over the last several years with varying results[106-109]. Preliminary data, from patients with acute coronary syndromes without ST elevation, show that low dose infusion results in only a marginal benefit[110]. At higher doses excess bleeding has led to premature discontinuation of the drug[111]. A large trial is now underway evaluating the effects of moderate doses of hirudin on the basis of favorable results observed in pilot studies [106].

More selective antithrombotic therapies are evolving targeting factors such as glycoprotein 1b/IX and inactive fragments of von Willebrand factor. Other therapeutic targets include the TF-factor VII complex, the tenase complex (direct inhibitors of factor Xa), and amplification of endogenous anticoagulants such as heparin cofactor 2 and recombinant activated protein C [46].

Thrombolytic therapy represents a substantial advance in the reduction of mortality after acute MI[95, 96]. However, thrombolysis has not proven effective in the treatment of unstable angina [97]. Unstable angina is felt to depend mainly on platelet-mediated mechanisms of thrombosis[98]. As a result, unstable angina is less responsive to fibrinolytic therapies than to antiplatelet strategies such as aspirin and the GP IIb/IIIa antagonists.

The most recent breakthrough in treatment modalities used in the acute coronary syndromes utilizes glycoprotein IIb/IIIa receptor antagonists[112]. Direct occupancy of the receptor by monoclonal antibody or by synthetic compounds mimicking the fibrinogen binding sequence prevents platelet aggregation. Abciximab, a monoclonal antibody against the IIb/IIIa receptor, eptifibatide, a peptidic inhibitor and the nonpeptides, lamifiban and tirofiban, are now available for intravenous use. The effects of these drugs are highly specific at therapeutic doses. Recent data has indicated an improved outcome in patients receiving these agents in the setting of acute coronary syndromes[113, 114]. Like aspirin, abciximab, a glycoprotein IIb/IIIa antagonist, has proven effective at reducing cardiac events after coronary interventions in the setting of acute coronary syndromes[114, 115]. Therapy with antiplatelet agents has been associated with an increased risk of bleeding [95]. However, bleeding risk with abciximab as an adjunct to percutaneous intervention has improved substantially with dose modification and other improvements[114, 115].

Trials with abciximab have demonstrated its efficacy in preventing death, MI and abrupt closure associated with coronary angioplasty[114]. Because of the preponderance of supportive data, these agents are now routinely used for percutaneous coronary interventions. Recent trials have shown that Glycoprotein IIb/IIIa receptor antagonists combined with aspirin improve the reperfusion rate and decrease the incidence of recurrent cardiac events[116, 117]. Experimental data suggests that in addition to requiring lower doses of fibrinolytic agents in the presence of Glycoprotein IIb/IIIa receptor antagonists, these agents also prevent reocclusion of the coronary arteries after using thrombolytics[118-120].

CONCLUSIONS

Over the last two decades, our understanding of the biology of the atherosclerotic lesion has broadened considerably. As scientists and physicians identified more effective methods to diagnose coronary artery disease and characterized factors leading to plaque instability, the ability to prevent the complications of coronary disease has improved. The multiple factors involved in the acute coronary syndromes suggest the need to target these syndromes at several levels. Both basic and clinical investigation continue to increase our knowledge about the underlying events occurring in the acute coronary syndromes. Through increased understanding of the atherosclerotic process we can continue to identify novel targets for the prevention, diagnosis and treatment of atherosclerotic heart disease.

Acknowledgments

Portions of this chapter were modified from the following article: Fischer A, Gutstein DE, Fuster V. Thrombosis and coagulation abnormalities in the acute coronary syndromes. Cardiol Clin, in press

REFERENCES.

1. Goldberg RJ, Gorak EJ, Yarzebski J, et al. A communitywide perspective of sex differences and temporal trends in the incidence and survival rates after acute myocardial infarction and out-of-hospital deaths caused by coronary heart disease. Circulation 1993; 87:1947-53.
2. Gillum RF. Trends in acute myocardial infarction and coronary heart disease death in the United States. J Am Coll Cardiol 1994; 23:1273-7.
3. Gheorghiade M, Ruzumna P, Borzak S, Havstad S, Ali A, Goldstein S. Decline in the rate of hospital mortality from acute myocardial infarction: impact of changing management strategies. Am Heart J 1996; 131:250-6.
4. Thom TJ, Epstein FH. Heart Disease, cancer, and stroke mortality trends and their interpretations: an international perspective. Circulation 1994; 90:574-82.
5. Naylor CD, Chen E. Population-wide mortality trends among patients hospitalized for acute myocardial infarction: the Ontario experience, 1981 to 1991. J Am Coll Cardiol 1994; 24:1431-8.
6. Dellborg M, Eriksson P, Riha M, Swedberg K. Declining hospital mortality in acute myocardial infarction. European Heart Journal 1994; 15:5-9.
7. Behar S, Barbash GI, Copel L, Gottlieb S, Goldbourt U. Improved survival of hospitalized patients with acute myocardial infarction from 1981-1983 to 1992 in Israel. Coronary Artery Disease 1994; 5:1001-7.
8. Gottleib S, Goldbourt U, Boyko V, et al. Improved outcome of elderly patients (≥75 years of age) with acute myocardial infarction from 1981-1983 to 1992-1994 in Israel. Circulation 1997; 95:342-50.
9. Stary HC, Chandler AB, Dinsmore RE, et al. A definition of advanced types of atherosclerotic lesions and a histologic classification of atherosclerosis: a report from the Committee on Arteriosclerosis, American Heart Association. Circulation 1995; 92:1355-74.
10. Fuster V, Fallon JT, Nemerson Y. Coronary thrombosis. Lancet 1996; 348 (Suppl):s7-s10.
11. Gutstein DE, Fuster V. The pathophysiology and clinical significance of atherosclerotic plaque rupture. Cardiovasc Res in press.
12. Richardson PD, Davies MJ, Born GV. Influence of plaque configuration and stress distribution on fissuring of coronary atherosclerotic plaques. Lancet 1989; 2:1462-3.
13. Ambrose JA, Tannenbaum M, Alexpoulos D, et al. Angiographic progression of coronary artery disease and the development of myocardial infarction. J Am Coll Cardiol 1988; 12:56-62.
14. Fuster V. Lewis A. Conner Memorial Lecture. Mechanisms leading to myocardial infarction: insights from studies of vascular biology. Circulation 1994; 90:2126-46.
15. Fuster V, Badimon L, Badimon JJ, Chesebro JH. The pathogenesis of coronary artery disease and the acute coronary syndromes. N Engl J Med 1992; 326:310-318.
16. Ross R. The Pathogenesis of Atherosclerosis: A perspective for for the 1990's. Nature 1993; 362:801-808.
17. Steinberg D. Antioxidants and atherosclerosis: a current assessment. Circulation 1991; 84:1420-1425.
18. Steinberg D. Antioxidants in the prevention of human atherosclerosis. Circulation 1992; 85:2338.
19. Rosenfeld ME, Pestel E. Cellularity of atherosclerotic lesions. Cor Art Dis 1994; 5:189-197.
20. Navab M, Hama SY, Nguyen TB, Fogelman AM. Monocyte adhesion and transmigration in atherosclerosis. Cor Art Dis 1994; 5:198-204.
21. van der Wal AC, Becker AE, van der Loos CM, Das PK. Site of intimal rupture or erosion of thrombosed coronary atherosclerotic plaques is characterized by an inflammatory process irrespective of the dominant plaque morphology. Circulation 1994; 89:36-44.

22. Moreno PR, Falk E, Palacios IF, Newell JB, Fuster V, Fallon JT. Macrophage infiltration in acute coronary syndromes: implications for plaque rupture. Circulation 1994; 90:775-8.

23. Falk E, Shah PK, Fuster V. Coronary plaque disruption. Circulation 1995; 92:657-71.

24. Shah PK, Falk E, Badimon JJ, et al. Human monocyte-derived macrophages induce collagen breakdown in fibrous caps of atherosclerotic plaques: potential role of matrix-degrading metalloproteinases and implications for plaque rupture. Circulation 1995; 92:1565-9.

25. Galis ZS, Sukhova GK, Kranzhofer R, Clark S, Libby P. Macrophage foam cells from experimental atheroma constitutively produce matrix-degrading proteinases. Proc Natl Acad Sci USA 1995; 92:402-6.

26. Libby P. Molecular basis of the acute coronary syndromes. Circulation 1995; 91:2844-50.

27. Rajagopalan S, Meng XP, Ramasamy S, Harrison DG, Galis ZS. Reactive oxygen species produced by macrophage-derived foam cells regulate the activity of vascular matrix metalloproteinases in vivo: implications for atherosclerotic plaque stability. J Clin Invest 1996; 98:2572-9.

28. Schecter AD, Rollins BJ, Zhang YJ, et al. Tissue factor is induced by monocyte chemoattractant protein-1 in human aortic smooth muscle and THP-1 cells. J Biol Chem 1997; 272:28568-73.

29. Bjorkerud S, Bjorkerud B. Apoptosis is abundant in human atherosclerotic lesions, especially in inflammatory cells (macrophages and T cells), and may contribute to the accumulation of gruel and plaque instability. Am J Pathol 1996; 149:367-80.

30. Melnick JL, Adam E, DeBakey ME. Possible role of cytomegalovirus in atherogenesis. JAMA 1990; 263:2204-7.

31. Pasceri V, Cammarota G, Patti G, et al. Association of virulent Helicobacter pylori strains with ischemic heart disease. Circulation 1998; 97:1675-79.

32. Campbell LA, O'Brien ER, Cappuccio AL, et al. Detection of Chlamydia pneumoniae TWAR in human coronary atherectomy tissues. J Infect Dis 1995; 172:585-8.

33. Gupta S, Leatham EW, Carrington D, Mendall MA, Kaski JC, Camm AJ. Elevated Chlamydia pneumoniae antibodies, cardiovascular events, and azithromycin in male survivors of myocardial infarction. Circulation 1997; 96:404-7.

34. Gurfinkel E, Bozovich G, Daroca A, Beck E, Mautner B, Group ftRS. Randomized trial of roxithromycin in non-Q-wave coronary syndromes: ROXIS pilot study. Lancet 1997; 350:404-7.

35. Wang P, Ba ZF, Chaudry IH. Administration of tumor necrosis factor-α in vivo depresses endothelium-dependent relaxation. Am J Physiol 1994; 266:H2535-41.

36. Bhagat K, Moss R, Collier J, et al. Endothelial 'stunning' following a brief exposure to endotoxin: a mechanism to link infection and infarction? Cardiovasc Res 1996; 32:822-9.

37. Smith PD, Saini SS, Raffeld M, Manischewitz JF, Wahl SM. Cytomegalovirus induction of tumor necrosis factor-α by human monocytes and mucosal macrophages. J Clin Invest 1992; 90:1642-1648.

38. Witzum JL, Steinberg D. Role of oxidized low density lipoprotein in atherogenesis. J Clin Invest 1991; 88:1785-92.

39. Lapenna D, de Gioia S, Ciofani G, et al. Glutathione-related antioxidant defenses in human atherosclerotic plaques. Circulation 1998; 97:1930-4.

40. Han DKM, Haudenschild CC, Hong MK, Tinkle BT, Leon MB, Liau G. Evidence for apoptosis in human atherogenesis and in a rat vascular injury model. Am J Pathol 1995; 147:267-77.

41. Kockx MM, De Meyer GRY, Muhring J, Jacob W, Bult H, Herman AG. Apoptosis and related proteins in different stages of human atherosclerotic plaques. Circulation 1998; 97:2307-15.

42. Geng YJ, Wu Q, Muszynski M, Hansson GK, Libby P. Apoptosis of vascular smooth muscle cells induced by in vitro stimulation with interferon-γ, tumor necrosis factor-α, and interleukin-1β. Arterioscler Thromb Vasc Biol 1996; 16:19-27.

43. Kockx MM, De Meyer GR, Buyssens N, Knaapen MW, Bult H, Herman AG. Cell composition, replication, and apoptosis in atherosclerotic plaques after 6 months of cholesterol withdrawal. Circ Res 1998; 83:378-87.

44. Fernandez-Ortiz A, Badimon JJ, Falk E, et al. Characterization of the relative thrombogenicity of atherosclerotic plaque components: implications for consequences of plaque rupture. J Am Coll Cardiol 1994; 23:1562-9.

45. Banner DW, D'Arcy A, Chene C, et al. The crystal structure of the complex of blood coagulation factor VIIa with soluble tissue factor. Nature 1996; 380:41-6.

46. Theroux P, Fuster V. Acute coronary syndromes: unstable angina and non-Q-wave myocardial infarction. Circulation 1998; 97:1195-1206.

47. Braunwald E, Jones RH, Mark DB, et al. Diagnosing and managing unstable angina. Circulation 1994; 90:613-22.

48. Aguirre FV, Younis LL, Chaitman BR, et al. Early and 1-year clinical outcome of patients evolving non-Q-wave versus Q-wave myocardial infarction after thrombolysis: results from the TIMI II study. Circulation 1995; 91:2541-48.

49. Zareba W, Moss AJ, Raubertas RF. Risk of subsequent cardiac events in stable convalescing patients after first non-Q-wave and Q-wave myocardial infarction. Coron Artery Dis 1994; 5:1009-18.

50. Braunwald E. Unstable angina: a classification. Circulation 1989; 80:410-4.

51. Davies MJ, Thomas A. Thrombosis and acute coronary artery lesions in sudden cardiac ischemic death. N Engl J Med 1984; 310:1137-40.

52. Demirovic J, Myerburg RJ. Epidemiology of sudden coronary death: an overview. Prog Cardiovasc Dis 1994; 37:39-48.

53. Janse MJ, Wit AL. Electrophysiological mechanisms of ventricular arrhythmias resulting from myocardial ischemia and infarction. Physiol Rev 1989; 69:1049-1169.

54. Opitz CF, Mitchell GF, Pfeffer MA, Pfeffer JM. Arrhythmias and death after coronary occlusion in the rat: continuous telemetric ECG monitoring in conscious, untethered rats. Circulation 1995; 92:253-61.

55. Davies MJ. Anatomic features in victims of sudden coronary death: coronary artery pathology. Circulation 1992; 85(Suppl I):I-19-I-24.

56. Vanantiz JM, Becker AE. Sudden cardiac death and acute pathology of coronary arteries. Eur Heart J 1986; 7:987-91.

57. Warnes CA, Roberts WC. Sudden cardiac death: comparison of patients with to those without coronary thrombosis at necropsy. Am J Cardiol 1984; 54:1206-11.

58. Burke AP, Farb A, Malcom GT, Liang Y, Smialek J, Virmani R. Effect of risk factors on the mechanism of acute thrombosis and sudden coronary death in women. Circulation 1998; 97:2110-6.

59. Gheorghiade M, Bonow RO. Chronic heart failure in the United States: a manifestation of coronary artery disease. Circulation 1998; 97:282-89.

60. Pedersen TR, Kjekshus J, Berg K, et al. Cholesterol lowering and the use of healthcare resources: results of the Scandinavian Simvastatin Survival Study. Circulation 1996; 93:1796-802.

61. Bots ML, Hoes AW, Koudstaal PJ, Hofman A, Grobbee DE. Common carotid intima-media thickness and risk of stroke and myocardial infarction: the Rotterdam Study. Circulation 1997; 96:1432-7.

62. O'Leary DH, Polak JF, Kronmal RA, Manolio TA, Burke GL, Wolfson SKJ. Carotid-artery intima and media thickness as a risk factor for myocardial infarction and stroke in older adults. N Engl J Med 1999; 340:14-22.

63. Vallabhajosula S, Fuster V. Atherosclerosis: imaging techniques and the evolving role of nuclear medicine. J Nucl Med 1997; 38:1788-96.

64. Ambrose JA. Angiographic correlations of advanced coronary lesions in acute coronary syndromes. In: Fuster V, ed. Syndromes of atherosclerosis: correlations of clinical imaging and pathology. Armonk, NY: Futura Publishing Co., Inc., 1996:105-22.

65. Feld S, Ganim M, Cavell ES, et al. Comparison of angioscopy intra-vascular ultrasound imaging and quantitative coronary angiography in predicting clinical outcome after coronary intervention in high-risk patients. J Am Coll Cardiol 1996; 28:97-105.

66. Taylor AJ, O'Mally PG. Self-referral of patients for electron-beam computed tomography to screen for coronary artery disease. N Engl J Med 1998; 339:2018-9.

67. Budoff MJ, Georgiou D, Brody A, et al. Ultrafast computed tomography as a diagnostic modality in the detection of coronary artery disease: a multicenter study. Circulation 1996; 93:898-904.

68. Rumberger JA, Sheddy PE, Breen JF, Schwartz RS. Electron beam computed tomographic coronary calcium score cutpoints and severity of associated angiographic lumen stenosis. J Am Coll Cardiol 1997; 29:1542-8.

69. Achenbach S, Moshage W, Ropers D, Nossen J, Daniel WG. Value of electron-beam computed tomography for the noninvasive detction of high-grade coronary-artery stenosis and occlusions. N Engl J Med 1998; 339:1964-71.

70. Callister TQ, Raggi P, Cooil B, Lippolis NJ, Russo DJ. Effect of HMG-CoA reductase inhibitors on coronary artery disease as assessed by electron-beam computed tomography. N Engl J Med 1998; 339:1972-8.

71. Fiorino AS. Electron-beam computed tomography, coronary artery calcium, and evaluation of patients with coronary artery disease. Ann Intern Med 1998; 128:839-47.

72. Celermajer DS. Noninvasive detection of atherosclerosis. N Engl J Med 1998; 339:2014-5.

73. Wexler L, Brundage B, Crouse J, et al. Coronary artery calcification: pathophysiology, epidemiology, imaging methods, and clinical implications: a statement for health professionals from the American Heart Association. Circulation 1996; 94:1175-92.

74. Fayad ZA, Fallon JT, Shinnar M, et al. Noninvasive in vivo high-resolution magnetic resonance imaging of atherosclerotic lesions in genetically engineered mice. Circulation 1998; 98:1541-7.

75. Toussaint JF, Southern JF, Fuster V, Kantor HL. T_2-weighted contrast for NMR characterization of human atherosclerosis. Arterioscler Thromb 1995; 15:1533-42.

76. Toussaint JF, LaMuraglia GM, Southern JF, et al. Magnetic resonance images lipid, fibrous, calcified, hemorrhagic and thrombotic components of human atherosclerosis in vivo. Circulation 1996; 1994:932-8.

77. Skinner MP, Yuan C, Mitsumori L, et al. Serial magnetic resonance imaging of experimental atherosclerosis detects lesion fine structure, progression and complications in vivo. Nat Med 1995; 1:69-73.

78. Pennell DJ, Bogren HG, Keegan J, et al. Assessment of coronary stenosis by magnetic resonance imaging. Heart 1996; 75:127-33.

79. Fayad ZA, Nahar T, Badimon JJ, et al. In-Vivo MR characterization of plaques in the thoracic aorta. Circulation 1998; 98:I-515.

80. Shepherd J, Cobbe SM, Ford I, et al. Prevention of coronary heart disease with pravastatin in men with hypercholesterolemia: West of Scotland Coronary Prevention Study Group. N Engl J Med 1995; 333:1301-7.

81. Scandinavian Simvastatin Survival Study Group. Randomised trial of cholesterol lowering in 4444 patients with coronary heart disease: the Scandinavian Simvastatin Survival Study (4S). Lancet 1994; 344:1383-89.

82. The Cholesterol and Recurrent Events (CARE) Trial Investigators. The effect of pravastatin on coronary events after myocardial infarction in patients with average cholesterol levels. N Engl J Med 1996; 335:1001-9.

83. Fuster V, Badimon JJ. Regression or stabilization of atherosclerosis means regression or stabilization of what we don't see in the arteriogram. Eur Heart J 1995; 16:6-12.

84. Waters D. Review of cholesterol-lowering therapy: coronary angiographic and events trials. Am J Med 1996; 101 (suppl 4A):34S-39S.

85. Gotto AM. Cholesterol management in theory and practice. Circulation 1997; 96:4424-30.

86. Fuster V, Fallon JT, Badimon JJ, Nemerson Y. The unstable atherosclerotic plaque: clinical significance and therapeutic intervention. Thromb Haemost 1997; 78:247-55.

87. Small DM, Bond MG, Waugh D, Prack M, Sawyer JK. Physicochemical and histological changes in the arterial wall of nonhuman primates during progression and regression of atherosclerosis. J Clin Invest 1984; 73:1590-605.

88. Kaplan JR, Manuck SB, Adams MR, Williams JK, Register TC, Clarkson TB. Plaque changes and arteriet alnlargement in atherosclerotic monkeys after manipulation of diet and societ alnvironment. Arterioscler Thromb 1993; 13:254-63.

89. Aikawa M, Rabkin E, Okada Y, et al. Lipid lowering by diet reduces matrix metalloproteinase activity and increases collagen content of rabbit atheroma: a potential mechanism of lesion stabilization. Circulation 1998; 97:2433-44.

90. Ryan TJ, Anderson JL, Antman EM, et al. ACC/AHA guidelines for the management of patients with acute myocardial infarction: a report of the American College of Cardiology/American Heart Association Task Force on Practice Guidelines (Committee on Management of Acute Myocardial Infarction). J Am Coll Cardiol 1996; 28:1328-428.

91. The E.P.S.I.M. Research Group. A controlled comparison of aspirin and oral anticoagulants in prevention of death after myocardial infarction. N Engl J Med 1982; 307:701-8.

92. The Coumadin Aspirin Reinfarction Study (CARS) Investigators. Randomised double-blind trial of fixed low-dose warfarin with aspirin after myocardial infarction. Lancet 1997; 350:389-96.

93. Prentice CRM. Antithrombotic therapy in the secondary prevention of myocardial infarction. Am J Cardiol 1993; 72:175G-180G.

94. Gutstein DE, Fuster V. Pathophysiologic bases for adjunctive therapies in the treatment and secondary prevention of acute myocardial infarction. Clin Cardiol 1998; 21:161-8.

95. ISIS (Second International Study of Infarct Survival) Collaborative Group. Randomised trial of intravenous streptokinase, oral aspirin, both or neither among 17,187 cases of suspected acute myocardial infarction: ISIS-2. Lancet 1988; 2:349-60.

96. Gruppo Italiano per lo Studio della Streptochinasi Nell'Infarto Miocardico (GISSI). Effectiveness of intravenous thrombolytic treatment in acute myocardial infarction. Lancet 1986; 1:397-402.

97. TIMI IIIB Investigators. Effects of tissue plasminogen activator and a comparison of early invasive and conservative strategies in unstable angina and non-Q-wave myocardial infarction: results of the TIMI IIIB trial. Circulation 1994; 89:1545-56.

98. Mizuno K, Satomura K, Miyamoto A, et al. Angioscopic evaluation of coronary artery thrombi in acute coronary syndromes. N Engl J Med 1992; 326:287-91.

99. Antiplatelet Trialists' Collaboration. Collaborative overview of randomised trials of antiplatelet therapy-I: prevention of death, myocardial infarction, and stroke by prolonged antiplatelet therapy in various categories of patients. BMJ 1994; 308:81-106.

100. Theroux P, Ouimet H, McCans J, et al. Aspirin, heparin or both to treat acute unstable angina. N Engl J Med 1988; 319:1105-11.

101. The RISC Group. Risk of myocardial infarction and death during treatment with low dose aspirin and intravenous heparin in men with unstable coronary disease. Lancet 1990; 336:827-30.

102. Lewis HD, Davis JW, Archibald DG, et al. Protective effects of aspirin against myocardial infarction and death in men with unstable angina. N Engl J Med 1983; 309:396-403.

103. Cairns JA, Gent M, Singer J, et al. Aspirin, sulfinpyrazone, or both in unstable angina. N Engl J Med 1985; 313:1369-75.

104. Cohen M, Adams PC, Parry G, et al. Combination antithrombotic therapy in unstable angina and non-Q-wave infarction in nonprior aspirin users. Circulation 1994; 89:81-8.

105. Oler S, Whooley MA, Oler J, Grady D. Adding heparin to aspirin reduces the incidence of myocardial infarction and death in patients with unstable angina. JAMA 1996; 276:811-5.

106. Organization to Assess Strategies for Ischemic Syndromes (OASIS) Investigators. Comparison of the effects of two doses of recombinant hirudin compared with heparin in patients with acute myocardial ischemia without ST elevation: a pilot study. Circulation 1997; 96:769-77.

107. White HD, Aylward PE, Frey MJ, et al. Randomized, double-blind comparison of hirulog versus heparin in patients receiving streptokinase and aspirin for acute myocardial infarction (HERO). Circulation 1997; 96:2155-61.

108. Cohen M, Demers C, Gurfinkel EP, et al. A comparison of low-molecular-weight heparin with unfractionated heparin for unstable coronary artery disease. N Engl J Med 1997; 337:447-52.

109. Fragmin during Instability in Coronary Artery Disease (FRISC) Study Group. Low-molecular-weight heparin during instability in coronary artery disease. Lancet 1996; 347:561-8.

110. The Global Use of Strategies to Open Occluded Coronary Arteries (GUSTO) IIb Investigators. A comparison of recombinant hirudin with heparin for the treatment of acute coronary syndromes. N Engl J Med 1996; 335:775-82.

111. The Global Use of Strategies to Open Occluded Coronary Arteries (GUSTO) IIa Investigators. Randomized trial of intravenous heparin versus recombinant hirudin for acute coronary syndromes. Circulation 1994; 90:1631-7.

112. Coller BS. Blockade of platelet GP IIb/IIIa receptors as an antithrombotic strategy. Circulation 1995; 92:2373-80.

113. Use of a monoclonal antibody directed against the platelet glycoprotein IIb/IIIa receptor in high-risk coronary angioplasty: The EPIC Investigation. N Engl J Med 1994; 330:956-61.

114. The CAPTURE Investigators. Randomised placebo-controlled trial of abciximab before and during coronary intervention in refractory unstable angina: The CAPTURE Study. Lancet 1997; 349:1429-35.

115. The EPIC Investigators. Use of a monoclonal antibody directed against the platelet glycoprotein IIb/IIIa receptor in high-risk coronary angioplasty. The EPIC Investigation. N Engl J Med 1994; 330:956-61.

116. Nicolini FA, Lee P, Rios G, Kottke-Marchant K, Topol EJ. Combination of platelet fibrinogen receptor antagonist and direct antithrombin inhibitor at low doses markedly improves thrombolysis. Circulation 1994; 89:1802-9.

117. Ohman EM, Kleiman NS, Gacioch G, et al. Combined accelerated tissue-plasminogen activator and platelet glycoprotein IIb/IIIa integrin receptor blockade with integrilin in acute myocardial infarction. Circulation 1997; 95:846-54.

118. Shebuski RJ, Stabilito IJ, Sitko GR, Polokoff MH. Acceleration of recombinant tissue-type plasminogen activator-induced thrombolysis and prevention of reocclusion by the combination of heparin and the Arg-Gly-Asp-containing peptide bitistatin in a canine model of coronary thrombosis. Circulation 1990; 82:169-77.

119. Coller BS. Inhibitors of the platelet glycoprotein IIb/IIIa receptor as conjunctive therapy for coronary artery thrombolysis. Coron Artery Dis 1992; 3:1016-29.

120. Gold HK, Coller BS, Yasuda T, et al. Rapid and sustained coronary artery recanalization with combined bolus injection of recombinant tissue-type plasminogen activator and monoclonal antiplatelet GP IIb/IIIa antibody in a canine preparation. Circulation 1988; 77:670-7.

121. Toschi V, Gallo R, Lettino M, et al. Tissue factor predicts the thrombogenicity of human atherosclerotic plaque components. Circulation 1997; 95:594-9.

5 PREVENTION OF ATHEROSCLEROSIS: ENDOTHELIAL FUNCTION, CHOLESTEROL, AND ANTIOXIDANTS

Robert A. Vogel, M.D.
University of Maryland School of Medicine

INTRODUCTION

Although age-adjusted mortality from atherosclerosis-related diseases has declined significantly in the United States and some European countries over the past four decades, it has recently become the world's leading cause of death, exceeding infectious diseases. Considerable epidemiologic, clinical, and experimental data suggest a causative relationship between coronary risk factors, especially hypercholesterolemia, and atherosclerotic cardiovascular disease.[1-9] Coronary and other atherosclerosis have traditionally been thought to result from cholesterol deposition, modification, and macrophage uptake leading to vascular smooth muscle cell proliferation and matrix formation.[10-12] Cardiovascular events subsequently arise from plaque rupture or ulceration with ensuing partial or complete vessel occlusion. Recently, the vasculature has been found to be an active and complex organ rather than a passive conduit. The endothelium is now known to be an important regulator of vascular tone, lipid breakdown, thrombogenesis, inflamation, and vessel growth.[13-141] In the presence of risk factors such as hypercholesterolemia, the endothelium promotes atherosclerosis through vasoconstriction, monocyte and platelet adhesion, thrombogenesis, and growth factor release. This dysfunctional state appears before the earliest anatomic evidence of atherosclerosis. Hypercholesterolemia and the other risk factors have been shown to reduce nitric oxide availability, the predominate endothelium-derived vasodilator. Experimentally, reduced nitric oxide availability leads to a proatherogenic state.[19-21] Improvements in endothelium-dependent vasodilation have been demonstrated by several cholesterol lowering and other risk factor modification trials. Although considerable evidence supports increased nitric oxide destruction in the presence of risk factors by superoxide anion, other data point to decreased nitric oxide production.[22] Antioxidant vitamins, especially vitamin E, have been found to be inversely correlated with coronary heart disease risk in observational studies.[142] Although most prospective trials of antioxidant vitamin therapy have not shown significant beneficial effects, a single vitamin E trial and several fruit and vegetable-rich diet trials have shown dramatic reductions in cardiovascular events.[143-155] One mechanism by which antioxidant vitamins may reduce atherosclerotic events is through improvement in endothelial function, possibly by increasing nitric oxide availability and decreasing adhesion molecule expression.[156-163] At least short-term improvements in endothelial function have be demonstrated with antioxidant therapy, supporting the concept of increased nitric oxide destruction. These observations suggest that atherosclerosis is at least in part due to endothelial dysfunction which may be improved by antioxidant therapy. This new understanding helps to explain the early and substantial reductions in major cardiovascular events associated with risk factor modification and underscore the importance of this therapy. This chapter reviews the evidence that risk factors produce endothelial dysfunction, perhaps through increased oxidative stress, leading to the development of atherosclerosis.

HYPERCHOLESTEROLEMIA AND CORONARY HEART DISEASE

Following early identification of the presence of cholesterol in atheroma, Anitschkow observed that atherosclerotic lesions could be induced in susceptible animals by a high saturated fat and cholesterol diet, and that lesions regressed when a low fat and cholesterol diet was resumed.[1] The landmark Framingham Heart Study, initiated in 1948, followed more than 5,000 men and women who were initially without cardiovascular disease.[2] This study demonstrated that hypercholesterolemia increases the risk of cardiovascular events and originated the concept of coronary risk factors. The Seven Countries Study and the Multiple Risk Factor Intervention Trial found continuous, graded relationships between serum cholesterol and coronary heart disease risk, although societies appear to lie on different cholesterol-risk curves.[3,4] The strongest evidence that dyslipidemias are causally related to the development of coronary heart disease is derived from clinical lipid lowering trials.[5-9] The Lipid Research Clinics Coronary Primary Prevention Trial and the Helsinki Heart Trial found 19-34% reductions in cardiovascular events in hypercholesterolemic men treated with cholestyramine and gemfibrozil, repectively.[5-7] During the past two decades, numerous coronary angiographic trials ulilizing different means of cholesterol lowering have consistently found reductions in disease progression and appearance of new lesions and an increases in disease regression.[164-168] Major cardiovascular events have also been found to decrease within months of starting treatment, despite the one to two years necessary to demonstrate anatomic changes. This association supports the concept of plaque stabilization possibly brought about by improvements in endothelial function.[8] In the past five years, three large secondary prevention trials (Scandinavian Simvastatin Survival Study, Cholesterol and Recurrent Events Trial, Long-Term Intervention with Pravastatin in Ischemic Disease Trial) and two large primary prevention trials (West of Scotland Coronary Prevention Study, AFCAPS/TexCAPS Study) employing HMG-CoA reductase inhibitors found major cardiovascular event reductions ranging from 24% to 40%.[9,169-172]

PATHOPHYSIOLOGY OF ATHEROSCLEROSIS

In broad terms, coronary atherosclerosis is an initially slow process of endothelial dysfunction, intimal lipid, monocyte and T lymphocyte accumulation leading to the migration and proliferation of smooth muscle cells and elaboration of collagen and matrix in the subintimal layer (Figure 1).[10-12,173-190] In its more advanced stages, this process is punctated by acute episodes of plaque disruption, thrombosis, and vessel reorganization, which underlie the clinical syndromes of unstable angina and acute myocardial infarction.[176-178,181,182,185,187]

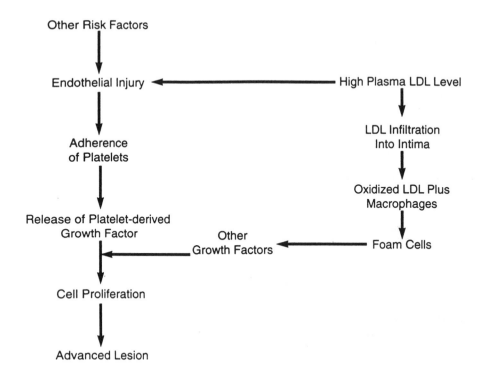

Figure 1. Pathophysiology of atherosclerosis demonstrating the endothelium-dependent and cholesterol-dependent mechanisms.

The disease, beginning in the first few decades of life, remains asymptomatic until significant lumen compromise develops or sudden occlusion occurs. In the former circumstance, stable exertional angina may be the presenting symptom, although this occurs in only 26% of men and 47% of women. Unstable angina, urgent need for coronary revascularization, acute myocardial infarction, and sudden death together make up the majority of the initial presenting symptoms of coronary heart disease. Important early pathophysiologic processes include endothelial dysfunction caused by coronary risk factors, mechanical trauma, infections (possibly chlamydia, CMV and herpes viruses[183,186]), and autoimmune processes, and the progressive modification of LDL, predominantly by oxidation.[11,179] Once atherosclerotic plaques develop, the combined factors of local plaque inflamation, dissolution of internal plaque collagen, and vasomotion lead to plaque disruption, with ensuing partial or complete vessel thrombosis. Cholesterol lowering has been shown to both slow the progression of coronary atherosclerosis and reduce plaque rupture. It may also decrease platelet adhesion to the denudated or ruptured vessel wall.[190]

ENDOTHELIUM-DEPENDENT VASOREGULATION

Although the endothelium was long considered to be simply a passive semipermeable membrane, it is now known to have key regulatory vascular functions, including conduit and resistance vessel tone, platelet activation, monocyte adhesion, thrombogenesis, lipid processing, and vessel growth (Table 1).[13-18,23-30]

Table 1.

Key Regulatory Functions of the Vascular Endothelium

semipermeable membrane
vascular tone
platelet aggregation and adhesion
thrombosis and thrombolysis
monocyte adhesion
inflamation
vessel remodeling and growth
lipoprotein metabolism and uptake

In performing these regulatory functions, the endothelium appears to be centrally involved in the development of atherosclerosis, hypertension, and heart failure. The process of vasoregulation provides an important means for assessing nitric oxide availability. Vasoregulation is accomplished by a balance among endothelium-derived relaxing factors and contracting factors released in response to local mechanical stimuli (e.g. shear stress, stretch), metabolic conditions (e.g. oxygen tension), platelet and coagulation derived products (e.g. thrombin), and receptor-mediated agonists (e.g. acetylcholine, bradykinin, serotonin, substance P) (Table 2).

Table 2:   Endothelium-dependent Stimuli and Products

Stimuli	Products
shear stress	nitric oxide
stretch	prostacyclin
hypoxia	hyperpolarizing factor
acetylcholine	endothelin-1
bradykinin	thromboxane A_2
serotonin	prostaglandin A_2
substance P	superoxide anion
thrombin	angiotensin converting enzyme
adenosine diphosphate	heparan sulfate
arachidonic acid	protein S
calcitonin gene-related peptide	von Willebrand factor
ergonovine	tissue factor
fatty acids	tissue plasminogen activator
histamine	plasminogen activator inhibitor
insulin	lipoprotein lipase
leukotrienes	LDL receptors
norepinephrine	antigens
vasoactive intestinal polypeptide	E-selectins
vasopressin	integrins
cholecystokinin	cytokines
	platelet derived growth factor
	basic fibroblast growth factor
	insulin-like growth factor
	transforming growth factor
	colony-stimulating factor

Vasorelaxing factors generally have antithrombogenic and antiproliferative effects and the reverse is true for contracting factors. The predominate relaxing factor is nitric oxide or a nitric oxide adduct, possibly in the form of a nitrosothiol or nitrosoheme. Prostacyclin and endothelium-derived hyperpolarizing factor are secondary vasodilators. Nitric oxide is derived from the amino acid L-arginine by the oxidation of the guanidine-nitrogen terminal through the action of nitric oxide synthase, leaving citrulline as a by-product. Nitric oxide synthase exists in several isoforms in endothelial cells, platelets, macrophages, vascular smooth muscle cells, nerves, and the brain. Gene expression of endothelial nitric oxide synthase is constitutively activated, calcium dependent, and can be upregulated by shear stress and estrogen. The activity of nitric oxide synthase is inhibited by the circulating amino acid asymmetrical dimethylarginine (ADMA), the levels of which are increased in hypercholesterolemia, peripheral atherosclerosis, and renal failure. Nitric oxide synthase can be pharmacologically inhibited by analogues of L-arginine such as L-N^G-monomethyl arginine (L-NMMA) and L-nitroarginine methylester (L-NAME), which compete on the catalytic site of the enzyme with L-arginine. Infusions of nitric oxide synthase inhibitors produces vasoconstriction, decreased blood flow, and sustained hypertension, although the effects are regionally variable. Nitric oxide is a diffusible free radical with a half-life of only a few seconds. Nitric oxide vasodilates locally by activating smooth muscle cell guanylate cyclase, leading to increased production of cyclic-3',5'-guanosine monophosphate.

Endothelial cells also release prostacyclin and a hyperpolarizing factors in response to the same stimuli that release nitric oxide.[13-18,31,32] These factors activate cyclic 3',5'-adenosine monophosphate and adenosine triphosphate-sensitive potassium channels, respectively. Prostacyclin contributes predominantly to platelet inactivation although its inhibitory effects are synergistically enhanced by nitric oxide. The existence of an endothelium-dependent hyperpolarizing factor has been postulated because vascular smooth muscle cells become hyperpolarized during nitric oxide-independent relaxation. Hyperpolarizing factor appears to be a labile arachidonic acid metabolite.

Endothelium-Derived Contracting Factors. The endothelium also releases several contracting factors, including endothelin-1, the vasoconstrictor prostanoids thromboxane A$_2$ and protaglandin H$_2$, oxygen free radicals such as superoxide anion, and angiotensin II through the activity of angiotensin converting enzyme.[13-18,33-35] Endothelial cells exclusively produce one of three isoforms of endothelin. At low concentrations, endothelin-1 is a vasodilator, but at higher concentrations, it is a potent vasoconstrictor. In general, vasomotor tone is regulated by the endothelium as a balance between nitric oxide and endothelin-1 and angiotensin II production. The endothelium also produces thromboxane A$_2$ and prostaglandin H$_2$ through the cyclooxygenase pathway. Receptors for these substances are found on both vascular smooth muscle cells and platelets, the stimulation of which tends to counteract the effects of nitric oxide. Angiotensin-converting enzyme (ACE) which both converts angiotensin I to angiotensin II and inactivates bradykinin is also expressed on the endothelial cell membrane. Angiotensin II has several proatherosclerotic effects, including the promotion of LDL oxidation, macrophage activation, smooth muscle cell proliferation, matrix formation, and thrombogenesis. Angiotensin II also stimulates the production of endothelin-1 and plasminogen activator inhibitor-1. An important vasocontracting product of both endothelial and smooth muscle cells is the oxygen free radical superoxide anion. In the presence of hypercholesterolemia, cigarette smoking, atherosclerosis, and hypertension, superoxide anion production is increased. This appears to lead to a decrease in nitric oxide availability through the combination of superoxide anion with nitric oxide, which procedes more rapidly than the reaction of superoxide anion with superoxide dismutase. A major source of vascular superoxide anion and hydrogen peroxide, another reactive oxygen species, is a membrane-bound, reduced nicotinamide-adenine dinucleotide-dependent oxidase, which is upregulated by angiotensin II. This effect may be an important link between hypertension and atherosclerosis.

Thrombosis. As with vasoregulation, the endothelium is an important modulator of platelet activation, thrombosis, and thrombolysis.[13,16,25,27-30,191-194] There is a complex interaction of these processes within the endothelial environment that involves platelets, coagulation factors, thrombomodulin, thrombin, proteins C and S, heparin, antithrombin III, plasminogen, and plasminogen activators and inhibitors. The endothelial surface has specific binding sites which play an important role in these enzymatic cascades. The actions of plasminogen and tissue plasminogen activator (tPA) are enhanced by this mechanism.

Normally, the endothelium provides a nonthrombogenic surface through the release of nitric oxide, prostacyclin, tissue plasminogen activator (tPA), and heparin sulfates.[13,16,28-30] Impaired endothelium promotes platelet aggregation through lessened nitric oxide and prostacyclin availability and thrombogenicity through an increased release of plasminogen activator inhibitor (PAI-1) and von Willebrand factor.[28,30] The endothelial surface has a high-affinity ligand for thrombin-thrombomodulin that catalyzes the thrombin activation of protein C, an inhibitor of coagulation factors V and VIII.[13] Intact endothelium also produces protein S, which is a cofactor for protein C. Dysfunctional human endothelial cells in culture exhibit a prothrombotic state, characterized by increased tissue-factor activity.[30] Activated platelets are directly cytotoxic to the endothelium. Shear stress has been shown to activate platelets which are repelled by the endothelium's negative surface charge which is mediated by hyperpolarizing factor.[13] Intact endothelium lessens shear through vasodilation and decreases platelet activation in stenotic or injured endothelium.[13]

Adhesion, Growth and Inflamatory Factors. The adhesion of circulating cells onto the endothelial surface and their transmigration through the vessel wall is modulated by adhesion receptors, cytokines, and chemotactic factors.[13,25,28,30,195-197] Endothelial adhesion molecules fall into three varieties: immunoglobulin antigen-specific receptors of T and B lymphocytes, selectins through which lymphocytes and neutophils interact with the endothelium (e.g. endothelial leukocyte adhesion molecule [ELAM-1]), and integrins involved in platelet adhesion and cell migration. Integrins include platelet glycoprotein IIb/IIIa, leukocyte membrane proteins, and matrix protein receptors for collagen, fibronectin, laminin, and vitronectin. Platelet adhesion also involves interaction with von Willebrand's factor and the nonintegrin glycoprotein Ib complex.

Inflamatory chemotactic factors such as platelet-activating factor, leukotriene B$_4$, and complement C5a facilitate inflamatory cell binding to the endothelium. The cytokines IL-1 and tumor necrosing factor (TNF$_\alpha$) enhance leukocyte binding by increasing expression of ELAM-1 and intercellular cell adhesion molecule (ICAM-1).[28]

The endothelium and vascular smooth muscle cells produce several growth regulating factors such as platelet-derived growth factor (PDGF), basic fibroblast growth factor (bFGF), insulin-like growth factor (IGF-1), transforming growth factor (TGF-β), colony-stimulating factor (CSF-1), interleukin-1, nitric oxide, prostacyclin, endothelin-1, and angiotensin II.[13,16,18,28-30,198-200] The adhesion, growth, and inflamatory factors are integral to the processes of vascular remodelling, such as occurs with increased blood flow or pressure, and atherosclerosis. Important remodeling processes include cellular proliferation and apoptosis and matrix synthesis and breakdown which may result in vessel enlargement, vessel wall hypertrophy, or lumenal obliteration.[18,28,29] Coagulation factors are also involved in vessel remodeling. The serine protease plasmin both initiates fibrinolysis and is involved in extracellular matrix restructuring.[28,192,201] Plasmin activates endothelium-dependent collagenase and other matrix proteinases and activates transforming growth factor-β which can either stimulate or inhibit smooth muscle cell growth.[199,200] In general, the endothelium-dependent vasodilators, such as nitric oxide, inhibit cell proliferation and the vasocontractors, such as endothelin-1 and angiotensin II promote cellular proliferation. Angiotensin II is especially important in the development of atherosclerosis.[16,28,29,34,35,202] Its actions include the promotion of LDL oxidation, macrophage activation, smooth muscle cell proliferation, matrix formation, and thrombogenesis and the reduction of vascular cell apotosis.

Vessel Growth and Atherosclerosis. Increased shear stress releases nitric oxide and prostacyclin, increases expression of nitric oxide synthase and reduces production on endothelin-1 and adhesion molecules.[28,203] Over a period of minutes to hours, the endothelial cells undergo realignment in the direction of flow and increase pinocytosis and LDL receptor expression.[204-206] Thrombogenicity is concurrently reduced through increased expression of tissue plasminogen activator and extracellular matrix composition is altered through decreased fibronectin synthesis. If increased shear stress is sustained, growth factors are released with resultant abluminal vascular remodeling.[29,174]

Administration of the nitric oxide precursor, L-arginine, has been used as a means for evaluating the role of nitric oxide in atherogenesis.[24,46,88,124-128,130,132,134,135,139] In humans, intracoronary L-arginine administration has been shown to improve endothelium-dependent vasodilation in dysfunctional coronary segments in patients with atherosclerosis or coronary risk factors.[88,124,125] Similar findings have been reported in patients with microvascular angina (syndrome X).[46] In healthy men, the oral administration of L-arginine was found to improve platelet aggregation, but not endothelium-dependent vasodilation.[127] A lack of improvement in coronary endothelial function after L-arginine infusion has also been reported in patients with advanced atherosclerosis.[128] L-arginine administration also reduces monocyte adhesion molecule expression (ICAM-1) in cultured cells and cigarette smokers.[130,131] Inhibition of nitric oxide synthase by L-NMMA has been shown to increase adhesion molecule expression.[130]

MEASUREMENT OF NITRIC OXIDE AVAILABILITY

Although reponsible for numerous regulatory actions, endothelial function is most commonly assessed as the vasodilatory response to pharmacologic or mechanical stimuli.[23,36-43] Numerous endothelium-dependent agonists have been identified, including acetylcholine, serotonin, bradykinin, thrombin, and substance P.[31] Each acts through a membrane receptor with signal transduction operating through G-proteins. Alternatively, increased blood flow (shear stress) has been used as a mechanical means for stimulating the endothelium. In vitro, endothelial function in most commonly measured as vascular ring tension in response to varying concentrations of acetylcholine or other endothelial stimuli.

Clinically, vasoregulation has been measured in both the coronary and peripheral circulations using changes in vessel diameter as an index of conduit vessel endothelial function and changes in blood flow as an index of resistance vessel endothelial function.[36-43] The three most common clinical techniques are: 1. quantitative angiographic measurement of changes in coronary artery diameter and/or blood flow in response to intracoronary infusions of varying concentrations of acetylcholine, serotonin, or substance P, 2. ultrasound measurement of changes in brachial artery diameter following induction of hyperemia with blood pressure cuff occlusion (flow-mediated), and 3. venous plethysmographic measurement of forearm blood flow following intraarterial infusion of a cholinergic stimulus (e.g. methacholine). Acetylcholine-induced coronary vasodilation has been shown to correlate weakly, but significantly, with flow-mediated brachial artery vasodilation.[44] The normal coronary artery response to acetylcholine is vasodilation. In the presence of endothelial dysfunction, vasoconstriction is observed, probably due to an unopposed direct smooth muscle cell response to the acetylcholine. Distal coronary artery infusions of a vasodilator (e.g. adenosine) to increase blood flow with measurement of changes in proximal coronary artery diameter have also been used to assess flow-mediated endothelial function.[37,38] Flow-mediated vasoconstriction has been demonstrated in the coronary circulation during exercise and is thought to be an important cause of ischemia in the setting of coronary heart disease and syndrome X.[45,46]

Flow-mediated vasodilation has also been assessed noninvasively in peripheral arteries. As a manifestation of shear stress induced nitric oxide release, the brachial artery normally dilates 5%-15% following release of an arterial occlusion (flow-mediated vasodilation).[42,43] Nitric oxide synthase inhibition completely eliminates this vasodilatory response in the peripheral arteries, but may have a lesser effect in coronary resistance vessels.[47,48] An abnormal response consists of lesser vasodilatation or occasionally vasoconstriction. Flow-mediated brachial artery vasodilatory responses vary inversely with arterial diameter. The normal response of a 3 mm artery is about 15% vasodilation, whereas a 5 mm artery may normally vasodilate only about 5%. The use of 5 minutes of upper arm occlusion produces more post-occlusion hyperemia and flow mediated vasodilation than does 5 minutes of lower arm occlusion. The upper arm occlusion technique appears to better separate patients with and without risk factors, including hypercholesterolemia.

Measurements of endothelial function vary depending on technique and location. In conduit vessels including the coronary circulation, distal arteries tend to be more vasoactive than more proximal, larger vessels.[40,49-51] Especially in the setting of atherosclerosis, endothelium-dependent responses tend to vary regionally, even in the same vessel.[52-54] Nitric oxide appears to contribute significantly to basal tone in conduit and resistance vessels, but may have a lesser effect on endothelium-dependent agonist response in resistance vessels.[49] Nitric oxide also appears to contribute to the sustained hyperemia observed after ischemic stimulus, but has little effect during peak hyperemia.[55] Finally, risk factors may affect the endothelial response to one agonist, but may not affect the response to another agonist. For example, hypercholesterolemia impairs the vasodilatory response to acetylcholine, but not to bradykinin.[50]

RISK FACTORS AND ENDOTHELIAL FUNCTION

All of the the traditional coronary risk factors have been shown to be associated with abnormal endothelial function in patients with and without atherosclerotic disease by angiography and ultrasound.[13-15,56-69] Moreover, endothelial function has been demonstrated to improve rapidly even in patients with coronary artery disease following risk factor modification in the form of cholesterol lowering, smoking cessation, exercise, estrogen replacement, homocysteine lowering, and ACE-inhibition in atherosclerotic vessels (Table 3).[70-74]

Table 3.
Factors Associated with Endothelial Dysfunction and Interventions Demonstrated to Improve Endothelial Function

Factors Associated with Endothelial Dysfunction	Interventions Improving Endothelial Function
increased age	L-arginine
male gender	estrogen
family history CHD	antioxidants
smoking	smoking cessation
increased cholesterol	cholesterol lowering
low HDL-cholesterol	ACE-inhibitors
hypertension	exercise
diabetes mellitus	homocysteine lowering
obesity	
high fat meal	
increased homocysteine	
atherosclerosis	
congestive heart failure	

Adapted from Vogel RA and Corretti MC.[78]
    Abbreviations: ACE = angiotensin converting enzyme, CHD = coronary heart disease
HDL = high density lipoprotein

Both coronary and brachial artery endothelial dysfunction have been observed to correlate in multivariate analysis with the presence of traditional risk factors, including advanced age, male gender, hypercholesterolemia, cigarette smoking, hypertension, diabetes mellitus, high homocysteine levels, high fat diet, inactivity, and family history of premature coronary heart disease. The magnitude of endothelial dysfunction has been shown to correlate with the number of risk factors present.[58,65] Aging is an independent risk factor for endothelial dysfunction. A decline in flow-mediated endothelial function has been noted in men more than about 40 years old and in women more than about 55 years old. Endothelial cells survive about 30 years and regenerated cells appear to have reduced function.

Hypercholesterolemia. Considerable experimental and clinical data suggest that elevated total and LDL-cholesterol levels are associated with impaired endothelium-dependent vasodilation, independent of the presence of coronary artery disease.[58,74-80] Hypercholesterolemia impairs both conduit and resistance vessel function.

Clinical investigations have found inverse relationships between cholesterol and both coronary and peripheral endothelium-dependent vasodilation that extends down to a cholesterol level of about 170 mg/dl (Figure 2). Even short periods of hypercholesterolemia have been found to impair vascular function. Feeding rabbits a high cholesterol diet for two weeks has been found to impair endothelium-dependent vasodilation and increase ischemic myocardial damage.[74] In this study, adverse effects of the diet were substantially reduced by concomitant lovastatin administration. Modified (oxidized) LDL impairs endothelial function more than does native LDL based on in vitro vasodilator responses. [81-86] The offending component of LDL appears to be lysolecithin. Certain types of LDL are more prone to oxidation. Small, dense LDL as occurs in the metabolic syndrome of insulin resistance, dyslipidemia, hypertension, and truncal obesity tends to have a low vitamin E content, oxidizes easily, and is rapidly taken up by macrophages. Oxidized lipoprotein(a) impairs endothelial function more than does oxidized native LDL. Clinical studies assessing both coronary and peripheral endothelium-mediated vasodilation have shown an impaiment of nitric oxide availability in the presence of borderline and elevated cholesterol.[48,87,88] The susceptibility of LDL to oxidation correlates better with impairment in endothelial function than does the cholesterol level.[84,86] High-density lipoprotein (HDL) reduces the inhibitory effect of LDL on endothelium-mediated vasodilation and has been shown to vary inversely with clinical measures of endothelial function.[89,90] Hypercholesterolemia increases endothelial adhesion molecule expression and platelet aggregability and adhesion, as well as vasomotion.[91-94]

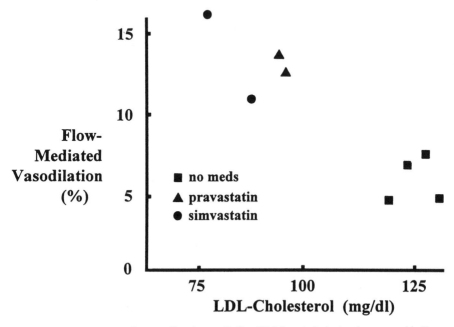

Figure 2. Brachial artery flow-mediated vasodilation (FMV) and cholesterol measured in 7 healthy, normocholesterolemic, middle-aged men before, during, and after simvastatin (10 mg/day) therapy.

Postprandial Triglycerides. A high fat diet impairs vascular function through at least three mechanisms: elevation of serum LDL and VLDL, direct impairment of endothelial function, and increased thrombogenicity. A single high-fat meal has recently been demonstrated to reduce flow-mediated brachial artery vasodilation during the 2 to 6 hour postprandial period (Figure 3).[95]

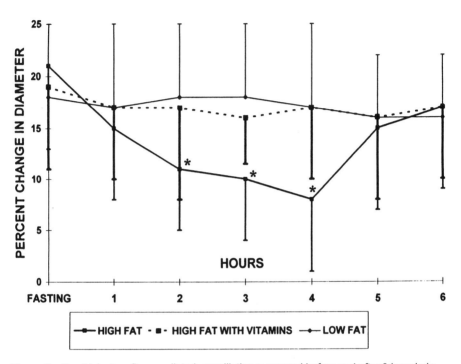

Figure 3. Brachial artery flow-mediated vasodilation measured before and after 3 isocaloric meals (high fat, high fat with vitamins C and E, and no fat) in 20 healthy, normocholesterolemic, young and middle-aged men and women. Adapted from Plotnick GD, et al.[96]

This adverse effect is substantially reduced by concomitant administration of vitamins C and E along with the high fat meal.[96] The offending lipid fraction appears to be triglyceride-rich chylomicron remnants, and monounsaturated, polyunsaturated, and saturated fats have been shown to have similar effects. Similar findings have been reported with intravenous triglyceride and free fatty acid administration.[97,98] An exception to this adverse effect of dietary fat on endothelial function is fish oil. Endothelial function has been reported to be improved by chronic fish oil administration in both experimental and clinical studies.[99,100] Fish oil has also been demonstrated to reduce endothelial superoxide production. Increases in coagulation factor VIIa have also been reported following dietary administration of most types of high fat meals.[101] The impact of fasting as opposed to postprandial hypertriglyceridemia remains controvertial. Fasting hypertriglyceridemia has been shown to be associated with reduced dipyridamole-induced coronary hyperemia, but not with acetylcholine-induced forearm hyperemia.however.[102,103]   Acute hyperglycemia (locally administered) also appears to impair forearm methacholine-induced vasodilation.[104]

VLDL Remnants. VLDL remnant lipoproteins have recently been shown to be associated with impairments of both coronary conduit and resistance vessel vasodilation to acetylcholine.[105,106] By multivariate analysis, remnant lipoproteins concentrations isolated by immunoaffinity mixed gel containing anti apo A-I and anti B-100 monoclonal antibodies correlated better with endothelial function than did LDL-cholesterol.

Cigarette smoking. Cigarette smoking profoundly impairs endothelial function, as well as being a major risk factor for coronary and other atherosclerosis. Endothelial function is reduced in both active and passive smokers in a dose-dependent fashion.[58,59,61,65,6,69] Smoking cessation is associated with improvement in endothelial function.[61] As in hypercholesterolemia, smoking appears to increase vascular oxidative stress and endothelial function in smokers may be improved by administration of antioxidant vitamin C.[131,153]   Other atherosclerotic effects of cigarette smoking are nicotine-induced direct vasocontriction, elevation of fibrinogen levels, increased platelet aggregability, increased blood viscosity, reduction in HDL-cholesterol, and increased oxidation of LDL-cholesterol.

Hypertension. Impaired endothelial function is associated with hypertension,[58-60,65,69] especially in the presence of high renin levels or left ventricular hypertrophy. Congestive heart failure is also associated with endothelial dysfunction.[207] Improvement in endothelial function has been variably reported following blood pressure reduction.[208-210]   Other atherosclerotic effects of hypertension include vascular remodeling of conduit arteries leading to decreased shear and stimulation and phenotypic change in smooth muscle cell growth by angiotensin II and other factors.

Age and Gender. Parallel to the risk of coronary heart disease, endothelial dysfunction increases in men and women after age 40 and 55, respectively, regardless of the presence or absence of other risk factors.[58,59,63-66,69] Although aging is generally associated with increased vasoconstriction[211] and/or reduced vasodilation, vascular beds and models vary and the specific cause of the decrease in endothelial function with age is unknown. Estrogen appears to be a major factor associated with gender differences in endothelial function. Intravenous estradiol improves endothelial function within a few minutes of administration, independent of its effects on lipoproteins.[212-215] Most studies have shown no improvement in endothelial function with estrogen administration in men or male mammalian cells, but transsexual men taking estrogen appear to have endothelium-dependent vasodilation at least as great as that of premenapausal women.[216,217]

Diabetes mellitus. Diabetes is clinically associated with impaired endothelial function[218] which is worsened by severe hyperglycemia. Additionally, the chronic hyperglycemia associated with diabetes modifies protein structure and function due to glycosylation of amino acid residues. Glycated proteins and local growth factors such as insulin stimulate the proliferation of smooth muscle cells. Diabetes is also associated with elevations of PAI-1, triglycerides and LDL-cholesterol and reductions in HDL-cholesterol.

MODIFICATIONS TO ENDOTHELIAL FUNCTION

Cholesterol Lowering Trials.   Following the initial demonstration that lovastatin improves endothelial function in cholesterol-fed rabbits, to date 15 clinical trials have reported the effect of cholesterol lowering on endothelial function using a variety of therapies in patients with a wide range of cholesterol (Table 4).[70-73,107-117,156] Methods of lowering cholesterol have included HMG-CoA reductase inhibitors, bile acid sequestrants, fibric acid derivatives, niacin, and LDL apheresis. Initial mean cholesterol levels in these studies have ranged from 195 to 354 mg/dl. Both angiographically normal and atherosclerotic vessels have been studied, with comparable improvements in both groups. Studies of flow-mediated brachial artery vasodilation following HMG-CoA reductase administration have found similar changes in groups with and without coronary artery disease (Figure 4).[73,109,117]

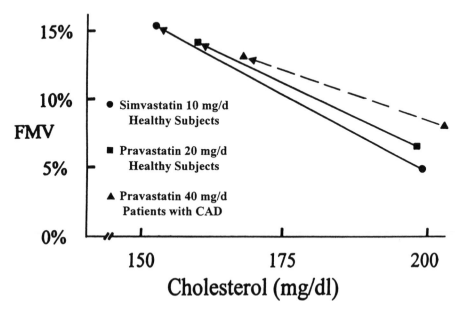

Figure 4. Changes in brachial artery flow-mediated vasodilation (FMV) and cholesterol measured in middle-aged subjects with and without coronary heart disease before and during simvastatin or pravastatin therapy.[73,109,117]

Table 4.   Studies of the Effect of Cholesterol Lowering on Endothelial
               Function

Study (Ref) Result	Result	CAD	Mean Chol	Tech	Intervention	Mo
Egashira (70)	(+)	Yes	272	CV	Prava	6
Anderson (71)	(±)	Yes	209	CV	Lova/Cho	12
Treasure (72)	(+)	Yes	226	CV	Lova	6
Seiler (110)	(+)	Yes	300	CV	Beza	7
Yeung (113)	(-)	Yes	230	CV	Simva	6
Drury (73)	(+)	Yes	209	BV	Prava	54
Tamai (114)	(+)	Yes	195	FP	Apheresis	1 hr
O'Driscoll (115)	(+)	Yes	254	FP	Simva	1
Andrews (116)	(-)	Yes	202	BV	Gem/Nia/Cho	30
Leung (108)	(+)	No	239	CV	Cho	6
Stroes (112)	(+)	No	354	FP	Simva/Coles	3
Vogel (109)	(+)	No	200	BV	Simva	0.5-3
Goode (111)	(+)	No	373	AR	Unspec	10
Vogel (117)	(-)	No	198	BV	Prava	1-7 day
						0.5-3
John (156)	(+)	No	273	FP	Fluva	6

Abbreviations: AR = excised arterial ring, Beza = bezafibrate, BV = brachial vasodilation, CAD = coronary artery disease, Cho = cholestyramine, Chol = cholesterol, Coles = colestipol, CV = coronary vasodilation, Fluva = fluvastatin, FP = forearm plethymography, Gem = gemfibrozil, Mo = months, Nia = niacin, Prava = pravastatin, Prob = probucol, Simva = simvastatin, Tech = technique, Unspec = unspecified drugs, (+) = significant improvement, (±) = borderline improvement (p=0.08) with lovastatin and cholestyramine, significant improvement with lovastatin and probucol, (-) = no improvement

Of the 15 trials, 12 have shown statistically significant improvements in endothelial function as measured by acetylcholine induced coronary vasodilation, flow-mediated brachial artery vasodilation, methacholine brachial artery plethysmography, or in vitro vascular ring vasodilation in excised vessels. The improvement in endothelial-dependent vasodilation has recently been demonstrated to be due to increased nitric oxide availability.[156] Of the three negative trials, one did not show an improvement with an HMG-CoA reductase inhibitor,[113] one did not show an improvement with combination therapy,[116] and one showed a trend toward improvement (p = 0.08) with cholesterol lowering alone (lovastatin + cholestyramine) which reached statistical significance in those subjects reiving both cholesterol lowering (lovastatin) and antioxidant therapy (probucol) (see below).[71] An improvement in endothelial function was found within one hour of cholesterol lowering by LDL apheresis and within two weeks of starting an HMG-CoA reductase inhibitor. Improvements in endothelial function have been reported to correlate better with decreased susceptibility of LDL to oxidation than LDL levels.[84,86] Improvements in endothelial function have been observed with reductions of borderline elevated cholesterol levels in the 200 mg/dl range with HMG-CoA reductase inhibitors, suggesting that this level is not ideal (193,199,207)[79,80109,114,117]. Whether HMG-CoA reductase inhibitors have direct vascular effects beyond cholesterol lowering remains a controversial issue. In vitro studies have demonstrated a direct effect of lovastatin on LDL susceptibility to oxidation and a reduction in cellular adhesion molecule expression.[118,119] Improvements in endothelial function with cholesterol lowering have also been shown to improve myocardial perfusion as measured by positron emission tomography, digital radiographiy, and ST segment monitoring.[120-123] Current opinion also holds that an improvement in endothelial function with cholesterol lowering is an important component of plaque stabilization thought to be a major factor in the decrease in cardiovascular events observed in the recent clinical trials.[8]

L-Arginine, L-NAME, and L-NMMA. Administration of the nitric oxide precursor L-arginine and the nitric oxide synthase inhibitors L-NAME and L-NMMA have been used as means for evaluating nitric oxide availability. In humans, intracoronary L-arginine administration has been shown to improve endothelium-dependent vasodilation in dysfunctional coronary segments in patients with atherosclerosis, coronary risk factors, and microvascular angina.[46,88,124-126] In healthy men, the oral administration of L-arginine was found to improve platelet aggregation, but not endothelium-dependent vasodilation.[127] A lack of improvement in coronary endothelial function after L-arginine infusion has also been reported in patients with advanced atherosclerosis.[128] Intravenously administered L-arginine has been reported to improve brachial artery flow-mediated vasodilation in hypercholesterolemic and cigarette smoking young subjects without established coronary heart disease, but not in diabetic subjects.[129] L-arginine administration also reduces monocyte adhesion molecule expression (ICAM-1) in cultured cells and cigarette smokers.[130,131] Inhibition of nitric oxide synthase by L-NMMA has been shown to increase adhesion molecule expression.[130]

The strongest evidence that nitric oxide is an antiatherosclerotic molecule[19-21,35,56,57,128-130, 132,133,135,136,139-141] comes from several experimental animal models of atherosclerosis in which nitric oxide availability has been either increased or decreased. The oral administration of L-arginine has been shown to decrease intimal thickening and atherosclerosis progression in LDL receptor knockout mice fed high cholesterol diets[132] and in hypercholesterolemic rabbits with[133-135] and without[136] balloon vascular injury. Associated improvements in vasodilator endothelial function have also been reported and have also been observed during dietary regression of atherosclerosis in monkeys.[137] Whether L-arginine may have long-term effects remains in question. Six months of oral L-arginine (9 g/day) administration has been shown to improve blood flow responses to acetylcholine in atherosclerotis subjects.[138] After 14 weeks of dietary L-arginine administration in a hypercholesterolemic rabbit model, however, no differences were observed in endothelium-dependent vasodilation and the progression of atherosclerosis was not reduced in female animals nor at certain vascular sites.[139] The chronic administration of nitric oxide synthase by L-NAME administration has been shown to accelerate neointimal formation and atherosclerosis progression in the chosterol-fed rabbit model.[140,141] Associated impairment of endothelial function was also found, which was not reversed by inhibition of thromboxane A_2 and prostaglandin H_2. These studies demonstrate that nitric oxide is a directly antiatherosclerotic molecule independent of changes in cholesterol.[19-21]

Antioxidants. Several observational studies of dietary and supplemental antioxidant intake have shown inverse correlations with coronary heart disease incidence.[142,219-221] This relationship is strongest for vitamin E, which attaches to both LDL and lipid membranes and prevents oxidation. Two large observational studies, the Health Professionals Follow-up Study (51,529 men) and the Nurses' Health Study (87,245 women) found respective 36% and 34% reductions in coronary heart disease risk in those taking at least 100 U/day for a minimum of one to two years.[220,221] The Iowa Women's Health Study of 34,486 postmenopausal women found a strong inverse correlation between dietary vitamin E intake and coronary heart disease risk, but no additional benefit from vitamin supplementation.[219] The strongest secondary prevention evidence for vitamin E comes from the Cambridge Heart Antioxidant Study (CHAOS) which found a 77% reduction in nonfatal myocardial infarction over three years, but no effect on overall mortality.[143] An D-alpha-tocopherol (natural vitamin E) dose of 400 U/day was found to reduce the susceptibility of LDL to oxidation as well as 800 IU/day. The event rate in those patients taking 400 IU/day was insignificantly less than those patients taking 800 IU/day. Vitamin C is of theoretical benefit in rejuvenating vitamin E. Only three of eight observation studies have found inverse relationships between vitamin C intake and coronary heart disease, however, and two randomized trials failed to show statistical benefit. No trials have shown an adverse effect of vitamin C. In contrast to vitamin E, β-carotene does not inhibit LDL oxidation and has not been found to decrease cardiovascular events in clinical trials.[145,222,223] Three of six observational studies of beta-carotene have shown a benefit for higher dietary intake, but the 29,133 male smoker ATBC Trial found an 8% increase in overall mortality in those randomized to 20 mg/day beta-carotene.[142] The potent antioxidant probucol was not found to reduce the progression of femoral atherosclerosis in the PQRST Trial.[155]

Supporting these observations are the results of the Lyon Diet Heart Trial which also demonstrated benefit for a Mediterranean diet high in fruits and vegetables.[143,144] The adverse event reduction in both of this and the CHAOS trial was unassociated with changes in serum cholesterol levels. These findings support the concept that coronary risk factors adversely affect the vasculature through an oxidative stress process. Coronary risk factors, including smoking, lack of exercise, increased body mass index, male gender, family history of premature coronary heart disease, and abstinence from alcohol, have been shown to be associated with elevated levels of oxidized LDL.[146] In turn, both endothelium-dependent (acetylcholine) and independent (dipyridamole) vasodilator responses correlate with the susceptibilty of LDL to oxidation.[81,84,86] Modification of proteins other than LDL also appear to be associated with atherosclerosis.[147]

In experimental models, a reduction in superoxide anion production by dietary cholesterol lowering has been shown in a cholesterol-fed rabbits.[148] Decreases in lipid peroxidation and slowing of the progression of atherosclerosis with both cholesterol lowering and antioxidant vitamin E administration have been reported.[118] In clinical studies, the combined administration of vitamins C and E and β-carotene reduces the susceptibility of LDL to oxidation,[149] but may not be superior to vitamin E administration alone.[150] Short-term studies of antioxidant vitamin administration have demonstrated improvements in endothelial function, but most long-term studies have reported negative results. Vitamin C infusion has been shown to reverse both brachial and coronary endothelial dysfunction in patients with coronary heart disease and hypertension.[151,152] Decreases in monocyte adhesion molecule expression have also been reported in smokers following 10 days of oral vitamin C supplementation.[153] In contrast, decreases in adhesion molecule expression have been found in smokers following administration of L-arginine, but not with vitamin C.[131] Similarly, an investigation employing plethysmographic measurement of forearm vasodilation did not find an improvement in hypercholesterolemic patients treated with vitamins C and E and β-carotene for 1 month.[154] Conflicting data also exist for the potent antioxidant probucol. Although probucol reduces the development of experimental atherosclerosis and improves endothelial function in combination with cholesterol lowering, it has not been found to decrease the progression of peripheral vascular disease.[71,155]

ENDOTHELIUM-LIPID INTERACTIONS

The endothelium and lipoproteins are involved in a several complex interactions. The endothelium is involved in lipid breakdown and uptake through the expression of LDL receptors and lipoprotein lipase. Through the hydrolysis of triglycerides, the latter releases free fatty acids. Triglyceride-rich chylomicrons remnants, free fatty acids, and VLDL remnants have recently been shown to impair endothelial function.[95-98,105,106] A decrease in nitric oxide availability appears to be the central defect in hypercholesterolemia based on the finding that nitric oxide synthase inhibition (L-NMMA) reduces endothelium-dependent vasodilation in normocholestolemic patients more than in hypercholesterolemic patients.[48,87,88] Cholesterol lowering in humans has been shown to increase nitric oxide availability.[156] *Evidence exists for alterations of both nitric oxide production and destruction in hypercholesterolemia.* In contrast to experimental atherosclerosis, in which nitric oxide production is increased, in human atherosclerotic aortic tissue, endothelial nitric oxide synthase expression and nitric oxide release have been shown to be reduced.[157,158] Oxidized LDL has been found to decrease the platelet uptake of L-arginine and reduce nitric oxide synthase expression.[118] L-arginine restores endothelial function induced by oxidized LDL suggesting an impairment in nitric oxide synthase and/or decreased L-arginine availablility.[118] In most but not all clinical studies, L-arginine infusion has been shown to improve impaired endothelium-dependent vasodilation, including that due to hypercholesterolemia.[125,126,159,160] The issue of nitric oxide synthase substrate availability in hypercholesterolemia remains controversial because the concentration of L-arginine exceeds the K_m of nitric oxide synthase. Several explanations have been offered for the improvement in endothelial function by L-arginine in hypercholesterolemia, including: inhibition of substrate availability by ADMA, decreased microdomain concentration of L-arginine, and insulin release by L-arginine with subsequent vasodilation. Hypercholesterolemia is associated with increases in ADMA, which decreases nitric oxide synthase activity.[16]

Increased superoxide radical production has been demonstrated in cholesterol-fed rabbits.[161] Removal of the endothelium increased superoxide production in the normocholesterolemic animals, but substantially reduced it in the hypercholesterolemic animals. Reduction in cholesterol feeding normalizes superoxide anion production.[162] Hypothetically, superoxide and other oxygen-free radicals such as hydrogen peroxide and hydroxl radical can combine with and deactivate nitric oxide. A major source of vascular superoxide anion and hydrogen peroxide, another reactive oxygen species, is a membrane-bound, reduced nicotinamide-adenine dinucleotide (NADH)-dependent oxidase, which is upregulated by angiotensin II.[22] The reaction between nitric oxide and superoxide radical is considerably faster than that between superoxide radical and superoxide dismutase, which may explain why the in vivo administration of superoxide dismutase was not found to improve endothelial function in hypercholesterolemic patients.[163] In vitro, superoxide has been shown to restore endothelial function in the presence of oxidized lipoprotein(a).[83] The concept that hypercholesterolemia and/or atherosclerosis associated endothelial dysfunction is due to increased nitric oxide destruction is supported by observations that nitric oxide production is not reduced in these conditions,[157] that changes in coronary endothelial function correlate with changes in susceptibility of LDL to oxidation,[84,86] that endothelial dysfunction and adhesion molecule production are improved by the administration of the antioxidant vitamin C,[96,151-154] and that the antioxidant drug probucol improves endothelial function beyond that achieved with cholesterol reduction.[71] Data opposing this concept exit, however. Nitric oxide production has been found to be reduced in human aortic atherosclerotic tissue.[156] Clinical trials have shown no improvement in endothelial function with administration of antioxidant vitamins[142] or superoxide dismutase[163] and no reduction in the progression of femoral atherosclerosis with probucol.[155] Reduced high-density cholesterol and elevated total to high-density cholesterol ratios have also been reported to be associated with endothelial dysfunction, possibly due to the antioxidant properties of high-density lipoprotein.[90]

These data underscore the close but complex relationship that exists between dyslipidemias and vascular biology. At the same time, they provide a mechanistic understanding of the impressive benefits that have been observed in the recent clinical trials of risk factor modification and underscore the need for aggressive lipid management, especially in those with established coronary heart disease. It is possible that ongoing antioxidant vitamin trials will also demonstrate clinical efficacy, which would confirm our evolving understanding of the balance between risk factor-induced oxidative stress and intrinsic and extrinsic antioxidants.

REFERENCES.

1. Anitschkow N: Experimental atherosclerosis in animals. In Cowdry EV (ed) Arteriosclerosis:ASurvey of the Problem. New York, Macmillan, 1933, pp 271–322.
2. Gordon T, Kannel WB. Premature mortality from coronary heart disease. The Framinghan Heart Study. JAMA 1971;215:1617-25.
3. Keys A, Araranis C, Blackburn H, et al. Epidemiologic studies related to coronary heart disease: Characteristics of men aged 40-59 in seven countries. Acta Med Scand 1967;180 (Suppl 460):1-392.
4. The Multiple Risk Factor Intervention Trial Research Group. Mortality rates after 10.5 years for participants in the Multiple Risk Factor Intervention Trial. Findings related to a priori hypothesis of the trial. JAMA 1990;263:1795-1801.
5. Lipid Research Clinics Program. The Lipid Research Clinics Coronary Primary Prevention Trial Result. I. Reduction in incidence of coronary heart disease. JAMA 1984;251:351-64.
6. Lipid Research Clinics Program. The Lipid Research Clinics Coronary Primary Prevention Trial Results. II. The relationship of reduction in incidence of coronary heart disease to cholesterol lowering. JAMA 1984;25:365-74.
7. Frick MH, Elo O, Haapa K, et al. Helsinki Heart Study: Primary-prevention trial with gemfibrozil in middle-aged men with dyslipidemia. Safety of treatment, changes in risk factors, and incidence of coronary heart disease. N Engl J Med 1987;317:1237-45.
8. Brown BG, Zhao X-Q, Sacco DE, Albers JJ. Lipid lowering and plaque regression. New insights into prevention of plaque disruption and clinical events in coronary disease. Circulation 1993;87:1781-89.
9. Gotto AM Jr. Results of recent large cholesterol-lowering trials and their implications for clinical management. Am J Cardiol 1997;79:1663-1669.
10. Ross R. The pathogenesis of atherosclerosis. N Engl J Med 1986;314:488-500.
11. Steinberg D, Parthasarathy S, Carew TE, Khoo JC, Witztum JL. Beyond cholesterol. Modifications of low-density lipoprotein that increase its atherogenicity. N Engl J Med 1989;320:915-24.
12. Segrest JP, Anantharamaiah GM. Pathogenesis of atherosclerosis. Curr Opinion Cardiol 1994;9:404-10.
13. McGorisk GM, Treasure CB. Endothelial dysfunction and coronary heart disease. Curr Opin Cardiol 1996;11:341-350.
14. Abrams J. Role of endothelial dysfunction in coronary artery disease. Am J Cardiol 1997;79(12B):2-9.
15. Vogel RA. Coronary risk factors, endothelial function, and atherosclerosis: a review. Clin Cardiol 1997;20:426-32.
16. Luscher TF, Barton M. Biology of the endothelium. Clin Cardiol 1997;20(suppl II):II-3-II-10.
17. Celermajer DS. Endothelial dysfunction: Does it matter? Is it reversible? J Am Coll Cardiol 1997;30:325-333.
18. Gibbons GH. Endothelial function as a determinant of vascular function and structure: a new theraputic target. Am J Cardiol 1997;79 (5A):3-8.
19. Cooke JP, Tsao PS. Is NO an endogenous antiatherosclerotic molecule? Arterioscler Thromb 1994;14:653-655.
20. Candipan RC, Wang B-Y, Buitrago R, Cooke JP. Regression or progression. Dependency on vascular nitric oxide. Arterioscler Thromb Vasc Biol 1996;16:44-50.
21. Wever RMF, Luscher TF, Cosentino F, Rabelink TJ. Atherosclerosis and the two faces of endothelial nitric oxide synthase. Circulation 1998;97:108-112.

22. Harrison DG. Endothelial function and oxidant stress. Clin Cardiol 1997;20(suppl II):II- 11-II-17.
23. Furchgott RF, Zawadzki JV. The obligatory role of endothelial cells in the relaxation of arterial smooth muscle by acetylcholine. Nature 1980;288:373-76.
24. Mocada S, Higgs A. The L-arginine-nitric oxide pathway. N Engl J Med 1993;329:2002-12.
25. Vane JR, Anggard EE, Botting RM. Regulatory functions of the vascular endothelium. NEngl J Med 1990;323:27-36.
26. Lerman A, Burnett JC Jr. Intact and altered endothelium in regulation of vasomotion. Circulation 1992;86 (suppl III):III-12-III-19.
27. Flavahan NA. Atherosclerosis or lipoprotein-induced endothelial dysfunction. Potential mechanisms underlying reduction in EDRF/nitric oxide activity. Circulation 1992;85:1927-38.
28. Dzau VJ, Gibbons GH, Cooke JP, Omoigui N. Vascular biology and medicine in the 1990's: scope, concepts, potentials, and perspectives. Circulation 1993;87:705-719.
29. Gibbons GH, Dzau VJ. The emerging concept of vascular remodeling. N Engl J Med 1994;330:1431-1438.
30. Levine GN, Keaney JF Jr, Vita JA. Cholesterol reduction in cardiovascular disease. Clinical benefits and possible mechanisms. N Engl J Med 1995;332:512-521.
31. Flavahan NA, Vanhoutte PM. Endothelium-derived hyperpolarizing factor. Blood Vessels 1990;27:238-245.
32. Cohen RA, Vanhouette PM. Endothelium-dependent hyperpolarization. Beyond nitric oxide and cyclic GMP. Circulation 1995;92:3337-3349.
33. Lerman A, Hildebrand FL Jr, Margulies KB, O'Murchu B, Perella MA, Heublin DM, Schwab TR, Burnett JC. Endothelin: a new cardiovascular regulatory peptide. Mayo Clin Proc 1990;65:1441-1455.
34. Yanagisawa M. The endothelin system. A new target for theraputic intervention. Circulation 1994:89:1320-1322.
35. Gibbons GH. Vasculoprotective and cardioprotective mechanisms of angiotensin-converting enzyme inhibition: the homeostatic balance between angiotensin II and nitric oxide. Clin Cardiol 1997;20 (suppl II):II-18-II-25.
36. Ludmer PL, Selwyn AP, Shook TL, Wayne RR, Mudge GH, Alexander RW, Ganz P. Paradoxical vasoconstriction induced by acetylcholine in atherosclerotic coronary arteries. N Engl J Med 1986;315:1046-51.
37 Cox DA, Vita JA, Treasure CB, Fish D, Alexander RW, Ganz P, Selwyn AP. Atherosclerosis impairs flow-mediated dilation of human coronary arteries. Circulation 1989;80:458-465
38. Drexler H, Zeiher AM, Wollschlager H, Meinertz T, Just H, Bonzel T. Flow-dependent coronary artery dilatation in humans. Circulation 1989;80:466-74.
39. Werns SW, Walton JA, Hsia HH, Nabel EG, Sanz ML, Pitt B. Evidence of endothelial dysfunction in angiographically normal coronary arteries of patients with coronary artery disease. Circulation 1989;79:287-91.
40. Vogel RA. Endothelium-dependent vasoregulation of coronary artery diameter and blood flow. Circulation 1993;88:325-27.
41. Celermajer DS, Sorensen KE, Gooch VM, Spiegelhalter DJ, Miller OI, Sullivan ID, Lloyd JK, Deanfield JE. Non-invasive detection of endothelial dysfunction in children and adults at risk of atherosclerosis. Lancet 1992;340:1111-15.
42. Corretti MC, Plotnick GD, Vogel RA. Technical aspects of evaluating brachial artery vasodilation using high-frequency ultrasound. Am J Physiol 1995;268 (Heart Circ Physiol 37):H1397-H1404.
43. Sorensen KE, Celermajer DS, Spiegelhalter DJ, et al. Non-invasive measurement of human endothelium dependent responses: accuracy and reproducibility. Br Heart J 1995;74:247-253.
44. Anderson TJ, Uehata A, Gerhard MD, et al. Close relationship of endothelial function in the human coronary and peripheral circulations. J Am Coll Cardiol 1995;26:1235-41.
45. Zeiher AM, Krause T, Schachinger V, Minners J, Moser E. Impaired endothelium-dependent vasodilation of coronary resistance vessels is associated with exercise-induced myocardial ischemia. Circulation 1995;91:2345-52.
46. Egashira K, Hirooka Y, Kuga T, Mohri M, Takeshita A. Effects of L-arginine supplementation on endothelium-dependent caronary vasodilation in patients with angina pectoris and normal coronary arteries. Circulation 1996;94:130-134.

47. Joannides R, Haefeli WE, Linder L, Richard V, Bakkali EH, Thuillez C, Luscher TF. Nitric oxide is responsible for flow-dependent dilatation of human peripheral conduit arteries in vivo. Circulation 1995;91:1314-1319.

48. Shiode N, Morishima N, Nakayama K, Yamagata T, Matsuura H, Kajiyama G. Flow-mediated vasodilation of human epicardial coronary arteries: effect of inhibition of nitric oxide synthesis. J Am Coll Cardiol 1996;27:304-310.

49. Lefroy DC, Crake T, Uren NG, Davies GJ, Maseri A. Effect of inhibition of nitric oxide synthesis on epicardial coronary artery caliber and coronary blood flow in humans. Circulation 1993;88:43-54.

50. Gilligan DM, Guetta V, Panza JA, Garcia CE, Quyyumi AA, Cannon RO III. Selective loss of microvascular endothelial function in human hypercholesterolemia. Circulation 1994;90:35-41.

51. Shiode N, Nakayama K, Morishima N, et al. Nitric oxide production by coronary conductance vessels in hypercholesterolemic patients. Am Heart J 1996;131:1051-57.

52. El-Tamimi H, Mansour M, Wargovich TJ, et al. Constrictor and dilator responses to intracoronary acetylcholine in adjacent segments of the same coronary artery in patients with coronary artery disease. Circulation 1994;89:45-51.

53. Penny WF, Rockman H, Long J, et al. Heterogeneity of vasomotor response to acetylcholine along the human coronary artery. J Am Coll Cardiol 1995;25:1046-55.

54. Kuo L, Davis MJ, Chilian WM. Longitudinal gradients for endothelium-dependent and independent vascular responses in the coronary microcirculation. Circulation 1995;92:518-25

55. Tagawa T, Imaizumi T, Endo T, Shiramoto M, Harasawa Y, Takeshita A. Role of nitric oxide in reactive hyperemia in human forearm vessels. Circulation 1994;90:2285-2290.

56. Reddy KG, Nair RN, Sheehan HM, Hodgson J McB. Evidence that selective endothelial dysfunction may occur in the absence of angiographic or ultrasound atherosclerosis in patients with risk factors for atherosclerosis. J Am Coll Cardiol 1994;23:833-43.

57. Mano T, Masuyama T, Yamamoto K, et al. Endothelial dysfunction in the early stage precedes appearance of intimal lesions assessable with intravascular ultrasound. Am Heart J 1996;131;231-38.

58. Vita JA, Treasure CB, Nabel EG, McLenachan JM, Fish D, Yeung AC, Vekshtein VI, Selwyn AP, Ganz P. Coronary vasomotor responses to acetylcholine relates to risk factors for coronary artery disease. Circulation 1990;81:491-97.

59. Seiler C, Hess M, Buechi M, Suter TM, Krayenbuehl HP. Influence of serum cholesterol and other coronary risk factors on vasomotion of angiographically normal coronary arteries. Circulation 1993;88 (part 1):2139-48.

60. Panza JA, Casino PR, Kilcoyne CM, et al. Role of endothelium-derived nitric oxide in the abnormal endothelium-dependent vascular relaxation of patients with essential hypertension. Circulation 1993;87:1468-74.

61. Celermajer DS, Sorensen KE, Georgakopoulos D, et al. Cigarette smoking is associated withdose-related and potentially reversible impairment of endothelium-dependent dilation in healthy young adults. Circulation 1993;88:2149-55.

62. Johnstone MT, Creager SJ, Scales KM, et al. Impaired endothelium-dependent vasodilation in patients with insulin-dependent diabetes mellitus. Circulation 1993;88:2510-16.

63. Egashira K, Inou T, Hirooka Y, et al. Effects of age on endothelium-dependent vasodilation of resistance coronary artery by acetylcholine in humans. Circulation 1993;88:77-81.

64. Celermaher DS, Sorensen KE, Spiegelhalter DJ, et al. Aging is associated with endothelial dysfunction in healthy men years before the age-related decline in women. J Am Coll Cardiol 1994;24:471-76.

65. Celermajer DS, Sorensen KE, Bull C, Robinson J, Deanfield JE. Endothelium-dependent dilation in the systemic arteries of asymptomatic subjects relates to coronary risk factors and their interaction. J Am Coll Cardiol 1994;24:1468-74.

66. Taddei S, Virdis A, Mattei P, et al. Aging and endothelial function in normotensive subjects and patients with essential hypertension. Circulation 1995;91:1981-87.

67. Celermajer DS, Adams MR, Clarkson P, et al. Passive smoking and impaired endothelium-dependent arteriial dilatation in healthy young adults. N Engl J Med 1996;334:150-54.

68. Heitzer T, Yla-Herttuala S, Kurz S, et al. Cigarette smoking potentiates endothelial dysfunction of forearm resistance vessels in patients with hypercholesterolemia. Role of oxidized LDL. Circulation 1996;1346-53.
69. Glasser SP, Selwyn AP, Ganz P. Atherosclerosis: risk factors and the vascular endothelium.   Am Heart J 1996;131:379-84.
70. Egashira K, Hirooka Y, Kai H, Sugimachi M, Suziki S, Inou T, Takeshita A.. Reduction in serum cholesterol with pravastatin improves endothelium-dependent coronary vasomotion in patients with hypercholesterolemia. Circulation 1994;89:2519-24.
71. Anderson TJ, Meredith IT, Yeung AC, Frei B, Selwyn AP, Ganz P. The effect of cholesterol-lowering and antioxidant therapy on endothelium-dependent coronary vasomotion. N Engl J Med 1995;332:488-93.
72. Treasure CB, Klein JL, Weintraub WS, Talley JD, Stillabower ME, Kosinski A, Zhang J, Boccuzzi SJ, Cedarholm JC, Alexander RW. Beneficial effects of cholesterol-lowering therapy on the coronary endothelium in patients with coronary artery disease. N Engl J Med 1995;332:481-87.
73. Drury J, Cohen JD, Veenendrababu B, et al. Brachial artery endothelium dependent vasodilation in patients enrolled in the cholesterol and recurrent events (CARE) study. Circulation 1996;94(suppl I):I-402 (abstr).
74. Osborne JA, Siegman MJ, Sedar AW, Mooers SU, Lefer AM. Lack of endothelium-dependent relaxation in coronary resistance arteries of cholesterol-fed rabbits. Am J Physiol 1989;256:C591-C597.
75. Shimokawa AH, Vanhoutte PM. Hypercholesterolemia causes generalized impairment of endothelium-dependent relaxation to aggregating platelets in porcine arteries. J Am Coll Cardiol 1989;13:1402-1408
76. Kugiyama K, Kerns SA, Morisett JD, et al. Impairment of endothelium-dependent-relaxation by lysolecithin in modified low-density lipoproteins. Nature 1990;334:160-62.
77. Creager MA, Cooke JP, Mendelsohn ME, Gallagher SJ, Coleman SM, Loscalzo J, Dzau VJ. Impaired vasodilation of forearm resistance vessels in hypercholesterolemic humans.   J Clin Invest 1990;86:228-34.
78. Vogel RA, Corretti MC. Estrogens, progestins, and heart disease. Can endothelial function devine the benefit? Circulation 1998;97:1223-1226.
79. Steinberg HO, Bayazeed B, Hook G, Johnson A, Cronin J, Baron AD. Endothelial dysfunction is associated with cholesterol levels in the high normal range in humans. Circulation 1997;96:3287-3293.
80. Creager MA, Selwyn A. When "normal" cholesterol levels injure the endothelium. Circulation 1997;96:3255-3257.
81. Simon BC, Cunningham LD, Cohen RA. Oxidized low density lipoproteins cause contraction and inhibit endothelium-dependent relaxation in the pig coronary artery. J   Clin Invest 1990;86:75-79.
82. Chin JH, Azhan S, Hoffman BB. Inactivation of endothelial derived relaxing factor by oxidized lipoproteins. J Clin Invest 1992;89:10-18.
83. Galle J, Bengen J, Schollmeyer P, Wanner C. Impairment of endothelium-dependent dilation in rabbit renal arteries by oxidized lipoprotein(a). Role of oxygen-derived radicals. Circulation 1995;92:1582-1589.
84. Anderson TJ, Meredith IT, Charbonneau F, Yeung AC, Frei B, Selwyn AP, Ganz P. Endothelium-dependent coronary vasomotion relates to the susceptibility of LDL to oxidation in humans. Circulation 1996;93:1647-50.
85. Chen LY, Mehta P, Mehta JL. Oxidized LDL decreases L-arginine uptake and nitric oxide protein expression in human platelets. Relevance of the effect of oxidized LDL on platelet function. Circulation 1996;93:1740-1746.
86. Raitakari OT, Pitkanen O-P, Lehtimaki T, et al. In vivo low density lipoprotein oxidation relates to coronary reactivity in young men. J Am Coll Cardiol 1997;30:97-102.
87. Casino PR, Kilcoyne CM, Quyyumi AA, Hoeg JM, Panza JA. The role of nitric oxide in endothelium-dependent vasodilation of hypercholesterolemic patients. Circulation 1993;88:2541-2547.
88. Quyyumi AA, Mulcahy D, Andrews NP, Husain S, Panza JA, Cannon RO III. Coronary vascular nitric oxide activity in hypertension and hypercholesterolemia. Circulation 1997;95:104-110.

89.   Matsuda Y, Hirata K, Inoue N, et al. High density lipoprotein reverses inhibitory effect of oxidized low density lipoprotein on endothelium-dependent arterial relaxation. Circ Res 1993;72:1103-1109.
90.   Kuhn FE, Mohler ER, Reagan K, Reagan K, Lu DY, Rackley CE. Effects of high-density lipoprotein on acetylcholine-induced coronary vasoreactivity. Am J Cardiol 1991;68:1425-1430.
91.   Hackman A, Abe Y, Insull W, Pownall H, Smith L, Dunn K, Gotto AM Jr, Ballantyne CM. Levels of soluble adhesion molecules in patients with dyslipidemia. Circulation 1996;93:1334-1338.
92.   Sampietro T, Tuomi M, Ferdeghini M, Ciardi A, Marraccini P, Prontera C, Sassi G, Taddei M, Bionda A. Plasma cholesterol regulates soluble cell adhesion molecule expression in familiar hypercholesterolemia. Circulation 1997;96:1381-1385.
93.   Lacoste L, Lam JYT, Hung J, et al. Hyperlipidemia and coronary disease. Correction of the increased thrombogenic potential with cholesterol reduction. Circulation 1995;92:3172-3177
94.   Nofer J-R, Tepel M, Kehrel B, et al. Low-density lipoproteins inhibit the Na^+/H^+ antiport in human platelets. A novel mechanism enhancing platelet activity in hypercholesterolemia. Circulation 1997;95:1370-77.
95.   Vogel RA, Corretti MC, Plotnick GD. Effect of a single high-fat meal on endothelial function in healthy subjects. Am J Cardiol 1997;79:350-54.
96.   Plotnick GD, Corretti MC, Vogel RA. Effect of antioxidant vitamins on the transient impairment of endothelium-dependent vasoactivity following a single high-fat meal. JAMA   1997;278:1682-1686.
97.   Lundman P, Eriksson M, Schenck-Gustafsson K, Karpe F, Tornvall P. Transient triglyceridemia decreases vascular reactivity in young, healthy men without risk factors   for coronary heart disease. Circulation 1997;96:3266-3268.
98.   Steinberg HO, Tarshoby M, Monestel R, Hook G, Cronin J, Johnson A, Bayazeed B, Baron AD. Elevated circulating free fatty acids impair endothelium-dependent vasodilation. J Clin Invest 1997;100:1230-1239
99.   Malis CD, Leaf A, Varadarajan GS, Newell JB, Weber PC, Force T, Bonventre JV. Effects of dietary ω3 fatty acids on vascular contractility in preanoxic and postanoxic aortic rings. Circulation 1991;84:1393-1401.
100.   Goode GK, Garcia S, Heagerty AM. Dietary supplementation with marine fish oil improves in vitro small artery endothelial function in hypercholesterolemic patients, Circulation 1997;96:2802-2807.
101.   Larsen LF, Bladbjerg E-E, Jespersen J, Markmann P. Effects of dietary fat quality and quantity on postprandial activation of blood coagulation factor VII. Arterioscl Thromb Vasc Biol 1997;17:2904-2909.
102.   Chowienczyk PJ, Watts GF, Wierzbicki AS, Cockcroft JR, Brett SE, Ritter JM. Preserved endothelial function in patients with severe hypertriglyceridemia and low functional lipoprotein lipase activity. J Am Coll Cardiol 1997;29:964-968.
103.   Yokoyama I, Ohtake T, Momomura S-I, Yonekura K, Nishikawa J, Sasaki Y, Omata M. Impaired myocardial vasodilation during hyperemic stress with dipyridamole in hypertriglyceridemia. J Am Coll Cardiol 1998;31:1568-1574.
104.   Williams SB, Goldfine AB, Timimi FK, Ting HH, Roddy M-A, Simonson DC, Creager MA. Acute hyperglycemia attenuates endothelium-dependent vasodilation in humans in vivo. Circulation 1998;97:1695-1701.
105.   Kugiyama K, Doi H, Motoyama T, Soejima H, Misumi K, Kawano H, Nakagawa O, Yoshimura M, Ogawa H, Matsumura T, Sugiyama S, Nakano T, Nakajima K, Yasue H. Association of remnant lipoprotein levels with impairment of endothelium-dependent vasomotor function in human coronary arteries. Circulation 1998;97:2519-2526.
106.   Masuoka H, Ishikura K, Kamei S, Obe T, Seko T, Okuda K, Koyabu S, Tsuneoka K, Tamai T, Sugawa M, Nakano T. Predictive value of remnant-like particles cholesterol/high-density lipoprotein cholesterol as a new indicator of coronary artery disease. Am Heart J 1998;136:226-230.

107.   Osborne JA, Lento PH, Siegfried MR, Stahl GL, Fusman B, Lefer AM. Cardiovascular
        effects of acute hypercholesterolemia. Reversal with lovastatin treatment. J Clin Invest
        1989;83:465-473.
108.   Leung W-H, Lau C-P, Wong C-K. Beneficial effect of cholesterol-lowering therapy on
        coronary endothelium-dependent relaxation in hypercholesterolaemic patients. Lancet
        1993;341:1496-500.
109.   Vogel RA, Corretti MC, Plotnick GP. Changes in flow-mediated brachial artery vasoactivity
        with lowering of desirable cholesterol levels in healthy middle-aged men.   Am J Cardiol
        1996;77:37-40.
110.   Seiler C, Suter TM, Hess OM. Exercise-induced vasomotion of angiographically normal and
        stenotic coronary arteries improves after cholesterol-lowering drug therapy with bezafibrate.
        J Am Coll Cardiol 1995;26:1615-22.
111.   Goode GK, Heagerty AM. In vitro responses of human peripheral small arteries in
        hypercholesterolemia and effects of therapy. Circulation 1995;91:2898-2903.
112.   Stroes ESG, Koomans HA, de Bruin TWA, et al. Vascular function in the forearm of
        hypercholesterolaemic patients off and on lipid-lowering medication. Lancet 1995;346:467-
        71.
113.   Yeung A, Hodgson JMcB, Winniford M, et al. Assessment of coronary vascular
        reactivity after cholesterol lowering. Circulation 1996;94(suppl I):I-402 (abstr)
114.   Tamai O, Matsuoka H, Itabe H, Wada Y, Kohno K, Imaizumi T. Single LDL aphesesis
        improves endothelium-dependent vasodilatation in hypercholesterolemic humans.
        Circulation 1997;95:76-82.
115.   O'Driscoll G, Green D, Taylor RR. Simvastatin, an HMG-coenzyme A reductase
        inhibitor, improves endothelial function within 1 month. Circulation 1997;95:1126-1131.
116.   Andrews TC, Whitnet EJ, Green G, Kalenian R, Personius BE. Effect of gemfibrozil ± niacin
        ± cholestyramine on endothelial function in patients with serum low-density   lipoprotein
        cholesterol levels <160 mg/dl and high-density lipoprotein cholesterol levels < 40 mg/dl.
        Am J Cardiol 1997;80:831-835.
117.   Vogel RA, Corretti MC, Plotnick GD. The mechanism of improvement in endothelial
        function by pravastatin: direct effect or through cholesterol lowering. J Am Coll Cardiol
        1998;31:60A.
118.   Chen L, Haught WH, Yang B, Saldeen TGP, Parathasarathy S, Mehta J. Preservation of
        endogenous antioxidant activity and inhibition of lipid peroxidation as common mechanisms
        of antiatherosclerotic effects of vitamin E, lovastatin and amlodipine. J Am   Coll Cardiol
        1997;30:569-575
119.   Weber C, Erl W, Weber KSC, Weber PC. HMG-CoA reductase inhibitors decrease
        CD11b expression and CD11b-dependent adhesion to endothelium and reduce increased
        adhesiveness of monocytes isolated from patients with hypercholesterolemia. J Am Coll
        Cardiol 1997;30:1212-1217.
120.   Gould KL, Ornish D, Scherwitz L, et al. Changes in myocardial perfusion abnormalities by
        positron emission tomography afetr long-term, intense risk factor modification. JAMA
        1995;274:894-901.
121.   van Boven AJ, Jukema JW, Zwinderman AH, et al. Reduction of transient myocardial
        ischemia with pravastatin in addition to the conventional treatment in patients with
        angina   pectoris. Circulation 1996;94:1503-1505.
122.   Aengevaeren WRM, Uijen GRH, Jukema JW, Bruschke AVG, van der Werf T.
        Functional improvement by pravastatin in the regression growth evaluation statin study
        (REGRESS).   Circulation 1997;96:429-435.
123.   Andrews TC, Raby K, Barry J, et al. Effect of cholesterol reduction on myocardial
        ischemia in patients with coronary disease. Circulation 1997;95:324-28.
124.   Drexler H, Zeiher AM, Meinzer K, Just H. Correction of endothelial dysfunction in
        coronary microcirculation of hypercholesterolaemic patients by L-arginine. Lancet
        1991;338:1546-1550.
125.   Creager MA, Gallagher SJ, Girerd XJ, Coleman SM, Dzau VJ, Cooke JP. L-arginine
        improves endothelium-dependent vasodilation in hypercholesterolemic humans. J Clin
        Invest 1992;90:1248-1253.
126.   Quyyumi AA, Dakak N, Diodati JG, Gilligan DM, Panza JA, Cannon RO III. Effect of L-
        arginine on human coronary endothelium- dependent and physiologic vasodilation. J   Am
        Coll Cardiol 1997;30:1220-1227.

127.   Adams MR, Forsyth CJ, Jessup W, Robinson J, Celermajer DS. Oral L-arginine inhibits platelet aggregation but does not enhance endothelium-dependent vasodilation in healthy young men. J Am Coll Cardiol 1995;26:1054-1061.

128.   Otsuji S, Nakajima O, Waku S, et al. Attenuation of acetylcholine-induced vasoconstriction by L-arginine is related to the progression of atherosclerosis. Am Heart   J 1995;129:1094-1100.

129.   Thorne S, Mullen MJ, Clarkson P, Donald AE, Deanfield JE. Early endothelial dysfunction in adults at risk from atherosclerosis: different responses to L-arginine. J   Am Coll Cardiol 1998;32:110-116.

130.   Adams MR, Jessup W, Hailstones D, Celermajer DS. L-arginine reduces human monocyte adhesion to vascular endothelium and endothelial expression of cell adhesion molecules. Circulation 1997;95:662-668.

131.   Adams MR, Jessup W, Celermajer DS. Cigarette smoking is associated with increased human monocyte adhesion to endothelial cells: reversibility with oral L-arginine but not vitamin C. J Am Coll Cardiol 1997;29:491-497.

132.   Aji W, Ravalli S, Szabolcs M, Jiang X-C, Sciacca RR, Michler RE, Cannon PJ. L-arginine prevents xanthoma development and inhibits atherosclerosis in LDL recptor knockout mice. Circulation 1997;95:430-437.

133.   Cooke JP, Singer AH, Tsao P, Zera P, Rowan RA, Billingham ME. Anti-atherogenic effects of L-arginine in the hypercholestyerolemic rabbit J Clin Invest 1992;90:1168-1172.

134.   Wang B-W, Candipan RC, Arjomandi M, Hsiun PT, Tsao PS, Cooke JP. Arginine restores nitric oxide activity and inhibits monocyte accumulation after vascular injury in hypercholesterolemic rabbits. J Am Coll Cardiol 1996;28:1573-1579.

135.   Hamon M, Vallet B, Bauters C, Wernert N, McFadden EP, LaBlanche J-M, Dupuis B, Bertrand ME. Long-term administration of L-arginine reduces intimal thickening and enhances neoendothelium-dependent acetylcholine relaxation after arterial injury. Circulation 1994;90:1357-1362.

136.   Boger RH, Bode-Boger SM, Brandes RP, Phivthong-Ngam L, Bohme M, Nafe R, Mugge A, Frolich J. Dietary L-arginine reduces the progression of atherosclerosis in cholesterol-   fed rabbits. Circulation 1997;96:1282-1290.

137.   Benzuly KH, Padgett RC, Kaul S, Piegors DJ, Armstrong ML, Heistad DD. Functional improvement precedes structural regression of atherosclerosis. Circulation 1994;89:1810-18.

138.   Lerman A, Burnett JC, Higano ST, McKinley LJ, Holmes DR Jr. Long-term L-arginine supplementation improves small-vessel coronary endothelial function in humans. Circulation 1998;97:2123-2128.

139.   Jeremy RW, McCarron H, Sullivan D. Effects of dietary L-arginine on atherosclerosis   and endothelium-dependent vasodilation in the hypercholesterolemic rabbit. Response according to treatment duration, anatomic site, and sex. Circulation 1996;94:498-506.

140.   Cayette AJ, Palacino JJ, Cohen RA. Chronic inhibition of nitric oxide production accelerates neointimal formation and impairs endothelial function in hypercholesterolemic rabbits. Arterioscler Thromb 1994;14:753-59.

141.   Naruse K, Shimizu K, Muramatsu M, Toki Y, Miyazaki Y, Okumura K, Takayuki H. Long-term inhibition of NO synthesis promotes atherosclerosis in the hypercholesterolemic rabbit thoracic aorta. PGH_2 does not contribute to impaired endothelium-dependent relaxation. Arterioscler Thromb 1994;14:746-752.

142.   Jha P, Flather M, Lonn E, et al. The antoxidant vitamins and cardiovascular disease. A critical review of epidemiologic and clinical trial data. Ann Intern Med 1995;123:860-72.

143.   Stephens NG, Parsons A, Schofield P, et al. Randomised controlled trial of vitamin E in patients with coronary disease: Cambridge Heart Antioxidant Study (CHAOS). Lancet 1996;347:781-86.

144.   de Longeril M, Salen P, Martin J-L, Mamell N, Monjaud I, Touboul P, Delaye J. Effect of a mediterranean type of diet on the rate of cardiac complications in patients with coronary artery disease. Insights into the cardioprotective effects of certain nutriments. J

145.   .Diaz MN, Frei B, Vita JA, Keaney JF Jr. Antioxidants and heart disease. N Engl J Med 1997;337:408-416
        Am Coll Cardiol 1996;29:1103-1108.

146. Mosca L, Rubenfire M, Tarshis T, Tsai A, Pearson T. Clinical predictors of oxidized low-density lipoprotein in patients with coronary artery disease. Am J Cardiol 1997;80:825-830.

147. O'Brien KD, Alpers CE, Hokanson JE, Wang S, Chait A/ Oxidation-specific epitopes in human coronary atherosclerosis are not limited to oxidized low-density lipoprotein. Circulation 1996;94:1216-1225.

148. Ohara Y, Peterson TE, Sayegh HS, Subramanian RR, Wilcox JN, Harrison DG. Dietary correction of hypercholesterolemia in the rabbit normalizes endothelial superoxide anion production. Circulation 1995;92:898-903.

149. Mosca L, Rubenfire M, Mandel C, Rock C, Tarshis T, Tsai A, Pearson T. Antioxidant nutrient supplementation reduces the susceptibility of low density lipoprotein to oxidation in patients with coronary artery disease. J Am Coll Cardiol 1997;30:392-299.

150. Jilal I, Grundy SM. Effect of combined supplementation with α-tocopherol, ascorbate, and beta carotene on low-density lipoprotein oxidation. Circulation 1993;88:2780-2786.

151. Levine GN, Frei B, Koulouris SN, et al. Ascorbic acid reverses endothelial vasomotor dysfunction in patients with coronary artery disease. Circulation 1996;93:1107-13.

152. Solzbach U, Hornig B, Jeserich M, Just H. Vitamin C improves endothelial dysfunction of epicardial coronary arteries in hypertensive patients. Circulation 1997;96:1513-1519.

153. Weber C, Erl W, Weber K, et al. Increased adhesiveness of isolated monocytes to endothelium is prevented by vitamin C intake in smokers. Circulation 1996;93:1488-92.

154. Gilligan DM, Sack MN, Guetta V, et al. Effect of antioxidant vitamins on low density lipoprotein oxidation and impaired endothelium-dependent vasodilation in patients with hypercholesterolemia. J Am Coll Cardiol 1994;24:1611-17.

155. Walldius G, Erikson U, Olsson AG, et al. The effect of probucol on femoral atherosclerosis: the Probucol Quantitative Regression Trial (PQRST). Am J Cardiol 1994;74:875-83.

156. John S, Schlaich M, Langenfeld M, Weilprecht H, Schmitz G, Weidinger G, Schmeider RE. Increased bioavailability of nitric oxide after lipid-lowering in hypercholesterolemic patients. Circulation 1998;98:211-216.

157. Minor R Jr, Myers PR, Guerra R Jr, Batas JN, Harrison DG. Diet-induced atherosclerosis increases the release of nitrogen oxides from rabbit aorta. J Clin Invest 1990;86:2109-2116.

158. Oemar BS, Tschudi MR, Godoy N, Brovkovich V, Malinski T, Luscher TF. Reduced endothelial nitric oxide synthase expression and production in human atherosclerosis. Circulation 1998;97:2494-2498.

159. Casino PR, Kilcoyne CM, Quyyumi AA, Hoeg JM, Panza JA. Investigation of decreased availability of nitric oxide precursor as the mechanism for impaired endothelium-dependent vasodilation in hypercholesterolemic patients. J Am Coll Cardiol 1994;23:844-850.

160. Chauhan A, More RS, Mullins PA, Taylor GT, Petch MC, Schofield PM. Aging-associated endothelial dysfunction is reversed by L-arginine. J Am Coll Cardiol 1996;28:1796-1804.

161. Ohara Y, Pederson TE, Harrison DG. Hypercholesterolemia increases endothelial superoxide production. J Clin Invest 1993;91:2546-51.

162. Ohara Y, Peterson TE, Sayegh HS, Subramanian RR, Wilcox JN, Harrison DG. Dietary correction of hypercholesterolemia normalizes endothelial superoxide anion production. Circulation 1995;92:898-903.

163. Garcia CE, Kilcoyne CM, Cardillo C, Cannon RO III, AA, Panza JA. Evidence that endothelial function in patients with hypercholesterolemia is not due to increased extracellular nitric oxide breakdown by superoxide anions. Am J Cardiol 1995;76:1157-1161.

164. Cashin-Hemphill L, Mack WJ, Pogoda JM, et al. Beneficial effects of colestipol-niacin oncoronary atherosclerosis. A 4-year follow-up. JAMA 1990;264:3013-17.

165. Brown G, Albers JJ, Fisher LD, et al. Regression of coronary artery disease as a result of intensive lipid-lowering therapy in men with high levels of apolipoprotein B. N Engl J Med 1990;323:1289-98.

166. Ornish D, Brown SE, Scherwitz, et al. Can lifestyle changes reverse coronary heart disease? The Lefestyle Heart Trial. Lancet 1990;336:129-33.

167. Buchwald H, Varco RL, Matts JP, et al. Effect of partial ileal bypass surgery on mortality and morbidity from coronary heart disease in patients with hypercholesterolemia. Report of the Program on the Surgical Control of the Hyperlipidemias (POSCH). N Engl J Med 1990;323:946-55.

168. The Post Coronary Artery Bypass Graft Trial Investigators. The effect of aggressive lowering of low-density lipoprotein cholesterol levels and low-dose anticoagulation on obstructive changes in saphenous-vein coronary-artery bypass grafts. N Engl J Med 1997;336:153-162.

169. Scandinavian Simvastatin Survival Study Group. Randomised trial of cholesterol lowering in 4444 patients with coronary heart disease: the Scandinavian Simvastatin Survival Study (4S). Lancet 1994;344:1383-89.

170. Shepherd J, Cobbe SM, Ford I, et al. Prevention of coronary heart disease with pravastatin in men with hypercholesterolemia. N Engl J Med 1995;333:1301-7.

171. Sachs FM, Pfeffer MA, Moye LA, et al. The effect of pravastatin on coronary events after myocardial infarction in patients with average cholesterol. N Engl J Med 1996;335:1001-9.

172. Downs JR, Clearfield M, Whitney E, Shapiro DR, Beere PA, Langendorfer A, Stein EA, Kruyer W, Gotto AM Jr. Primary prevention of acute coronary events with lovastatin in menand women with average cholesterol levels. Results of AFCAPS/TexCAPS. JAMA 1998;279:1615-1633.

173. Fuster V, Steele PM, Chesebro JH. Role of platelets and thrombosis in coronary atherosclerotic disease and sudden death. J Am Coll Cardiol 1986;5:175B-184B.

174. Glagov S, Weisenberg E, Zarins CK, et al. Compensatory enlargement of human atherosclerotic coronary arteries. N Engl J Med 1987;316:1371-75.

175. Davies MJ. A macro and micro view of coronary vascular insult in ischemic heart disease. Circulation 1990;82(suppl II);II-38-II-46.

176. Fuster V, Stein B, Ambrose JA, et al. Atherosclerotic plaque rupture and thrombosis - evolving concepts. Circulation 1990;82(suppl II):II-47-II-59.

177. Ip JH, Fuster V, Badimon L, et al. Syndromes of accelerated atherosclerosis: Role of vascular injury and smooth muscle cell proliferation. J Am Coll Cardiol 1990;15:1667- 87.

178. Fuster V, Badimon L, Badimon JJ, Chesebro JH. The pathogenesis of coronary artery disease. N Engl J Med 1992;326:242-50 and 326;310-18.

179. Witstum JL. Role of oxidized low density lipoprotein in atherosclerosis. Br Heart J 1993:69(suppl):S12-S18

180. Clarkson TB, Pritchard RW, Morgan TM, Remodeling of coronary arteries in human and nonhuman primates. JAMA 1994;271:289-94.

181. Libby P. Molecular basis of the acute coronary syndromes. Circulation 1995;91:2844- 50.

182. Falk E, Shah PK, Fuster V. Coronary plaque disruption. Circulation 1995;92:657-71.

183. Grayston JT, Kuo C, Coulson AS, et al. Chlamydia pneumoniae (TWAR) in atherosclerosisof the carotid artery. Circulation 1995;92:3397-3400.

184. Nishioka T, Luo H, Eigler NL, et al. Contribution of inadequate compensatory enlargement to development of human coronary artery stenosis: An in vitro intravascular ultrasound study. J Am Coll Cardiol 1996;27:1571-6.

185. Farb A, Burke AP, Tang AL, et al. Coronary plaque erosion without rupture into a lipid core. A frequent cause of coronary thrombosis in sudden coronary death. Circulation 1996;93:1354-63.

186. Zhou YF, Leon MB, Waclawiw MA, et al. Association between prior cytomegalovirus infection and the risk of restenosis after coronary atherectomy. N Engl JMed 1996;335:624-30.

187. Mann JM, Davies MJ. Vulnerable plaque. Relation of characteristics to degree of stenosis in human coronary arteries. Circulation 1996;94:928-31.

188. Burke AP, Farb A, Malcom GT, et al. Coronary risk factors and plaque morphology in menwith coronary disease who die suddenly. N Engl J Med 1997;336:1276-82.

189. Ridker PM, Cushman M, Stampfer MJ, et al. Inflamation, aspirin, and the risk of cardiovascular disease in apparently healthy men. N Engl J Med 1997;336:973-79.

190. Nofer J-R, Tepel M, Kehrel B, et al. low-density lipoproteins inhibit the Na^+/H^+ antiport inhuman platelets. A novel mechanism enhancing platelet activity in hypercholesterolemia. Circulation 1997;95:1370-77.

191. Hajjar KA, Hamel NM, Harpel PC, Nachman RL. Binding of tissue plaminogen activator to cultured human endothelial cells. J Clin Invest 1987;80:1712-1719.

192. Saksela O, Rifkin DB. Cell-associated plasminogen activation: Regulation and physiological functions. Ann Rev Cell Biol 1988;4:93-126.

193. Hajjar KA, Gavish D, Breslow JL, Nachman RL. Lipoprotein(a) modulation of endothelial cell surface fibrinolysis and its potential role in atherosclerosis. Nature 1989;339:303-305.

194. Shimokawa H, Aarhus LL, Vanhoutte PM. Porcine coronary arteries with regenerated endothelium have a reduced endothelium-dependent responsiveness to aggregating platelets and serotonin. Circ Res 1989;64;900-914.

195. Springer TA. Adhesion receptors of the immune system. Nature 1990;346:425-434.

196. Hsieh HJ, Li NQ, Frangos JA. Shear stress increases endothelial platelet-derived growth factor mRNA levels. Am J Physiol 1991;260:H642-H646.

197. Tsao PS, Buitrago R, Chan JR, Cooke JP. Fluid flow inhibits endothelial adhesiveness. Nitric oxide and transcriptional regulation of VCAM-1. Circulation 1996;94:1682-1689.

198. Rifkin DB, Moscatelli D. Recent developments in the cell biology of basic fibroblast growth factor. J Cell Biol 1989;109:1-6.

199. Battegay EJ, Raines EW, Seifert RA, Bowen-Pope DF, Ross R. TGF-β induces bimodal proliferation of connective tissue cells via complex control of autocrine PDGF loop. Cell 1990;63:515-524.

200. Gimbrone MA Jr, Bevilacqua MP, Cubulsky MI. Endothelial-dependent mechanisms of leukocyte adhesion in inflamation and atherosclerosis. Ann N Y Acad Sci 1990;598:77- 85.

201. Knudsen BS, Nachman RL. Matrix plasminogen activator inhibitor. Modulation of the extracellular proteolytic environment. J Biol Chem 1988;263:9476-9481.

202. Vanhoutte PM, Boulanger CM, MoJV. Endothelium-derived relaxing factor and converting enzyme inhibition. Am J Cardiol 1995;76:3E-12E

203. Tsao PS, Buitrago R, Chan JR, Cooke JP. Fluid flow inhibits endothelial adhesiveness. Nitric oxide and transcriptional regulation of VCAM-1. Circulation 1996;94:1682-1689.

204. Davies PF, Dewey CF, Bussolari SR, Gordon EJ, Gimbrone MA. Influence of hemodynamic forces on vascular endothelial function: In vitro studies of shear stress and pinocytosis in bovine aortic cells. J Clin Invest 1984;73:1121-1129.

205. Sprague PR, Steinbach BC, Nerem RM, Schwartz CJ. Influence of laminar steady-state fluid imposed wall shear stress on the binding, internalization, and degredation of low density lipoprotein by cultured arterial endothelium. Circulation 1987;76:648-656.

206. Davies PF, Dull RO. How does the arterial endothelium sense flow? Hemodynamic forces   and signal transduction. Adv Exp Med Biol 1990;273:281-293.

207. Katz SD, Biasucci L, Sabba C, et al. Impaired endothelium-mediated vasodilation in the peripheral vasculature of patients with congestive heart failure. J Am Coll Cardiol 1992;19:918-25.

208. Luscher TF, Vanhouette PM, Rau L. Antihtpertensive treatment normalizes decreased endothelium-dependent relaxations in rats with salt-induced hypertension. Hypertension1987; 9(suppl III):III-193-III-197.

209. Panza JA, Casino PR, Kilcoyne CM, et al. Role othelium-derived nitric oxide in the abnormal endothelium-dependent vascular relaxation of patients with essential hypertension. Circulation 1993;87:1468-74.

210. Panza JA, Quyyumi AA, Callahan TS, et al. Effect of antihypertensive treatment on endothelium-dependent vascual relaxation in patients with essential hypertension. J Am CollCardiol 1993;21:1145-51.

211. Taddei S, Virdis A, Mattei P, et al. Aging and endothelial function in normotensive subjects and patients with essential hypertension. Circulation 1995;91:1981-87.

212. Liberman EH, Gerhard MD, Uehata A, et al. Estrogen improves endothelium-dependent, flow-mediated vasodilation in post menopausal women. Ann Intern Med 1994:121:936 -41.

213. Gilligan DM, Badar DM, Panza JA, et al. Acute vascular effects of estrogen in postmenopausal women. Circulation 1994;90:786-91.

214. Reis SE, Gloth ST, Blumenthal RS, et al. Ethinyl estradiol acutely attenuates abnormal coronary vasomotor responses to acetylcholine in postmenopausal women. Circulation 1994;89:52-60.

215. Collins P, Rosano GMC, Sarrel PM, et al. 17B-estradiol attenuates acetylcholine-induced coronary arterial constriction in women but not in men with coronary heart disease. Circulation 1995;92:24-30.

216. McCrohon JA, Walters WAW, Robinson JTC, McCredie RJ, Turner L, Adams MA, Handelsman DJ, Celermajer DS. Arterial reactivity is enhanced in genetic males taking highdose estrogen. J Am Coll Cardiol 1997;29:1432-1436.

217. New G, Timmins KL, Dufy SJ, Tran BT, O'Brien RC, Harper RW, Meredith IT. Long-term therapy improves vascular function in male to female transsexuals. J Am Coll Cardiol 1997;29:1437-1444.

218. Johnstone MT, Creager SJ, Scales KM, et al. Impaired endothelium-dependent vasodilation in patients with insulin-dependent diabetes mellitus. Circulation 1993;88:2510-16.

219. Kushi LH, Folsom AR, Prineas RJ, et al. Dietary antioxidant vitamins and death from coronary heart disease in postmenopausal women. N Engl J Med 1996;334:1156-62

220. Rim EB, Stampfer MJ, Ascherio A, et al. Vitamin E consumption and the rsk of coronary heart disease in men. N Engl J Med 1993;328:1450-66.

221. Stampfer MJ, Hennekens CH, Manson JE, et al. Vitamin E consumption and the risk of coronary disease in women. N Engl J Med 1993;328:1444-49.

222. Alpha-Tocopherol, Beta Carotene Cancer Prevention Study Group. ɪne effect of vitamin E and beta carotene on the incidence of lung cancer and other cancers in male smokers. NEngl J Med 1994;330:1029-35

223. Hennekens CH, Buring JE, Manson JE, et al. Lack of effect of long-term supplementation with beta carotene on the incidence of malignant neoplasms and cardiovascular disease. N Engl J Med 1996;334:1145-9

6 Physiologic and Pathophysiologic Effects of Angiotensin in the Heart and Vessel Wall

Richard E. Pratt, Ph.D.
Brigham and Women's Hospital

INTRODUCTION

Angiotensin II (Ang II) exerts a majority of its known cardiovascular activities through the AT_1 receptor. This receptor is a member of the 7-transmembrane superfamily and it exerts its actions via coupling to various G-proteins. Its downstream effectors include adenylate-cyclase, various phospholipases and ion channels. Moreover, various tyrosine kinase pathways have been reported to be activated by the AT_1 receptor which result in the stimulation of the early response genes controlling cell growth. This action has been observed in several cell lines including cardiac myocytes and vascular smooth muscle cells. Moreover, studies strongly implicate the renin angiotensin system in the initiation and progression of atherosclerosis. Therefore, blockade of this system should influence not only vascular tone but may also have dramatic effects on vascular and cardiac structure.

The function of the AT_2 receptor is still poorly understood. This receptor appears to be coupled to G proteins and stimulation of this receptor results in the activation of various tyrosine phosphatases, the stimulation of which counterbalances (or possibly opposes) the effects of AT_1 receptor stimulation. Thus, this receptor has been reported to result in vasodilatation, increased natriuresis, inhibition of proliferation and stimulation of apoptosis. The AT_2 receptor is transiently expressed at extraordinary levels during fetal life, however, low level expression of the receptor persists in several tissues, including the heart and vasculature. Moreover, re-expression of the receptor occurs in various pathologic situations, such as cardiac hypertrophy and vascular injury.

Data suggest that differences may exist between blockade of the renin-angiotensin system with an AT_1 receptor antagonist vs. an ACE inhibitor and it is still unclear if one approach will be more beneficial than the other. Clearly, long-term comparative studies are needed to better realize the potential differences between these two classes of drugs.

GROWTH PROMOTING EFFECTS OF ANGIOTENSIN II

In addition to its well known actions as a vasoconstrictor, angiotensin (Ang) II has been shown to be a potent inducer of growth [1-5]. Our laboratories, as well as several others, have studied the mechanism by which Ang II induces growth in smooth muscle. The results show that Ang II rapidly activates several growth associated kinase pathways including the MAP kinase pathway and JAK/STAT pathway [6-11]. Within minutes, Ang II induces the expression of the protooncogenes c-fos, c-jun and c-myc and within hours, the Ang II induced expression of several autocrine growth factors (PDGF, FGF, TGFβ, IGF) are observed [2-5, 12-14]. Several lines of evidence suggests that the interaction between these autocrine growth factors mediate the induction of hyperplastic or hypertrophic growth, depending on the exact culture conditions.

Ang II has also been implicated in the control of smooth muscle cell growth in vivo. Early studies demonstrated that hypertensive animals exhibited vascular hypertrophy and that treatment of the animals to decrease the hypertension would in many cases, decrease or prevent the hypertrophy [15]. Interestingly, blockade of the renin angiotensin system with ACE inhibitors had a greater effect on the vascular hypertrophy than other treatments such as hydralazine or propranolol [16] suggesting that the effect of the ACE inhibitor on vascular structure was not due to the effects on pressure alone.

Consistent with the above conclusions, continuous in vivo infusion of Ang II markedly enhances VSMC proliferation in the normal and injured arterial wall [17, 18] and it appears that this action is independent of blood pressure [18]. Similar to what is observed with cultured smooth muscle cells [5], investigations have shown that this induction of growth is dependent in part on the action of Ang II induced growth factors. Su et al [19] treated rats with Ang II alone or in combination with an antibody specific for basic FGF. The results indicated that the Ang II increase in DNA synthesis in normal and balloon injured vessels was blunted by the antibody administration but not by administration of a control IgG.

Further evidence indicates that Ang II can induce growth of vascular smooth muscle cells in vivo. Balloon injury of the rat carotid artery induces a well-described increase in smooth muscle cell proliferation and migration, and results in the development of a neointima. Early studies from our laboratory demonstrated that the development of the neointima was associated with an increase in components of the tissue renin angiotensin system [20-22], most dramatically angiotensin converting enzyme [21, 22]. Treatment with ACE inhibitors blocked neointimal proliferation after balloon injury [21, 23]. These growth inhibitory effects of Ang II are due, in part, to the decrease in Ang II production since Ang II receptor blockade will also blunt the smooth muscle cell growth response to injury [24-26]. In addition to the inhibition of Ang II formation by ACE inhibitors this protective effect may be due to an increase in bradykinin and nitric oxide levels [27, 28].

It is interesting to note that several studies have shown that basic FGF is important in the proliferation of smooth muscle following injury [29-31]. Moreover, evidence suggests that FGF can induce ACE activity in vivo [32]. Thus, one can envision a vicious loop where vascular injury leads to the release of FGF from cellular and extracellular stores, contributes to the induction of smooth muscle proliferation and contributes to the induction of ACE expression in the smooth muscle. The induction of ACE expression results in the increased production of Ang II in the injured vessel which further contributes to the proliferation of the smooth muscle both directly as well as via the induction of other growth factors, particularly FGF.

ANGIOTENSIN II AND THE INITIATION AND PROGRESSION OF ATHEROSCLEROSIS

The above studies provide evidence that Ang II may contribute to the growth of vascular smooth muscle, but these studies have focused mainly on rodents and have involved an artificial system for the induction of vascular growth. However, there is evidence that Ang II may also play a role in the development of atherosclerosis, a situation with a more obvious clinical relevance. Atherosclerosis is a complex disease under the influence of both genetic and environmental factors. Pathological examination of atherosclerotic lesions reveal the presence of several cell types including smooth muscle cells, T-lymphocytes, macrophages, and fibroblasts. While previous studies have concentrated on the role of lipids, cholesterol and lipoproteins in the initiation and progression of the atherosclerotic plaque, the contribution of cytokines, growth factors and vasoactive substances to the pathobiology of atherosclerotic vascular disease have recently generated significant interest.

Chobanian and co-workers [33, 34] were among the first to demonstrate that treatment of Watanabe heritable hyperlipidemic rabbits with the ACE inhibitor captopril resulted in a marked reduction in aortic atherosclerosis as measured by a reduced area of involvement and reduced cholesterol content as well as a decrease in the cellularity of the lesion with an increase matrix deposition. This action was not dependent on the reduction in blood pressure since several other antihypertensive agents failed to influence lesion characteristics in this model [33, 34]. Similar responses have been reported in hypercholesterolemic rabbits and hamsters as well as in cholesterol fed minipigs and cynomologus monkeys. Moreover, this effect is seen with several different ACE inhibitors and at doses comparable with those used clinically.

An emerging body of evidence suggests that ACE may also play an important pathogenic role in the progression of human coronary artery atherosclerosis. For example, recent genetic studies [35] have identified a deletion polymorphism in the ACE gene as a potent risk factor for myocardial infarction in humans. While controversial, these data do suggest a link between ACE activity and coronary heart disease. Interestingly, this deletion polymorphism is associated with increased plasma and cellular levels of ACE. The potential clinical significance is suggested by the findings of the Survival and Ventricular Enlargement (SAVE) and Studies Of Left Ventricular Dysfunction (SOLVD) trials showing that ACE inhibitors reduced the incidence of recurrent myocardial infarction [36-38]. These data are constant with the postulate that ACE inhibition may alter the natural history of human coronary atherosclerosis.

EXPRESSION OF ACE IN THE VESSEL WALL

ACE has been shown to exist both as a cell membrane associated ectoenzyme as well as a circulating enzyme. Plasma ACE levels represents a small fraction of the total body ACE which is mostly present on tissue endothelial cells throughout the body and in the parenchymal cells of certain tissues. Interestingly, circulating levels of Ang II are several orders of magnitude below the Km for the receptor and studies suggest that the primary site of ACE inhibitor action is within the vasculature [39, 40]. The importance of tissue ACE was demonstrated recently by Bernstein and co-workers [41]. Recombinant mice were produced which lack the carboxyl terminal domain of ACE, including the transmembrane anchor. Thus, all ACE is secreted into the plasma with no tissue bound ACE detected. These animals exhibit a low blood pressure and an inability to concentrate urine, a phenotype similar to that observed in recombinant mice harboring a complete disruption of the ACE gene. Thus, the loss of tissue ACE was functionally similar to the total loss of the ACE gene.

The expression of ACE in the vasculature plays an important role in the regulation of vascular growth. As stated above, we have shown that it is necessary to block tissue ACE activity in the intimal lesion [21, 22] in order to inhibit lesion development in the balloon injured rat carotid artery. Further proof that tissue ACE is the rate limiting enzyme in the local production of Ang II was provided by a gene transfer protocol in which an ACE expression vector was transfected into the vessel wall [42]. The results demonstrated the increase in smooth muscle cell growth that was independent of any alterations in the circulating renin angiotensin system.

With these issues in mind, we examined the expression of ACE within human atherosclerotic coronary arteries [43]. In nonatherosclerotic coronary arteries, ACE immunoreactivity was found in luminal endothelial cells and those of adventitial vasa vasorum. However, in early and immediate stage atherosclerotic lesions, ACE was detected prominently in fat laden macrophages in the cholesterol rich portion of the lesion and in association with T lymphocytes and smooth muscle cells. In advanced lesions, in addition to macrophages, ACE immunoreactivity was localized to the endothelium of the microvasculature throughout the plaques. Immunoreactive angiotensin (Ang) II was also detected in these areas. The mechanism of ACE expression in macrophages was suggested by in vitro experiments with THP1 cells, a monocytoid cell line. We observed that ACE activity was induced 3 fold following differentiation of THP1 cells into macrophages. ACE activity was further increased after stimulation of the THP1 cells with acetylated LDL. These observations demonstrate that intimal macrophages and endothelial cells of plaque microvessels are significant sources of tissue ACE in atherosclerotic plaques of human coronary arteries. Viewed in light of the clinical data, these results suggest that ACE within the plaque may play a role in the local production of angiotensin II that contributes to the pathobiology of coronary artery disease.

The expression of ACE in atherosclerotic lesions and in macrophages has been confirmed in several studies. Moreover, Ang II has been detected in isolated human monocytes by immunocytochemistry and radioimmunoassay [44]. Recently, the expression of vascular ACE in atherosclerotic lesions has been confirmed in hypercholesterolemic rabbits [45, 46] and in humans [47]. In rabbits, the increase in ACE expression preceded lesion development [46], lending support for the hypothesis that ACE may play a role in the initiation of the lesion. The vascular ACE expression was related to the levels of cholesterol in the diet and at 17 weeks, were correlated with the severity of lesion [45]. Moreover, the increased expression of ACE was restricted to vascular beds susceptible to lesion formation [45] and was associated with an increase in tissue Ang II levels [46]. In patient samples, ACE was detected by immunohistochemistry in macrophages, smooth muscle cells and fibroblasts [47]. Moreover, the level of expression correlated with the risk for restenosis and for the severity of vessel wall damage. Furthermore, Yang et al [48] has recently shown that Ang II receptors are increased 5 fold in atherosclerotic lesions of the hypercholesterolemic rabbit. Thus, accumulating evidence support a role for ACE and Ang II in the initiation and progression of the atherosclerotic lesion.

The uptake of LDL by the vessel wall with the subsequent oxidation and uptake by macrophages is central to the development of the atherosclerotic lesion. Several reports have demonstrated that infusions of Ang II into rats or rabbits increases the vascular uptake of LDL [49-51]. The uptake was rapid, being observed during the first hour of Ang II infusion [51]; however, it is unclear if the increased uptake is independent of the vasopressor responses. On the one hand, elevation of pressure by infusion of adrenergic agents or by blockade of NO synthase is also accompanied by increased vascular influx of LDL. Moreover, infusion of Ang II at doses that yield only transient increases in pressure induce LDL influx only during the pressor phase [51]. On the other hand, this latter point is controversial and in a comparison of SHR with vehicle or Ang II infused Wistar rats, only the Ang II treated animals exhibited the increased LDL influx [49]. Thus, the role of pressure in the increased influx is unclear. Nevertheless, these results demonstrate that Ang II can induce increased LDL influx into the vessel wall. Furthermore, evidence also indicates that Ang II can stimulate the oxidation of LDL [52-54] and stimulates the uptake of LDL by the macrophage [55].

Ang II has also been shown to induce attraction of monocytes to the vessel wall and the binding of monocytes to the endothelial cells. In rabbits, an early event in response to an atherogenic diet is the increase in the expression of monocyte chemoattractant factor-1 (MCP-1) within the vessel wall, resulting in the attraction of monocytes to the endothelial surface and migration of monocytes into the vessel wall. Treatment of the rabbits with an ACE inhibitor decreases both the expression of MCP-1 and monocyte accumulation as well as lesion formation [56]. Moreover, Mervaala et al [57] recently demonstrated that a double transgenic rat, expressing both human angiotensinogen and human renin, exhibits monocyte infiltration and overexpression of several adhesion molecules in the vessel wall. Treatment of these animals with either an ACE inhibitor or an angiotensin receptor antagonists blocked both adhesion molecule expression and the adhesion of monocytes. Further evidence that this is an Ang II mediated event was provided by exposing cultured monocytes and smooth muscle cells to Ang II. Both cell types responded with an increase in MCP-1 expression. Not only does Ang II induce the expression of MCP-1 in the vessel wall, thus attracting the monocytes, but it also stimulates the adhesion of the monocyte to the endothelial layer. Cultured human coronary artery endothelial cells, treated with increasing concentrations of Ang II, exhibited a dose-dependent increase in monocyte adhesion and E-selectin expression [58]. Treatment of the cells with an antibody specific for E-selectin abolished the monocyte binding, suggesting a causal link. This increased E-selectin expression and monocyte adhesiveness was an AT_1 mediated event since blockade of the AT_1 receptor but not blockade of the AT_2 receptor, greatly attenuated monocyte adhesiveness.

Endothelial cell activation with expression of adhesion molecules and subsequent adhesion of monocytes is thought to be one of the initiating events in atherosclerosis. Thus, the ability of Ang II to induce adhesion molecule expression in human endothelial cells and to stimulate the production of the potent monocyte chemotactic agent, MCP-1, suggests that Ang II may play a role in these initiating events in atherosclerosis. Moreover, Ang II has been shown to induce NADH and NADPH oxidase activity with resulting superoxide production in cultured VSMC and in the vessel wall [59] as well as in macrophage [60]. Superoxide radicals have numerous effects on cell function promoting atherosclerotic plaque formation including induction of growth of VSMC [61, 62], lipid peroxidation, inactivation of nitric oxide and stimulation of adhesion molecule expression. Moreover, oxidative stress activates the transcription factor NF-kB [63, 64] that may induce the expression of ACE in the endothelium since the ACE gene contains two potential NF-kB binding sites that correspond exactly to the consensus NF-kB binding site. Thus Ang II, in conjunction with other pro-atherogenic stimuli, may initiate a positive loop, resulting in increased oxidative stress and increased Ang II production.

In addition to its pro-atherogenic actions via the production of Ang II, ACE may also participate in the initiation/progression of atherosclerosis by a second mechanism, the decrease in NO production (Figure 1). ACE will degrade bradykinin, a potent inducer of NO release. In addition to its vasodilatory actions, NO has several anti-atherogenic effects including the inhibition of endothelial-monocyte adhesion, reduction in oxidative stress and inhibition of NF-kB [65-68]. Indeed, dietary supplimentation with L-arginine, the precursor to NO will inhibit lesion formation in the hypercholesterolemic rabbit . Thus, ACE may participate in atherogenesis by the activation of a pro-atherogenic pathway (Ang II) and the inhibition of an anti-atherogenic pathway (NO).

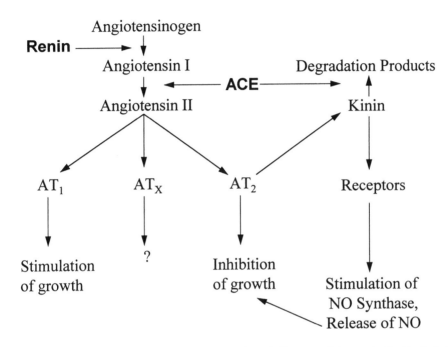

Figure 1. Action of the Angiotensin and the Angiotensin Receptor Subtypes in the Control of Cellular Growth. Angiotensinogen, a liver derived protein that is also expressed in extra-hepatic tissues, is cleaved by renin to produce Ang I. Ang I is then cleaved by Angiotensin Converting Enzyme (ACE), generating Ang II. ACE also cleaves kinins producing inactive degradation products. Ang II acts via the AT_1 and AT_2 receptor subtypes to stimulate or inhibit growth, respectively. (Other angiotensin receptors, indicated as AT_X, may also exist and may contribute to the actions of Ang II in the vessel and the heart.) Kinins, acting via the B2 receptors, result in an increased production of nitric oxide that may also inhibit cellular growth. Recent evidence suggest that, in addition to a direct inhibition of growth, the AT_2 receptor may function via the induction of NO. (See the text for details and references.)

ANGIOTENSIN II RECEPTOR SUBTYPES

Over the years, multiple lines of evidence have suggested the existence of Ang II receptor subtypes, but it was only in the last decade that at least two distinct receptor subtypes were defined, based on their differential pharmacological and biochemical properties and designated as type-1 (AT_1) and type-2 (AT_2) receptors [69, 70]. Ang II does not discriminate between these two receptors, neither does the non-selective ligand Sar1, Ile8-Ang II. However, the AT_1 and AT_2 receptor subtypes can be distinguished using the AT_1 specific ligands (losartan, candesartan, valsartan, etc.) and PD123319 and CGP42112A which bind specifically to the AT_2

but not the AT_1 receptor.

The availability of specific angiotensin receptor antagonists has allowed the more detailed study of role of the renin angiotensin system in the alterations leading to the development of vascular lesions and allowing one to ask if the antiatherogenic effects of the ACE inhibitors are due to the inhibition of Ang II generation or to some other action such as the stabilization of bradykinin (Figure 1). As stated earlier, the growth promoting effects of Ang II on vascular smooth muscle cells in culture are mediated by the AT_1 receptor. Moreover, the growth of smooth muscle following balloon injury of the carotid or aorta is also inhibited by AT_1 receptor blockade. The effects of Ang II on the oxidation and macrophage uptake of LDL occurred in response to infused Ang II, suggsting a direct effect while the binding of monocytes to endothelial cells could be blocked by AT_1 receptor blockade. Thus, evidence suggests that the effects of ACE inhibitors on atherosclerosis are due, at least in part, to a direct effect of Ang II via the AT_1 receptor. Consistent with this, several reports suggest that blockade of the AT_1 receptors will inhibit atherosclerosis [71, 72]; however, this is not a consistent finding [28, 73]. Clearly, more work is needed to clarify this important point.

ROLE OF THE AT_2 RECEPTOR IN REMODELLING

If many of the vascular effects of Ang II are mediated by the AT_1 receptor, what then is the role of the AT_2 receptor? Cloning of the AT_1 receptor has revealed that it belongs to a seven-transmembrane, G protein-coupled receptor family [74, 75]. To date, extensive pharmacological evidence indicates that most of the known effects of Ang II in adult tissues are attributable to the AT_1 receptor, through its ability to activate the phosphoinositide/calcium pathway, or to inhibit adenylate cyclase activity [74-77]. In contrast, much less is known about the structure and function of the AT_2 receptor. It is abundantly and widely expressed in fetal tissues, but present only in scant levels in tissues in the adult including adrenal gland, brain, uterine myometrium, and atretic ovarian follicles [69, 70, 78-81]. When examined in cells with endogenous AT_2 receptor expression, this receptor does not appear to involve any known classical intracellular signaling pathways. Moreover, coupling to G proteins has been difficult to determine [80, 82]. Using an expression cloning strategy, we and Inagami's group independently reported the cloning of the AT_2 receptor from a rat expression library [83 84]. Sequencing revealed that this receptor also belongs to the seven-transmembrane, G protein-coupled receptor family.

The AT_2 receptor is widely and abundantly expressed in fetal tissues, including the neonatal and embryonic vessels [85] with lower but detectable levels in the adult vessels. Interestingly, following vascular injury and the development of proliferative vascular lesions, we and others have shown that the AT_2 receptor is re-expressed, constituting ~10% of the total Ang II receptor mRNA [86]. Initially, this pattern of expression during periods of rapid smooth muscle cell growth led to the speculation that this receptor might be involved in growth or migration since Ang II is known to be a trophic factor for many cell types in vivo as well as in vitro. However, all of the demonstrated growth promoting effects of Ang II have been shown to be inhibitable by AT_1 receptor blockade. It must be remembered that many other processes occur during development such as differentiation and apoptosis (programmed cell death). Thus, it is entirely conceivable that Ang II via the AT_2 receptor may be involved in these events.

We hypothesized that the AT_2 receptor modulates cellular growth responses to AT_1 receptor or other growth stimuli either by an antiproliferative effect or by way of its actions on differentiation, migration and/or apoptosis. The availability of the cloned AT_2 receptor has allowed us to carry out preliminary studies on the in vivo and in vitro effects of the AT_2 receptor on growth. Using in vivo gene transfer of the rat AT_2 receptor into an injured rat carotid artery, we have demonstrated an attenuation of neointimal hyperplasia resulting from AT_2 receptor transgene overexpression [87]. Indeed, a 70% decrease in neointimal area was observed. Treatment of the animals with AT_2 receptor antagonist, PD123319, abolished this protective effect of the AT_2 receptor. Thus, these results suggest that the AT_1 and AT_2 receptors exert opposing actions on growth. Similar conclusions were obtained using endothelial cells in culture (which express the endogenous AT_2 receptor) by Unger and colleagues [88] and in cardiomyocytes in culture [89]. In the latter study, Booz and colleagues demonstrated that the hypertrophic effects of Ang II on the myocyte, which is mediated by the AT_1 receptor, can be counteracted by the AT_2 receptor. Consistent with this finding, Bartunek et al [90] have demonstrated using ex vivo studies that the AT_2 receptor counteracts the growth promoting effects of the AT1 receptor in hypertrophied but not normal hearts.

Consistent with this in vivo observation, proliferating cultured VSMC in vitro, transfected with the AT_2 receptor expression vector also exhibit decreased rates of cell accumulation. We examined the effects of expression of the AT_2 receptor in cultured vascular smooth muscle cells (VSMC). Rat aortic VSMC, isolated from 3 month old rats, were transfected with an AT_2 receptor expression vector. Ang II significantly increased the cell number in the control vector transfected VSMC. This increase was abolished with the AT_1 receptor antagonist, DuP753, demonstrating that AT_1 receptor activation enhances VSMC growth in this culture. In the cells expressing the AT_2 receptor on the other hand, Ang II treatment had little or no effect on cell number. However, in AT_2 receptor-expressing cells treated with the AT_2 receptor antagonist, PD123319, Ang II increased the cell number to that observed in the control vector transfected cells. DuP 753 did not affect the antigrowth effect of the AT_2 receptor. Taken together, these experiments strongly suggest that the AT_2 receptor mediates an antigrowth effect on vascular smooth muscle cells.

We have also examined another model of vascular growth, embryonic aortic development. Cook et al [91] demonstrated that during embryonic development, a transition exists where the rates of DNA synthesis drop from a very high level (~75% daily labeling index) to 30-40% labeling index over the course of two days (embryonic day e17-e18, gestation is 21 days). Interestingly, this is the point where the AT_2 receptor becomes abundantly expressed in the vasculature. We have shown that rat vascular AT_2 receptor mRNA is expressed at very low levels in the rat aorta during early rat embryonic development (up to embryonic day 15, E15) but at high levels during the later stages of development (E16-21) and in the neonatal rat [86, 87]. Therefore, we examined if the AT_2 receptor may play a role during this transition phase. To examine the functional significance of the prenatal expression of the AT_1 and AT_2 receptors, we examined the effects the specific antagonists, DuP753 and PD123319, on DNA synthesis in the aorta. Drugs were administered maternally using Alzet minipumps for 4 days before tissue harvest. On the last day, bromodeoxyuridine (BrdU) was administered maternally by intraperitoneal injection. BrdU is incorporated into replicating DNA in place of thymidine and can be detected immunohistochemically. As shown previously [91], a developmentally regulated decrease in DNA synthesis, as evidenced by an increase in BrdU incorporation, was observed. During early gestation (E15), 73% of the aortic nuclei displayed positive immunoreactivity for BrdU following an 18 hour exposure to the compound, demonstrating the rapid growth of the embryonic aorta. This rate dropped progressively such that on E21, the rate of DNA synthesis was 37%. This developmentally regulated decrease in DNA synthesis is mediated, in part, by the action of the AT_2 receptor. At days E18, E19, and E21, administration of the AT_2 receptor blockade increased DNA synthesis towards the maximum rate observed on day E15. In contrast, AT_1 receptor blockade had opposing effects on DNA synthesis. A significant decrease in BrdU incorporation was observed with infusion of the AT_1 receptor antagonist on days E18, E19, and E21. Interestingly, in animals receiving both receptor antagonists, the rates of DNA synthesis were indistinguishable from the rates observed in the AT_2 receptor antagonist treated animals, suggesting that the antiproliferative effects of the AT_1 receptor blockade may be mediated, in part, by the unopposed action of Ang II at the AT_2 receptor.

Evidence suggest that the AT_2 receptor may also influence tissue structure by other mechanisms, including the induction of cell death by apoptosis. Recently, apoptosis (or programmed cell death) has been highlighted in studies of the cardiovascular system. Apoptosis is an energy-requiring process, distinguished from necrosis by a lack of inflammation, that plays an important role during development of many structures. At the molecular level, apoptosis is best characterized by the internucleosomal cleavage of DNA which results in the generation of DNA fragments of multiples of ~200 bp (the size of a nucleosome). This DNA laddering can easily be observed by gel electrophoretic analysis of the DNA isolated from apoptotic tissues or cells. This process occurs in the adult as well as during development. Processes as diverse as the elimination of self-recognizing T cells, regulation of hematopoesis, turnover of the gut epithelium and atresia of the ovarian follicles all depend on apoptotic events. Several reports have highlighted apoptosis in cardiac and vascular biology [92-107]. Our colleagues have demonstrated that the AT_2 receptor, under certain conditions, may initiate a pro-apoptotic signal. In several different cell types which express an endogenous AT_2 receptor, Ang II can induce apoptosis in an AT_2 dependent manner [108-110] while the AT_1 receptor signaling pathway can inhibit apoptosis [99]. This induction of apoptosis can be blocked by AT_2 receptor blockade but not by AT_1 receptor blockade and can be blocked by pertussis toxin. While the AT_2 receptor dependent apoptosis is controversial [106, 107, 111] and requires further study, these results have added an additional dimension to the mechanisms by which Ang II may influence cardiovascular structure. Consistent with the idea that the AT_2 receptor may induce apoptosis, Ichikawa and colleagues [112] have observed a decreased apoptosis in the kidneys of AT_2 knockout animals.

The signaling pathway(s) for the AT_2 receptor are not well understood. Typically, the seven transmembrane receptors are coupled to heterotrimeric GTP-binding (G) proteins. These heterotrimers, made of α, β and γ subunits, direct the appropriate signaling from the receptor. At one time, the signaling was thought to be directed exclusively by the α subunit, however, reports over the last several years have shown that the $\beta\gamma$ dimer is, in fact, responsible for much of the intracellular signaling and may be important in the induction of MAP kinase activity by Gi pathway [113]. We have examined the potential the G protein coupling of the AT_2 receptor [114] in rat fetal membranes. An antibody which binds several G_α subunits immunoselected Ang II receptor-G_α complexes. In addition, $G_{i\alpha}1$-3 antibody, which recognizes $G_{i\alpha}1$, $G_{i\alpha}2$ and $G_{i\alpha}3$, also co-immunoselect the AT_2 receptor. Anti-$G_{i\alpha}2$ and anti-$G_{i\alpha}3$ antibodies were both able to co-immunoselected AT_2 receptor-$G_{i\alpha}$ complexes but, consistent with the lack of $G_{i\alpha}1$ in the fetal extracts, anti-$G_{i\alpha}1$ antibodies did not immunoselect Ang II binding sites. In addition, no other G protein-directed antisera immunoselected Ang II binding sites . The finding that AT_2 receptor couples to both $G_{i\alpha}2$ and $G_{i\alpha}3$ raises the possibility that selective interactions between AT_2 receptor and different G proteins may result in specific cellular effects mediated by AT_2 stimulation. Consistent with the coupling to $G_{i\alpha}$, many of the actions of the AT_2 receptor can be blocked with pertussis toxin.

We next examined the downstream signaling pathway which may be affected by the actions of the AT_2 receptor . Treatment of the control vector transfected vascular smooth muscle cells with Ang II resulted in an AT_1 receptor mediated increase in MAP kinase activity. Conversely, in cells transfected with the AT_2 receptor expression vector, the AT_1 mediated increase in MAP kinase activity was greatly attenuated as compared to the control vector transfected cells [87]. Furthermore, in the presence of the AT_2 receptor antagonist PD123319, Ang II stimulated MAP kinase activity in the AT_2 receptor expression vector transfected cells to a value indistinguishable from the Ang II treated control cells. These results have been confirmed in several cell types; furthermore, our colleagues have observed that antisense oligonucleotide to MAP kinase phosphatase-1 (MKP-1) inhibited the AT_2 receptor mediated MAP kinase dephosphorylation [108, 110]. Taken together, these results demonstrate that the two Ang II receptor subtypes exert opposing effects on MAP kinase activity and confirm that the AT_2 receptor may mediate an antigrowth effect.

The growth inhibitory actions of the AT_2 receptor are particularly intriguing. A large body of literature presented by numerous laboratories demonstrate that many seven transmembrane receptors induce MAP kinase activity and in some cases, induce cellular growth. For example, we and others have shown that the AT_1 receptor can induce growth in smooth muscle cells and that this induction of growth may play an important role in physiologic and patho-physiologic conditions [4, 5, 12, 21, 22]. The fact that the AT_2 receptor antagonizes the MAP kinase induction and growth stimulatory effects of the AT_1 receptor as well as the effects of the polypeptide growth factors may indicate a heretofore unappreciated characteristic of these receptors since few reports on the growth inhibitory actions of the seven transmembrane receptors exist. Clearly, this area requires further study. Nevertheless, based on these observations, we hypothesize that the AT_2 receptor belongs to a subfamily of receptors which may play a fundamental role in the commitment or fate of specific cells in response to growth or hormonal stimuli. However, the exact pathway by which the receptor induces intracellular signals is still unclear.

Other cellular effects of AT_2 receptor stimulation are becoming apparent and may contribute to and help to explain the actions of the receptor signaling cascade. Several lines of investigation suggest that Ang II induces the generation of cGMP via activation of the AT_2 receptor. Siragy and Carey [115, 116] have shown that, in sodium depleted rats, Ang II, via the AT_2 receptor, increases cGMP in the kidney. In the blood vessel, Unger and coworkers [117] have recently shown that losartan acutely administered to rats increased aortic concentrations of cGMP. This increased cGMP accumulation was independent of the effects on pressure and could be blocked by simultaneous treatment with AT_2 receptor blockade. Furthermore, blockade of the bradykinin B2 receptor with icatibant (HOE 140) also abolished the increased accumulation of cGMP as did L-NAME, the nitric oxide synthase (NOS) inhibitor. These results suggesting that the signaling through the AT_2 receptor may involve the production of bradykinin and stimulation of NOS, production of NO and activation of soluble guanylyl cyclase. Since several investigators have shown that activation of either soluble or particulate guanylyl cyclase inhibits growth of numerous cell lines including cardiac myocytes and vascular smooth muscle cells, this pathway may play a role in the AT_2 receptor mediated inhibition of cellular growth; however, a direct connection has yet to be demonstrated. This intriguing possibility is deserving of further study.

A direct link between the AT_2 receptor-bradykinin-NO-cGMP pathway and a biological effect has been demonstrated in the heart. In this study, Carretero and colleagues [118] have examined the effects of AT_1 receptor blockade and ACE inhibitors on cardiac function when administered 2 months following a coronary artery ligation in rats. As expected, ACE inhibitors improved cardiac performance as measured by LVEDV, LVESV and LVEF; and this improvement could be blunted by blockade of the B2 receptors, demonstrating that the cardioprotective effects of ACE inhibitors are due to a combination of the decreased actions of Ang II and the increased action of bradykinin. Interestingly, AT_1 receptor blockade could also improve cardiac function and this improvement could be blunted by AT_2 receptor antagonists, PD123319, as well as by the B 2 receptor antagonist, HOE 140. Thus, again, these results suggest a pathway involving the AT_2 receptor-bradykinin-NO-cGMP.

SUMMARY

Over the past decade, it has become increasingly apparent that the renin angiotensin system exerts actions on the cardiovascular system that go far beyond the acute regulation of vascular tone and homeostasis. The discovery that Ang II could act as a trophic factor for smooth muscle cells and cardiac myocytes opened several areas of research that continue to the current time. Recent data on the role of Ang II in the initiation and progression of atherosclerosis will insure that further studies into the actions of this system continue for years to come. Moreover, the actions of Ang II during vascular development (and perhaps the development of other tissues?) may have implications in normal physiology and the pathophysiology of numerous diseases of the cardiovascular system.

Acknowledgments

Work reviewed here was supported by NIH grants HL42663 and HL58516 in collaboration with Drs. Victor J. Dzau, Gary H. Gibbons and Masa Horiuchi.

REFERENCES

1. Geisterfer AA, Peach MJ, Owens GK. Angiotensin II induces hypertrophy, not hyperplasia, of cultured rat aortic smooth muscle cells. Circ Res 62:749-56, 1988.
2. Naftilan AJ, Pratt RE, Eldridge CS, Lin HL, Dzau VJ. Angiotensin II induces c-fos expression in smooth muscle via transcriptional control. Hypertension 13:706-11, 1989.
3. Naftilan AJ, Pratt RE, Dzau VJ. Induction of platelet-derived growth factor A-chain and c-myc gene expressions by angiotensin II in cultured rat vascular smooth muscle cells. J Clin Invest 83:1419-24, 1989.
4. Gibbons GH, Pratt RE, Dzau VJ. Vascular smooth muscle cell hypertrophy vs. hyperplasia. Autocrine transforming growth factor-beta 1 expression determines growth response to angiotensin II. J Clin Invest 90:456-61, 1992.
5. Itoh H, Mukoyama M, Pratt RE, Gibbons GH, Dzau VJ. Multiple autocrine growth factors modulate vascular smooth muscle cell growth response to angiotensin II. J Clin Invest 91:2268-74, 1993.
6. Duff JL, Marrero MB, Paxton WG, Schieffer B, Bernstein KE, Berk BC. Angiotensin II signal transduction and the mitogen-activated protein kinase pathway. Cardiovasc Res 30:511-7, 1995.
7. Berk BC. Angiotensin II signal transduction in vascular smooth muscle: pathways activated by specific tyrosine kinases [In Process Citation]. J Am Soc Nephrol 10 Suppl 11:S62-8, 1999.
8. Marrero MB, Schieffer B, Paxton WG, Heerdt L, Berk BC, Delafontaine P, Bernstein KE. Direct stimulation of Jak/STAT pathway by the angiotensin II AT1 receptor. Nature 375:247-50, 1995.
9. Marrero MB, Schieffer B, Paxton WG, Duff JL, Berk BC, Bernstein KE. The role of tyrosine phosphorylation in angiotensin II-mediated intracellular signalling. Cardiovasc Res 30:530-6, 1995.
10. Inagami T, Eguchi S, Numaguchi K, Motley ED, Tang H, Matsumoto T, Yamakawa T. Cross-talk between angiotensin II receptors and the tyrosine kinases and phosphatases [In Process Citation]. J Am Soc Nephrol 10 Suppl 11:S57-61, 1999.
11. Eguchi S, Iwasaki H, Inagami T, Numaguchi K, Yamakawa T, Motley ED, Owada KM, Marumo F, Hirata Y. Involvement of PYK2 in Angiotensin II Signaling of Vascular Smooth Muscle Cells. Hypertension 33:201-206, 1999.
12. Koibuchi Y, Lee WS, Gibbons GH, Pratt RE. Role of transforming growth factor-beta 1 in the cellular growth response to angiotensin II. Hypertension 21:1046-50, 1993.
13. Du J, Delafontaine P. Inhibition of vascular smooth muscle cell growth through antisense transcription of a rat insulin-like growth factor I receptor cDNA. Circ Res 76:963-72, 1995.
14. Delafontaine P, Lou H. Angiotensin II regulates insulin-like growth factor I gene expression in vascular smooth muscle cells. J Biol Chem 268:16866-70, 1993.
15. Owens GK. Differential effects of antihypertensive drug therapy on vascular smooth muscle cell hypertrophy, hyperploidy, and hyperplasia in the spontaneously hypertensive rat. Circ Res 56:525-36, 1985.
16. Owens GK. Influence of blood pressure on development of aortic medial smooth muscle hypertrophy in spontaneously hypertensive rats. Hypertension 9:178-87, 1987.

17. Daemen MJ, Lombardi DM, Bosman FT, Schwartz SM. Angiotensin II induces smooth muscle cell proliferation in the normal and injured rat arterial wall. Circ Res 68:450-6, 1991.
18. Su EJ, Lombardi DM, Siegal J, Schwartz SM. Angiotensin II induces vascular smooth muscle cell replication independent of blood pressure. Hypertension 31:1331-7, 1998.
19. Su EJ, Lombardi DM, Wiener J, Daemen MJ, Reidy MA, Schwartz SM. Mitogenic effect of angiotensin II on rat carotid arteries and type II or III mesenteric microvessels but not type I mesenteric microvessels is mediated by endogenous basic fibroblast growth factor. Circ Res 82:321-7, 1998.
20. Rakugi H, Jacob HJ, Krieger JE, Ingelfinger JR, Pratt RE. Vascular injury induces angiotensinogen gene expression in the media and neointima. Circulation 87:283-90, 1993.
21. Rakugi H, Wang DS, Dzau VJ, Pratt RE. Potential importance of tissue angiotensin-converting enzyme inhibition in preventing neointima formation. Circulation 90:449-55, 1994.
22. Rakugi H, Kim DK, Krieger JE, Wang DS, Dzau VJ, Pratt RE. Induction of angiotensin converting enzyme in the neointima after vascular injury. Possible role in restenosis. J Clin Invest 93:339-46, 1994.
23. Powell JS, Clozel JP, Muller RK, Kuhn H, Hefti F, Hosang M, Baumgartner HR. Inhibitors of angiotensin-converting enzyme prevent myointimal proliferation after vascular injury. Science 245:186-8, 1989.
24. Kawamura M, Terashita Z, Okuda H, Imura Y, Shino A, Nakao M, Nishikawa K. TCV-116, a novel angiotensin II receptor antagonist, prevents intimal thickening and impairment of vascular function after carotid injury in rats. J Pharmacol Exp Ther 266:1664-9, 1993.
25. Abe J, Deguchi J, Matsumoto T, Takuwa N, Noda M, Ohno M, Makuuchi M, Kurokawa K, Takuwa Y. Stimulated activation of platelet-derived growth factor receptor in vivo in balloon-injured arteries: a link between angiotensin II and intimal thickening. Circulation 96:1906-13, 1997.
26. Osterrieder W, Muller RK, Powell JS, Clozel JP, Hefti F, Baumgartner HR. Role of angiotensin II in injury-induced neointima formation in rats. Hypertension 18:II60-4, 1991.
27. Wiemer G, Scholkens BA, Wagner A, Heitsch H, Linz W. The possible role of angiotensin II subtype AT2 receptors in endothelial cells and isolated ischemic rat hearts. J Hypertens Suppl 11 Suppl 5:S234-5, 1993.
28. Schuh JR, Blehm DJ, Frierdich GE, McMahon EG, Blaine EH. Differential effects of renin-angiotensin system blockade on atherogenesis in cholesterol-fed rabbits. J Clin Invest 91:1453-8, 1993.
29. Lindner V, Lappi DA, Baird A, Majack RA, Reidy MA. Role of basic fibroblast growth factor in vascular lesion formation. Circ Res 68:106-13, 1991.
30. Lindner V, Reidy MA. Proliferation of smooth muscle cells after vascular injury is inhibited by an antibody against basic fibroblast growth factor. Proc Natl Acad Sci U S A 88:3739-43, 1991.
31. Lindner V, Olson NE, Clowes AW, Reidy MA. Inhibition of smooth muscle cell proliferation in injured rat arteries. Interaction of heparin with basic fibroblast growth factor. J Clin Invest 90:2044-9, 1992.
32. Fishel RS, Thourani V, Eisenberg SJ, Shai SY, Corson MA, Nabel EG, Bernstein KE, Berk BC. Fibroblast growth factor stimulates angiotensin converting enzyme expression in vascular smooth muscle cells. Possible mediator of the response to vascular injury. J Clin Invest 95:377-87, 1995.
33. Chobanian AV. The effects of ACE inhibitors and other antihypertensive drugs on cardiovascular risk factors and atherogenesis. Clin Cardiol 13:VII43-8, 1990.
34. Chobanian AV, Haudenschild CC, Nickerson C, Drago R. Antiatherogenic effect of captopril in the Watanabe heritable hyperlipidemic rabbit. Hypertension 15:327-31, 1990.
35. Cambien F, Poirier O, Lecerf L, Evans A, Cambou JP, Arveiler D, Luc G, Bard JM, Bara L, Ricard S, et al. Deletion polymorphism in the gene for angiotensin-converting enzyme is a potent risk factor for myocardial infarction [see comments]. Nature 359:641-4, 1992.
36. Pfeffer MA, Braunwald E, Moye LA, Basta L, Brown EJ, Jr., Cuddy TE, Davis BR, Geltman EM, Goldman S, Flaker GC, et al. Effect of captopril on mortality and morbidity in patients with left ventricular dysfunction after myocardial infarction. Results of the survival and ventricular enlargement trial. The SAVE Investigators [see comments]. N Engl J Med 327:669-77, 1992.
37. Effect of enalapril on mortality and the development of heart failure in asymptomatic patients with reduced left ventricular ejection fractions. The SOLVD Investigattors [published erratum appears in N Engl J Med 1992 Dec 10;327(24):1768] [see comments]. N Engl J Med 327:685-91, 1992.
38. Effect of enalapril on survival in patients with reduced left ventricular ejection fractions and congestive heart failure. The SOLVD Investigators [see comments]. N Engl J Med 325:293-302, 1991.
39. Kaplan HR, Taylor DG, Olson SC, Andrews LK. Quinapril--a preclinical review of the pharmacology, pharmacokinetics, and toxicology. Angiology 40:335-50, 1989.

40. Weishaar RE, Panek RL, Major TC, Simmerman J, Rapundalo ST, Taylor DG, Jr. Evidence for a functional tissue renin-angiotensin system in the rat mesenteric vasculature and its involvement in regulating blood pressure. J Pharmacol Exp Ther 256:568-74, 1991.

41. Esther CR, Marino EM, Howard TE, Machaud A, Corvol P, Capecchi MR, Bernstein KE. The critical role of tissue angiotensin-converting enzyme as revealed by gene targeting in mice. J Clin Invest 99:2375-85, 1997.

42. Morishita R, Gibbons GH, Ellison KE, Lee W, Zhang L, Yu H, Kaneda Y, Ogihara T, Dzau VJ. Evidence for direct local effect of angiotensin in vascular hypertrophy. In vivo gene transfer of angiotensin converting enzyme. J Clin Invest 94:978-84, 1994.

43. Diet F, Pratt RE, Berry GJ, Momose N, Gibbons GH, Dzau VJ. Increased accumulation of tissue ACE in human atherosclerotic coronary artery disease. Circulation 94:2756-67, 1996.

44. Kitazono T, Padgett RC, Armstrong ML, Tompkins PK, Heistad DD. Evidence that angiotensin II is present in human monocytes. Circulation 91:1129-34, 1995.

45. Mitani H, Bandoh T, Kimura M, Totsuka T, Hayashi S. Increased activity of vascular ACE related to atherosclerotic lesions in hyperlipidemic rabbits. Am J Physiol 271:H1065-71, 1996.

46. Hoshida S, Nishida M, Yamashita N, Igarashi J, Aoki K, Hori M, Kuzuya T, Tada M. Vascular angiotensin-converting enzyme activity in cholesterol-fed rabbits: effects of enalapril. Atherosclerosis 130:53-9, 1997.

47. Haberbosch W, Bohle RM, Franke FE, Danilov S, Alhenc-Gelas F, Braun-Dullaeus R, Holschermann H, Waas W, Tillmanns H, Gardemann A. The expression of angiotensin-I converting enzyme in human atherosclerotic plaques is not related to the deletion/insertion polymorphism but to the risk of restenosis after coronary interventions. Atherosclerosis 130:203-13, 1997.

48. Yang BC, Phillips MI, Mohuczy D, Meng H, Shen L, Mehta P, Mehta JL. Increased angiotensin II type 1 receptor expression in hypercholesterolemic atherosclerosis in rabbits. Arterioscler Thromb Vasc Biol 18:1433-9, 1998.

49. Cardona-Sanclemente LE, Medina R, Born GV. Effect of increasing doses of angiotensin II infused into normal and hypertensive Wistar rats on low density lipoprotein and fibrinogen uptake by aortic walls. Proc Natl Acad Sci U S A 91:3285-8, 1994.

50. Cardona-Sanclemente LE, Born GV. Increase by adrenaline or angiotensin II of the accumulation of low density lipoprotein and fibrinogen by aortic walls in unrestrained conscious rats. Br J Pharmacol 117:1089-94, 1996.

51. Nielsen LB, Stender S, Kjeldsen K, Nordestgaard BG. Effect of angiotensin II and enalapril on transfer of low-density lipoprotein into aortic intima in rabbits. Circ Res 75:63-9, 1994.

52. Keidar S, Kaplan M, Shapira C, Brook JG, Aviram M. Low density lipoprotein isolated from patients with essential hypertension exhibits increased propensity for oxidation and enhanced uptake by macrophages: a possible role for angiotensin II. Atherosclerosis 107:71-84, 1994.

53. Keidar S, Kaplan M, Hoffman A, Aviram M. Angiotensin II stimulates macrophage-mediated oxidation of low density lipoproteins. Atherosclerosis 115:201-15, 1995.

54. Scheidegger KJ, Butler S, Witztum JL. Angiotensin II increases macrophage-mediated modification of low density lipoprotein via a lipoxygenase-dependent pathway. J Biol Chem 272:21609-15, 1997.

55. Keidar S, Kaplan M, Aviram M. Angiotensin II-modified LDL is taken up by macrophages via the scavenger receptor, leading to cellular cholesterol accumulation. Arterioscler Thromb Vasc Biol 16:97-105, 1996.

56. Hernandez-Presa M, Bustos C, Ortego M, Tunon J, Renedo G, Ruiz-Ortega M, Egido J. Angiotensin-converting enzyme inhibition prevents arterial nuclear factor-kappa B activation, monocyte chemoattractant protein-1 expression, and macrophage infiltration in a rabbit model of early accelerated atherosclerosis. Circulation 95:1532-41, 1997.

57. Mervaala EM, M ller DN, Park JK, Schmidt F, Lohn M, Breu V, Dragun D, Ganten D, Haller H, Luft FC. Monocyte infiltration and adhesion molecules in a rat model of high human renin hypertension [In Process Citation]. Hypertension 33:389-95, 1999.

58. Grafe M, Auch-Schwelk W, Zakrzewicz A, Regitz-Zagrosek V, Bartsch P, Graf K, Loebe M, Gaehtgens P, Fleck E. Angiotensin II-induced leukocyte adhesion on human coronary endothelial cells is mediated by E-selectin [In Process Citation]. Circ Res 81:804-11, 1997.

59. Rajagopalan S, Kurz S, Munzel T, Tarpey M, Freeman BA, Griendling KK, Harrison DG. Angiotensin II-mediated hypertension in the rat increases vascular superoxide production via membrane NADH/NADPH oxidase activation. Contribution to alterations of vasomotor tone. J Clin Invest 97:1916-23, 1996.

60. Yanagitani Y, Rakugi H, Okamura A, Moriguchi K, Takiuchi S, Ohishi M, Suzuki K, Higaki J, Ogihara T. Angiotensin II type 1 receptor-mediated peroxide production in human macrophages [In Process Citation]. Hypertension 33:335-9, 1999.
61. Zafari AM, Ushio-Fukai M, Akers M, Yin Q, Shah A, Harrison DG, Taylor WR, Griendling KK. Role of NADH/NADPH oxidase-derived H2O2 in angiotensin II-induced vascular hypertrophy. Hypertension 32:488-95, 1998.
62. Ushio-Fukai M, Zafari AM, Fukui T, Ishizaka N, Griendling KK. p22phox is a critical component of the superoxide-generating NADH/NADPH oxidase system and regulates angiotensin II-induced hypertrophy in vascular smooth muscle cells. J Biol Chem 271:23317-21, 1996.
63. Khan BV, Harrison DG, Olbrych MT, Alexander RW, Medford RM. Nitric oxide regulates vascular cell adhesion molecule 1 gene expression and redox-sensitive transcriptional events in human vascular endothelial cells. Proc Natl Acad Sci U S A 93:9114-9, 1996.
64. Marui N, Offermann MK, Swerlick R, Kunsch C, Rosen CA, Ahmad M, Alexander RW, Medford RM. Vascular cell adhesion molecule-1 (VCAM-1) gene transcription and expression are regulated through an antioxidant-sensitive mechanism in human vascular endothelial cells. J Clin Invest 92:1866-74, 1993.
65. Candipan RC, Wang BY, Buitrago R, Tsao PS, Cooke JP. Regression or progression. Dependency on vascular nitric oxide. Arterioscler Thromb Vasc Biol 16:44-50, 1996.
66. Wang BY, Candipan RC, Arjomandi M, Hsiun PT, Tsao PS, Cooke JP. Arginine restores nitric oxide activity and inhibits monocyte accumulation after vascular injury in hypercholesterolemic rabbits. J Am Coll Cardiol 28:1573-9, 1996.
67. Tsao PS, Wang B, Buitrago R, Shyy JY, Cooke JP. Nitric oxide regulates monocyte chemotactic protein-1. Circulation 96:934-40, 1997.
68. Theilmeier G, Chan JR, Zalpour C, Anderson B, Wang BY, Wolf A, Tsao PS, Cooke JP. Adhesiveness of mononuclear cells in hypercholesterolemic humans is normalized by dietary L-arginine. Arterioscler Thromb Vasc Biol 17:3557-64, 1997.
69. Whitebread S, Mele M, Kamber B, de Gasparo M. Preliminary biochemical characterization of two angiotensin II receptor subtypes. Biochem Biophys Res Commun 163:284-91, 1989.
70. Chiu AT, Herblin WF, McCall DE, Ardecky RJ, Carini DJ, Duncia JV, Pease LJ, Wong PC, Wexler RR, Johnson AL, et al. Identification of angiotensin II receptor subtypes. Biochem Biophys Res Commun 165:196-203, 1989.
71. Sugano M, Makino N, Yanaga T. The effects of renin-angiotensin system inhibition on aortic cholesterol content in cholesterol-fed rabbits. Atherosclerosis 127:123-9, 1996.
72. Keidar S, Attias J, Smith J, Breslow JL, Hayek T. The angiotensin-II receptor antagonist, losartan, inhibits LDL lipid peroxidation and atherosclerosis in apolipoprotein E-deficient mice. Biochem Biophys Res Commun 236:622-5, 1997.
73. Fennessy PA, Campbell JH, Mendelsohn FA, Campbell GR. Angiotensin-converting enzyme inhibitors and atherosclerosis: relevance of animal models to human disease. Clin Exp Pharmacol Physiol 23:S30-2, 1996.
74. Sasaki K, Yamano Y, Bardhan S, Iwai N, Murray JJ, Hasegawa M, Matsuda Y, Inagami T. Cloning and expression of a complementary DNA encoding a bovine adrenal angiotensin II type-1 receptor. Nature 351:230-3, 1991.
75. Murphy TJ, Alexander RW, Griendling KK, Runge MS, Bernstein KE. Isolation of a cDNA encoding the vascular type-1 angiotensin II receptor. Nature 351:233-6, 1991.
76. Sasamura H, Hein L, Krieger JE, Pratt RE, Kobilka BK, Dzau VJ. Cloning, characterization, and expression of two angiotensin receptor (AT-1) isoforms from the mouse genome. Biochem Biophys Res Commun 185:253-9, 1992.
77. Iwai N, Inagami T. Quantitative analysis of renin gene expression in extrarenal tissues by polymerase chain reaction method. J Hypertens 10:717-24, 1992.
78. Grady EF, Sechi LA, Griffin CA, Schambelan M, Kalinyak JE. Expression of AT2 receptors in the developing rat fetus. J Clin Invest 88:921-33, 1991.
79. Millan MA, Jacobowitz DM, Aguilera G, Catt KJ. Differential distribution of AT1 and AT2 angiotensin II receptor subtypes in the rat brain during development. Proc Natl Acad Sci U S A 88:11440-4, 1991.
80. Pucell AG, Hodges JC, Sen I, Bumpus FM, Husain A. Biochemical properties of the ovarian granulosa cell type 2- angiotensin II receptor. Endocrinology 128:1947-59, 1991.

81. Tsutsumi K, Saavedra JM. Characterization and development of angiotensin II receptor subtypes (AT1 and AT2) in rat brain. Am J Physiol 261:R209-16, 1991.

82. Dudley DT, Hubbell SE, Summerfelt RM. Characterization of angiotensin II (AT2) binding sites in R3T3 cells. Mol Pharmacol 40:360-7, 1991.

83. Kambayashi Y, Bardhan S, Takahashi K, Tsuzuki S, Inui H, Hamakubo T, Inagami T. Molecular cloning of a novel angiotensin II receptor isoform involved in phosphotyrosine phosphatase inhibition. J Biol Chem 268:24543-6, 1993.

84. Mukoyama M, Nakajima M, Horiuchi M, Sasamura H, Pratt RE, Dzau VJ. Expression cloning of type 2 angiotensin II receptor reveals a unique class of seven-transmembrane receptors. J Biol Chem 268:24539-42, 1993.

85. Viswanathan M, Tsutsumi K, Correa FM, Saavedra JM. Changes in expression of angiotensin receptor subtypes in the rat aorta during development. Biochem Biophys Res Commun 179:1361-7, 1991.

86. Hutchinson HG, Hein L, Fuginaga M, Pratt RE. Modulation of vascular development and injury by angiotensin II. Cardiovascular Research In Press1998.

87. Nakajima M, Hutchinson HG, Fujinaga M, Hayashida W, Morishita R, Zhang L, Horiuchi M, Pratt RE, Dzau VJ. The angiotensin II type 2 (AT2) receptor antagonizes the growth effects of the AT1 receptor: gain-of-function study using gene transfer. Proc Natl Acad Sci U S A 92:10663-7, 1995.

88. Stoll M, Steckelings UM, Paul M, Bottari SP, Metzger R, Unger T. The angiotensin AT2-receptor mediates inhibition of cell proliferation in coronary endothelial cells. J Clin Invest 95:651-7, 1995.

89. Booz GW, Baker KM. Role of type 1 and type 2 angiotensin receptors in angiotensin II- induced cardiomyocyte hypertrophy. Hypertension 28:635-40, 1996.

90. Bartunek J, Weinberg EO, Tajima M, Rohrbach S, Lorell BH. Angiotensin II type 2 receptor blockade amplifies the early signals of cardiac growth response to angiotensin II in hypertrophied hearts [In Process Citation]. Circulation 99:22-5, 1999.

91. Cook CL, Weiser MC, Schwartz PE, Jones CL, Majack RA. Developmentally timed expression of an embryonic growth phenotype in vascular smooth muscle cells. Circ Res 74:189-96, 1994.

92. deBlois D, Tea BS, Than VD, Tremblay J, Hamet P. Smooth muscle apoptosis during vascular regression in spontaneously hypertensive rats. Hypertension 29:340-9, 1997.

93. Bennett MR, Evan GI, Schwartz SM. Apoptosis of rat vascular smooth muscle cells is regulated by p53- dependent and -independent pathways. Circ Res 77:266-73, 1995.

94. Cheng W, Kajstura J, Nitahara JA, Li B, Reiss K, Liu Y, Clark WA, Krajewski S, Reed JC, Olivetti G, Anversa P. Programmed myocyte cell death affects the viable myocardium after infarction in rats. Exp Cell Res 226:316-27, 1996.

95. Hamet P. Proliferation and apoptosis of vascular smooth muscle in hypertension. Curr Opin Nephrol Hypertens 4:1-7, 1995.

96. Isner JM, Kearney M, Bortman S, Passeri J. Apoptosis in human atherosclerosis and restenosis [see comments]. Circulation 91:2703-11, 1995.

97. Kajstura J, Cheng W, Reiss K, Clark WA, Sonnenblick EH, Krajewski S, Reed JC, Olivetti G, Anversa P. Apoptotic and necrotic myocyte cell deaths are independent contributing variables of infarct size in rats. Lab Invest 74:86-107, 1996.

98. Narula J, Haider N, Virmani R, DiSalvo TG, Kolodgie FD, Hajjar RJ, Schmidt U, Semigran MJ, Dec GW, Khaw BA. Apoptosis in myocytes in end-stage heart failure [see comments]. N Engl J Med 335:1182-9, 1996.

99. Pollman MJ, Yamada T, Horiuchi M, Gibbons GH. Vasoactive substances regulate vascular smooth muscle cell apoptosis. Countervailing influences of nitric oxide and angiotensin II. Circ Res 79:748-56, 1996.

100. Hamet P, deBlois D, Dam TV, Richard L, Teiger E, Tea BS, Orlov SN, Tremblay J. Apoptosis and vascular wall remodeling in hypertension. Can J Physiol Pharmacol 74:850-61, 1996.

101. Wu CF, Bishopric NH, Pratt RE. Atrial natriuretic peptide induces apoptosis in neonatal rat cardiac myocytes. J Biol Chem 272:14860-6, 1997.

102. Trindade P, Hutchinson HG, Pollman MJ, Gibbons GH, Pratt RE. Atrial Natriuretic Peptide (ANP) and C-type Natriuretic Peptide (CNP) induce apoptosis in vascular smooth muscle cells. Circulation 92:I-696 (Abstract), 1995.

103. Balligand JL, Cannon PJ. Nitric oxide synthases and cardiac muscle. Autocrine and paracrine influences. Arterioscler Thromb Vasc Biol 17:1846-58, 1997.

104. Colucci WS. Molecular and cellular mechanisms of myocardial failure. Am J Cardiol 80:15L-25L, 1997.

105. Geng YJ, Libby P. Evidence for apoptosis in advanced human atheroma. Colocalization with interleukin-1 beta-converting enzyme [see comments]. Am J Pathol 147:251-66, 1995.
106. Kajstura J, Cigola E, Malhotra A, Li P, Cheng W, Meggs LG, Anversa P. Angiotensin II induces apoptosis of adult ventricular myocytes in vitro. J Mol Cell Cardiol 29:859-70, 1997.
107. Pierzchalski P, Reiss K, Cheng W, Cirielli C, Kajstura J, Nitahara JA, Rizk M, Capogrossi MC, Anversa P. p53 Induces myocyte apoptosis via the activation of the renin- angiotensin system. Exp Cell Res 234:57-65, 1997.
108. Horiuchi M, Hayashida W, Kambe T, Yamada T, Dzau VJ. Angiotensin type 2 receptor dephosphorylates Bcl-2 by activating mitogen-activated protein kinase phosphatase-1 and induces apoptosis. J Biol Chem 272:19022-6, 1997.
109. Horiuchi M, Yamada T, Hayashida W, Dzau VJ. Interferon regulatory factor-1 up-regulates angiotensin II type 2 receptor and induces apoptosis. J Biol Chem 272:11952-8, 1997.
110. Yamada T, Horiuchi M, Dzau VJ. Angiotensin II type 2 receptor mediates programmed cell death. Proc Natl Acad Sci U S A 93:156-60, 1996.
111. Leri A, Claudio PP, Li Q, Wang X, Reiss K, Wang S, Malhotra A, Kajstura J, Anversa P. Stretch-mediated release of angiotensin II induces myocyte apoptosis by activating p53 that enhances the local renin-angiotensin system and decreases the Bcl-2-to-Bax protein ratio in the cell. J Clin Invest 101:1326-42, 1998.
112. Ma J, Nishimura H, Fogo A, Kon V, Inagami T, Ichikawa I. Accelerated fibrosis and collagen deposition develop in the renal interstitium of angiotensin type 2 receptor null mutant mice during ureteral obstruction. Kidney Int 53:937-44, 1998.
113. Koch WJ, Hawes BE, Allen LF, Lefkowitz RJ. Direct evidence that Gi-coupled receptor stimulation of mitogen- activated protein kinase is mediated by G beta gamma activation of p21ras. Proc Natl Acad Sci U S A 91:12706-10, 1994.
114. Zhang J, Pratt RE. The AT2 receptor selectively associates with Gialpha2 and Gialpha3 in the rat fetus. J Biol Chem 271:15026-33, 1996.
115. Siragy HM, Carey RM. The subtype 2 (AT2) angiotensin receptor mediates renal production of nitric oxide in conscious rats. J Clin Invest 100:264-9, 1997.
116. Siragy HM, Carey RM. The subtype-2 (AT2) angiotensin receptor regulates renal cyclic guanosine 3', 5'-monophosphate and AT1 receptor-mediated prostaglandin E2 production in conscious rats [see comments]. J Clin Invest 97:1978-82, 1996.
117. Gohlke P, Pees C, Unger T. AT2 receptor stimulation increases aortic cyclic GMP in SHRSP by a kinin-dependent mechanism. Hypertension 31:349-55, 1998.
118. Liu YH, Yang XP, Sharov VG, Nass O, Sabbah HN, Peterson E, Carretero OA. Effects of angiotensin-converting enzyme inhibitors and angiotensin II type 1 receptor antagonists in rats with heart failure. Role of kinins and angiotensin II type 2 receptors. J Clin Invest 99:1926-35, 1997.

7 REGULATION OF INFLAMMATION BY FAS LIGAND EXPRESSION ON THE VASCULAR ENDOTHELIUM

Kenneth Walsh, Ph.D
Masataka Sata, M.D.
Tufts University and
St. Elizabeth's Medical Center

INTRODUCTION

The monolayer of endothelial cells that coat the luminal surface of the vessel wall have numerous physiological functions including the prevention of coagulation, control of vascular permeability, maintenance of vascular tone, and regulation of leukocyte extravasation. While the vascular endothelium plays a pivotal role in recruiting inflammatory cells at the site of infection or wounding, the normal endothelium is believed to serve as a barrier to inflammation in the absence of inflammatory stimuli.

The vascular endothelial surface is in constant contact with circulating cellular constituents of the blood. Though much effort has been directed toward understanding the roles of pro-inflammatory proteins expressed by the vessel wall, such as cytokines, chemokines, co-stimulatory molecules, selectins and surface adhesion molecules, little is known about the mechanism by which endothelial cells may actively prevent inflammatory cell infiltration of the subendothelial space. Recently, functional Fas ligand expression was detected on the cell surface of endothelial cells and on the endothelial lining of blood vessels. Here, we review data suggesting that Fas ligand expressed by endothelial cells functions to negatively regulate the extravasation of inflammatory cells.

The inflammatory cytokine TNFα downregulates endothelial Fas ligand expression with an accompanying decrease in endothelial cell cytotoxicity toward Fas-bearing cells in co-culture. Endothelial Fas ligand expression in arteries is also downregulated by the local administration of TNFα, and this correlates with robust mononuclear cell infiltration of the subendothelial space. This TNFα-induced mononuclear cell infiltration can be inhibited by prior infection of the endothelium with a replication-defective adenovirus that constitutively expresses Fas ligand. Under these conditions, adherent leukocytes undergo apoptosis rather than extravasation. These findings suggest a novel function of vascular endothelium and may also provide a clue to pathogenic processes whereby endothelial dysfunction promotes excessive leukocyte infiltration. Furthermore, ectopic or augmented Fas ligand expression may have utility in treating inflammatory fibroproliferative vascular disorders.

FAS RECEPTOR AND FAS LIGAND

Fas ligand is a type II membrane protein that induces apoptotic cell death in cells that bear the Fas (CD95/Apo-1) receptor (1). The Fas receptor is a member of the TNF receptor family that is expressed on most cell types including leukocytes. Binding of the trimeric Fas ligand induces Fas receptor clustering, leading to the recruitment of the linker protein FADD (also referred to as MORT1) which binds to the Fas cytoplasmic domain, via its "death domain" (Figure 1). Caspase-8 (also referred to as FLICE and MACH) is then recruited to FADD/MORT1 by binding through its "death effector domain" (2,3) . Oligomerization of caspase-8 induces self-activation and triggers a proteolytic activation cascade of additional caspase family members. Activated caspase-8 also cleaves the Bcl-2 homologous protein Bid, which then translocates to the mitochondrial membrane and induces cytochrome c release and mitochondrial dysfunction (4,5). Cytoplasmic cytochrome c activates caspase-9 in the presence of Apaf-1 (for apoptosis activating factor-1) and dATP, leading to proteolytic activation of caspase-3 (CPP32-like protease). These activated caspases induce the morphological changes, such as cytoskeletal rearrangements and chromatin fragmentation, that accompany apoptosis (6). FLIP (for FLICE-inhibitory protein) is a recently identified cellular inhibitor of apoptosis (7-9). FLIP contains the FADD binding domain, but lacks an active-center cysteine residue. Thus, it appears to function as an inhibitor of caspase-8 activation, thus blocking Fas-mediated apoptosis (7-9). FLIP function is best understood in T cells where FLIP is expressed during the early stage of T-cell activation when these cells express both Fas and Fas ligand, but remain viable. However, as FLIP levels decline at later stages of T cell activation, cells become susceptible to Fas ligand-mediated apoptosis (7,10). Thus, these data provide correlative evidence that FLIP levels may be crucial in determining the sensitivity of the cells to Fas-mediated apoptosis.   In contrast to its receptor, Fas ligand is highly restricted in its expression. Cytotoxic T lymphocytes express Fas ligand, contributing to their cytotoxic function (1). Fas ligand expression has also been detected in tissues that are considered to be "immune privileged" such as eye and testis (11,12). It is believed that constitutive Fas ligand expression on these tissues prevents inflammatory leukocyte infiltration by inducing apoptotic cell death in Fas-expressing immune cells when they attempt to enter the tissue. Similarly, some tumor cells express Fas ligand, and this feature may contribute to their ability to evade immune response (13-15).

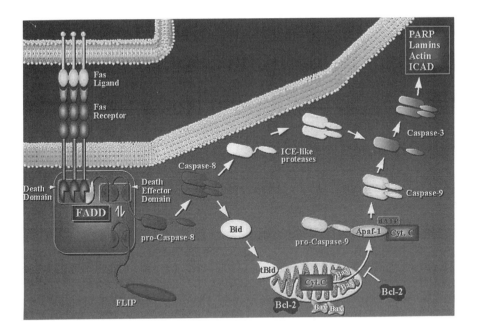

Figure 1. Apoptosis-inducing pathway induced by Fas-Fas ligand interaction. Fas ligand induces oligomerization of Fas, which recruits caspase-8 via the FADD adaptor protein. FADD interacts with Fas through the death domain (DD) and with caspase-8 through the death effector domain (DED). The oligomerization of caspase-8 results in self-activation of proteolytic activity and triggers proteolytic activation of other caspases family members. Activated caspase-8 also cleaves the Bcl-2 homologous protein Bid, which then translocates to the mitochondrial membrane and induces mitochondrial dysfunction and cytochrome c release. Cytosolic cytochrome c binds to Apaf-1 and dATP, leading to the activation of caspase-9. Activated caspases drive the morphological changes that accompany apoptosis including cytoskeletal rearrangements and chromatin fragmentation. FLIP is a homolog of caspase-8 that contains a DED, but lacks the active-center cysteine residue in a caspase-like domain. Thus, FLIP functions as an inhibitor of caspase-8, blocking the Fas death signal.

ROLE OF ENDOTHELIUM IN CONTROLLING LEUKOCYTE EXTRAVASATION

Leukocytes circulate within the network of blood vessels surveying tissues for pathogens, and rapidly accumulate at sites of infection and injury. To gain access to sites of infection, leukocytes pass the endothelial barrier and migrate out of blood vessels by a process known as extravasation (16). Extravasation involves tethering, firm adhesion, and the migration of leukocytes to the subendothelial space (diapedesis). Pathogen infection or injury leads to the release of cytokines, which induce the vascular endothelium to express selectins, intercellular adhesion molecules, and vascular cell adhesion molecule (VCAM-1) (17). These molecules serve to tether leukocytes to the vessel wall. Tethered leukocytes adhere firmly through interactions with the platelet-endothelial cell adhesion molecule (PECAM) expressed on the surface of the leukocyte and at the intercellular junctions of endothelial cells. These interactions ultimately enable leukocytes to pass between endothelial cells and penetrate the basement membrane aided by leukocyte derived proteolytic activity. Leukocytes then migrate through the subendothelial space to sites of inflammation under the influence of chemoattractant cytokines (16).

In the absence of infection, the endothelium functions as a barrier to inflammation. This barrier is breached in many vascular diseases, resulting in a detrimental chronic inflammatory response within vessels (18).

EXPRESSION OF FUNCTIONALFAS LIGAND ON CULTURED HUMAN ENDOTHELIAL CELLS

Regulated expression of Fas ligand on cultured human endothelial cells. Many vascular endothelial cell types express Fas ligand. Immunoblot analysis reveals Fas ligand expression by human umbilical vein endothelial cells (HUVECs), human aortic endothelial cells (HAECs), and human microvascular endothelial cells (HMVECs) (19). Flow cytometric analysis indicates that Fas ligand is expressed on the surface of these cell types. In contrast, cultured human smooth muscle cells are void of detectable Fas ligand expression, as are most other tissues in the body (20,21). Consistent with a potential function in regulating leukocyte extravasation, HUVEC cell surface expression of Fas ligand is markedly downregulated following activation by the inflammatory cytokine TNFα as determined by FACS analysis (Figure 2). Similar data have also been obtained with HAECs and HMVECs, suggesting that TNFα-mediated downregulation of Fas ligand is a feature exhibited by many endothelial cell types.

Fas ligand on endothelial cells kills co-cultured Fas-bearing cells. The functionality of the Fas ligand expressed on the endothelial cell surface was assessed by determining whether endothelial cells are capable of inducing apoptosis in Fas-positive target cells (19). In co-culture assays, endothelial cells induced DNA fragmentation, a marker of apoptotic cell death, in both a human T cell leukemia cell line (Jurkat cells) and a mastocytoma cell line overexpressing human Fas. The cytotoxicity of endothelial cells toward target cells was completely abrogated by the addition of a neutralizing anti-Fas ligand antibody, providing evidence that the cytotoxic activity is mediated by the Fas-Fas ligand interaction. The cytotoxicity of endothelial cells was also decreased by pretreating the endothelial cells with a dose of TNFα sufficient to downregulate Fas ligand expression. In contrast, endothelial cells pre-infected with an adenoviral vector constitutively expressing Fas ligand (Adeno-Fas ligand) promote very high levels of target cell DNA fragmentation that cannot be inhibited by TNFα treatment. Collectively, these experiments document that endothelial cells express functional Fas ligand on their cell surface, which is capable of killing an adjacent Fas-bearing cell.

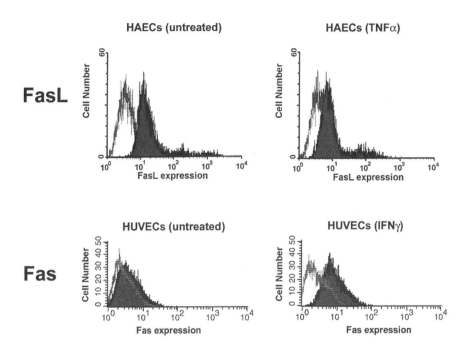

Figure 2. Regulated expression of Fas ligand and Fas expression on human endothelial cells.
Human aortic endothelial cells (HAECs) were treated with 25 ng/ml TNFα for 6 hours or 10 ng/ml
interferon γ (IFNγ) for 18 hours. Cell surface expression of Fas ligand and Fas was examined by flow
cytometry (filled curve). Isotype matched IgG was used as a negative control (open curve). A portion of
the data in this figure was reprinted with permission of *Nature Medicine*, Copyright 1998 (19).

Endothelial cells are resistant to Fas ligation. Endothelial cells express both Fas
receptor and Fas ligand on their cell surface (Figure 2). Despite simultaneous
expression of the ligand and receptor, these cells do not undergo Fas-mediated
apoptosis. Furthermore, endothelial cells are remarkably resistant to Fas-mediated
apoptosis induced by various experimental manipulations. For example, endothelial
cells do not undergo apoptosis when exposed to an anti-Fas antibody that can
function as a receptor agonist (19). Endothelial cells are also resistant to apoptosis
when cell surface Fas ligand is massively overexpressed by infection with Adeno-
Fas ligand. Endothelial cells are also refractory to Fas-mediated apoptosis under
conditions that upregulate the Fas death receptor (22), such as treatment of cells
with the cytokine interferon-γ (Figure 2).

Presumably, endothelial cells are resistant to Fas-mediated cell death
because they fail to transmit an apoptosis-inducing signal following the engagement
of Fas by Fas ligand. There are several mechanisms that may account for the
endothelial cell's lack of sensitivity to Fas-mediated cell death. For example,
endothelial cells may express relatively high levels of protective Bcl-2 family
proteins which have been shown to function as negative regulators of Fas-mediated
apoptosis in some (23,24) but not all (25,26) cell types. Another intriguing
possibility is that endothelial cells express high levels of FLIP (Figure 1), which can
inhibit the intracellular Fas-signaling pathway (7-9). Recently, we documented

FLIP expression in endothelial cells, and provided evidence that changes in FLIP expression may modulate viability under conditions of oxidized lipid-induced cell death (27).

In contrast to endothelial cells, Fas-bearing vascular smooth muscle cells (VSMCs) are highly sensitive to Fas ligand-induced apoptosis both *in vitro* and *in vivo*. Infection with Adeno-Fas ligand is sufficient to kill cultured rat (28) and human VSMCs (M.S. and K.W., unpublished observations) in a dose-dependent manner. Plasmid-mediated Fas ligand gene transfer is also sufficient to induce apoptosis in VSMCs. Others have also reported that cultured aortic human VSMCs undergo Fas-mediated cell death when exposed to an agonist anti-Fas antibody, but only when activated by cytokines (29). It appears paradoxical that the anti-Fas agonist antibody is not sufficient to kill VSMCs in the absence of cytokine stimulation, while transduction of the *Fas ligand* gene can kill in the absence of activation. A possible explanation for this apparent discrepancy is that *Fas ligand* gene transfer results in the insertion of Fas ligand in the cell membrane, thereby providing a more physiologically relevant presentation of the ligand to the target cell. In comparison, the agonist antibody is likely to be much less efficient in clustering Fas receptor molecules, a feature necessary for transmission of the death signal. Consistent with this interpretation, a soluble form of Fas ligand, like the agonist Fas antibody, is less efficient at engaging the Fas receptor (30,31).

REGULATED GAS LIGAND EXPRESSION IN VIVO

Fas ligand expression could be detected in the endothelium of the central artery of the rabbit ear by co-localization with CD31, an established marker for vascular endothelial cells (Figure 3). Regulation of Fas ligand expression *in vivo* was analyzed using a rabbit ear model of leukocyte extravasation (19). In this model, blood flow was temporarily interrupted in the ear by application of a tourniquet at the base, TNFα or saline was then infused into the lumen of the central artery. Following a 15 minute incubation, the tourniquet was removed to restore blood flow. At 30 hours post-treatment, tissue was harvested and analyzed for Fas ligand and VCAM-1 expression, and for T cell and monocyte/macrophage infiltrates. In arteries treated with TNFα, Fas ligand expression by the endothelium was markedly downregulated relative to the saline control. The TNFα-treated vessels also displayed an upregulation of VCAM-1 expression and robust infiltration of the arterial wall by T lymphocytes and macrophages (Figure 4).

CONSTITUTIVE FAS LIGAND EXPRESSION BY THE ENDOTHELIUM BLOCKS TNFα-INDUCED T CELL AND MONOCYTE INFILTRATION

To examine the functional significance of Fas ligand downregulation *in vivo*, the rabbit ear model of leukocyte extravasation was modified to accommodate adenovirus-mediated expression of the *Fas ligand* gene (19). In these experiments, a tourniquet was first applied at the base of the ear to allow infection of the endothelium of the central ear artery with Adeno-Fas ligand, or the control virus Adeno-βgal, for 15 minutes. After 12 hours, to permit adenovirus-mediated gene

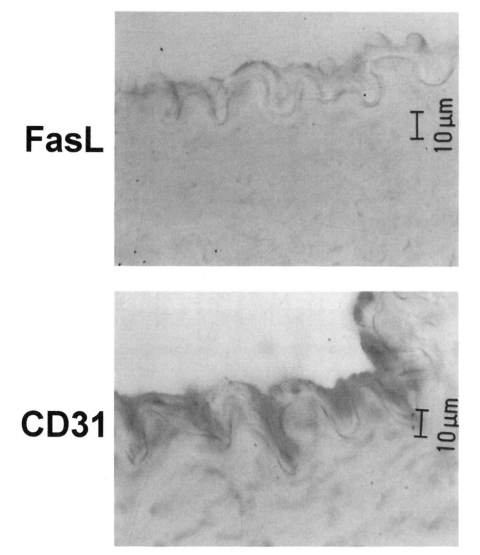

Figure 3. Fas ligand is expressed on the intact vascular endothelium. A cryosection of the central artery of an untreated rabbit ear was stained for Fas ligand and an adjacent section was stained for CD31, an antigen expressed by endothelial cells.

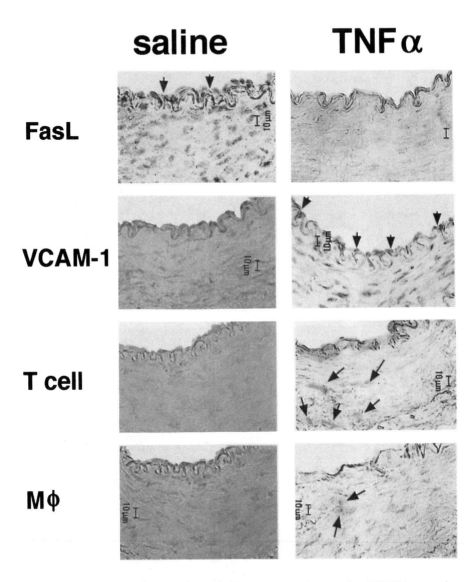

Figure 4. Effect of local administration of TNFα on Fas ligand expression, VCAM-1 expression and mononuclear cell infiltration. Central rabbit ear arteries were temporarily isolated by application of a tourniquet and incubated with either saline or TNFα (50 ng) for 15 minutes prior to the restoration of blood flow. Rabbits were then sacrificed 30 hours after treatment and the arteries were harvested and snap-frozen in embedding compound. Cryosections were stained for Fas ligand, VCAM-1, CD3 (T cells) or RAM 11 (macrophages, Mφ). Reprinted with permission of *Nature Medicine*, Copyright 1998 (19).

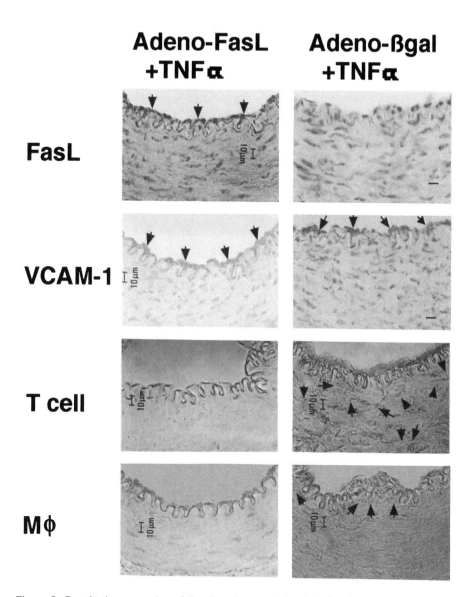

Figure 5. Constitutive expression of Fas ligand prevents TNFα-induced T cell and monocyte infiltration of the subendothelial space. Rabbit central ear arteries were isolated by application of a tourniquet and infected with either Adeno-Fas ligand (1×10^7 pfu) or the control adenovirus, Adeno-βgal (1×10^7 pfu), for 15 minutes prior to the restoration of blood flow. Adeno-βgal is a replication defective adenovirus expressing β-galactosidase. After 12 hours, the arteries were again isolated and incubated with TNFα (50 ng) for 15 minutes. Rabbits were sacrificed 30 hours after the TNFα treatment, and arteries were harvested. Cryosections were analyzed by immunohistochemical methods for Fas ligand, VCAM-1, T cells and macrophages (Mφ). Bar, 50 μm. Reprinted with permission of *Nature Medicine*, Copyright 1998 (19).

expression, the tourniquet was re-applied to allow infusion of TNFα or saline (incubation for 15 minutes). At 30 hours post-cytokine treatment, Fas ligand expression by the endothelium was readily detectable in Adeno-Fas ligand infected vessels, but not in vessels infected with Adeno-βgal (Figure 5). Despite increased VCAM-1 expression following treatment with TNFα, T cell and macrophage infiltration was markedly attenuated in vessels transduced with Adeno-Fas ligand but not in the Adeno-βgal-transduced vessels. In separate experiments, TUNEL staining of Adeno-Fas ligand-treated vessels at 4 hours post-cytokine treatment revealed mononuclear cells undergoing apoptosis at the luminal surface of endothelium, while mononuclear cell apoptosis was not detected in arteries pre-treated with Adeno-βgal (19). Thus, under conditions of constitutive Fas ligand expression, mononuclear cells adhere to the endothelium but undergo apoptosis rather than diapedesis. These findings indicate that Fas ligand expression by the vascular endothelium functions to prevent inflammatory cell migration to the sub-endothelial space and that Fas ligand downregulation may be an important feature of the normal inflammatory response to pathogen infection (Figure 6).

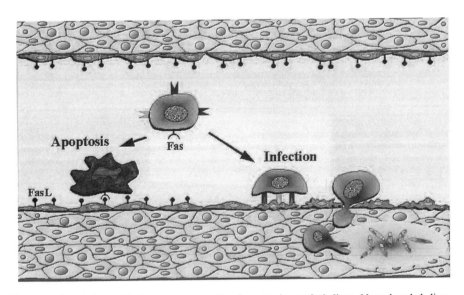

Figure 6. Regulation of leukocyte extravasation by vascular endothelium. Normal endothelium expresses Fas ligand which functions as an anti-inflammatory molecule by inducing apoptosis in leukocytes that attempt to infiltrate the vessel wall in the absence of inflammatory stimuli. Upon infection or injury, TNFα is released inducing endothelial cells to upregulate surface adhesion molecules and downregulate Fas ligand. Under these conditions, leukocytes adhere to activated endothelial cells, undergo successful diapedesis, and migrate to sites of inflammation.

IMPLICATIONS FOR ATHERSCLEROSIS

Atherosclerosis is believed to result from a chronic, detrimental immune response at localized regions within the vessel (18). Human atherosclerotic plaques contain large numbers of activated T lymphocytes and macrophages (18,32-36). TNFα is expressed by macrophage and smooth muscle cells at the sites of vascular injury, and this cytokine is thought to have an important role in the progression of atherosclerotic lesions (37,38). This is particularly evident in transplant arteriosclerosis, a robust form of atherosclerosis that is responsible for the majority of deaths in heart transplant recipients surviving for one or more years (39). In contrast with common atherosclerosis, the lesions of transplant-associated arteriosclerosis tend to be concentric rather than eccentric, and there is often less lipid accumulation (39). Leukocyte infiltration into the artery wall is more evident and cytokines are persistently expressed in the transplanted allografts (40). TNFα is thought to play a key role in this process, as it has been shown that a blockade of TNFα production reduces coronary artery neointimal formation in a rabbit model of cardiac transplant arteriosclerosis, while having no effect on the degree of myocardial rejection (41). Collectively, these findings indicate that the transplant-associated arteriosclerosis results in large part from the immune response to the grafted artery.

Based upon the above mentioned observations, it is tempting to speculate that Fas ligand expression by normal endothelium may fulfill an atheroprotective function by inhibiting leukocyte extravasation. Presumably, secretion of TNFα by activated cells within an early lesion (34,38,42) downregulates Fas ligand expression in adjacent endothelium, promoting increased leukocyte extravasation and growth of the atheroma. However, the etiology of atherosclerosis is complex, and detection of apoptotic Fas-positive smooth muscle cells in atherosclerotic plaques containing inflammatory cells suggests that Fas-mediated apoptosis may contribute to the sequelae of the lesion (29). Furthermore, recent observations that oxidized lipids increase the sensitivity of endothelial cells to death signals from the Fas receptor (43) suggest that Fas-mediated endothelial cell suicide may contribute to the atherosclerosis that results from exaggerated hyperlipidemia. Thus, further experimentation will be required to assess whether Fas ligand expression by the vessel wall has an overall positive or negative influence on atherogenesis, and these studies will likely provide new insights about the mechanisms that contribute to inflammatory-fibroproliferative disorders of the vessel wall.

IMPLICATION FOR POST-ANGIOPLASTY RESTENOSIS

Atherosclerotic lesions of the coronary artery are commonly treated by percutaneous transluminal coronary angioplasty, but a significant fraction of these procedures fail due to post-angioplasty restenosis (44,45). Restenosis results partly from inflammatory cell infiltration (46) and exuberant vascular smooth muscle cell proliferation (47). These pathological processes are particularly pronounced in the restenosis that occurs within stents (48,49), prosthetic devices inserted within vessels to prevent constrictive remodeling. Thus, much effort has been directed toward understanding the molecular pathways regulating vessel wall response to acute injury and development of strategies to block post-angioplasty restenosis. Some of these strategies have relied upon the transfer of cytotoxic or cytostatic genes to inhibit the proliferation of smooth muscle cells at sites of balloon angioplasty (50-52). Adenoviral vectors have shown considerable utility for vascular gene transfer by virtue of the following properties: 1. There is a high rate of transfection, 100-fold greater than can be achieved with liposome/DNA complexes (53); 2. High titers of purified virus are achievable, on the order of 10^{11} infectious units/ml; 3. Adenovirus is highly amphitrophic, infecting a wide range of cell types including quiescent populations; 4. Expression from adenovirus is transient in the vessel wall, peaking within 7 days, remaining half-maximal at 14 days, and slowly declining to low levels at 28 days; 5. The danger of mutagenesis is low since the adenoviral genome does not integrate into the host chromosome but remains extra-chromosomal. However, enthusiasm for adenoviral vectors remains guarded mainly because adenovirus-infected cells have been shown to trigger a cellular immune response which leads to the destruction of the transfected cell. This appears to be a significant limit on the duration of therapeutic effects (54).

Recent observations on the Fas system in the vasculature indicate that ectopic or augmented expression of Fas ligand may have utility for treating this disorder. First, Fas ligand induces apoptosis in Fas-bearing vascular smooth muscle cells (28), while endothelial cells are refractive to Fas ligand overexpression (19). Thus, the local delivery of Fas ligand to sites of balloon injury is predicted to reduce smooth muscle cell number by inducing apoptotic cell death, while this treatment would not inhibit the beneficial process of re-endothelialization at this same site. Second, local delivery of Fas ligand should also kill inflammatory cells infiltrating these lesions since these cells express Fas.

We have shown that adenovirus mediated delivery of the *Fas ligand* gene functions as a potent inhibitor of neointima formation when introduced locally to balloon-injured rat carotid arteries (28), a well characterized model that produces a vascular smooth muscle cell-derived lesion. In this model, the endothelium is denuded and Adeno-Fas ligand is applied to the medial layer of smooth muscle cells. Analysis of histological sections revealed decreased VSMC density at early time points in vessels infected with Adeno-Fas ligand. However, by 14 days post-injury the Adeno-Fas ligand-treated vessels appear normal with regard to size and cellularity, but the extent of neointima formation was significantly reduced. Fas ligand expression was no longer detectable after 14 days, presumably because the Fas ligand expressing VSMCs of the medial layer have themselves undergone apoptosis by this time. Adeno-Fas ligand inhibited intimal hyperplasia at a dose of 1×10^6 infectious units per vessel, more than 3 orders of magnitude less than the dose required to produce systemic toxicity. The effective dose of Adeno-Fas ligand is much lower than other adenovirally-mediated anti-proliferative approaches that typically require substantial transgene overexpression (for examples, see (55,56)) where effective doses typically range from 1 to 2×10^9 infectious units per vessel. The potency of Adeno-Fas ligand probably results from the ability of Fas ligand to induce apoptosis in a paracrine manner, thereby limiting smooth muscle cell proliferation and lesion formation.

Though its ability to achieve high gene transfer efficiency makes adenovirus a promising vector for gene therapy, a major limitation is a T cell-mediated immune response to adenoviral antigens that induces the destruction of the infected cells (57). Thus, repeated administration of recombinant virus is associated with a robust immune response and low gene transfer efficiency. Furthermore, a large portion of the potential patient population has a developed immunity to multiple adenovirus serotypes prior to treatment, and there is concern that even a one time administration of adenovirus may induce vascular inflammation.

Since Fas ligand functions to minimize immune response in some tissues (11,12), ectopic Fas ligand expression was tested for its ability to inhibit cellular immune responses to adenovirus in the carotid arteries of rats immunized by an intravenous injection of an adenoviral construct that lacked a transgene (28). The vessels of the immunized rats demonstrated robust inflammatory responses when control adenoviral constructs were delivered locally, but inflammation was markedly suppressed when Adeno-Fas ligand was delivered to the vessel wall. These findings demonstrated that localized expression of Fas ligand can minimize inflammatory cell infiltration in a balloon-injured vessel. In effect, this experiment demonstrated that transfer of the *Fas ligand* gene to the smooth muscle of the denuded vessels confers a property normally confined to the endothelium, an ability to inhibit inflammatory cell infiltration of the vessel wall. Thus ectopic Fas ligand expression in balloon-injured vessels may be particularly advantageous for the treatment of restenosis.

IMPLICATION FOR ANGIOGENESIS

The status of endothelial Fas ligand expression may also influence the formation of blood vessels from preexisting vessels, a process referred to as angiogenesis. Angiogenesis can occur in the adult organism during ischemia, wound healing, retinopathy, rheumatoid disease or tumorigenesis (58,59). Inflammatory cells, including monocytes/macrophages (60) and T lymphocytes (61), have been shown to be associated with adult angiogenesis (62), where they adhere to and extravasate from growing collateral vessels at the time of maximal endothelial proliferation (60,63). Attached leukocytes release growth factors essential for angiogenesis including basic fibroblast growth factor (bFGF) (60) and vascular endothelial cell growth factor (VEGF) (61). Although TNFα paradoxically inhibits endothelial cell proliferation *in vitro* (64), TNFα is a potent angiogenic factor *in vivo* (64,65). Presumably the angiogenic effect of TNFα is mediated by its ability to augment leukocyte extravasation. Consistent with this hypothesis, treatment of injured animals with lypopolysaccharide (LPS), a strong inducer of TNFα production in macrophages, facilitates monocyte extravasation and angiogenesis in ischemic rabbit hindlimb (60). Since endothelial Fas ligand functions as a negative regulator of leukocyte extravasation, it is possible that Fas ligand also negatively regulates angiogenesis by limiting the number of leukocytes available to supply angiogenic growth factors. From this line of reasoning it also follows that the downregulation of endothelial Fas ligand expression by TNFα may facilitate angiogenesis by permitting leukocyte extravasation.

CONCLUSIONS

Leukocyte extravasation is important in the inflammatory response to pathogens and the development of inflammatory-fibroproliferative diseases of the vessel wall. Recently, functional Fas ligand expression was detected on the endothelial lining of blood vessels where it appears to function as a negative regulator of leukocyte extravasation. This function is accomplished by its ability to induce apoptosis in mononuclear cells attempting to invade the vessel wall in the absence of normal stimuli. Future studies focusing on the regulation and function of the Fas system in the vasculature should continue to provide insights regarding the pathogenesis of vascular disease and may lead to novel therapies to treat these disorders.

ACKNOWLEDGMENTS

This work was supported by NIH Grants AG15052, HL50692 and AR40197 to K.W.

REFERENCES

1. Nagata S, Golstein P. The Fas death factor. Science 1995;267:1449-56.
2. Boldin MP, Goncharov TM, Goltsev YV, Wallach D. Involvement of Mach, a novel MORT1/FADD-interacting protease, in FAS/Apo-1 and TNF receptor-induced cell death. Cell 1996;85:803-15.
3. Muzio M, Chinnaiyan AM, Kischkel FC, O'Rouke K, Schevchenko A, Ni J, Scaffidi CC, Bretz JD, Zhang M, Gentz R, Mann M, Krammer PH, Peter ME, Dixit VM. FLICE, a novel, FADD-homologous ICE/CED-3-like protease is recruited to the CD95 (Fas/APO-1) death-inducing signaling complex. Cell 1996;85:817-27.
4. Li H, Zhu H, Xu C-J, Yuan J. Cleavage of BID by caspase8 mediates the mitochondrial damage in the Fas pathway of apoptosis. Cell 1998;94:491-501.
5. Luo X, Budihardjo I, Zou H, Slaughter C, Wang X. Bid, a Bcl2 interacting protein, mediates cytochrome c release from mitochondria in response to activation of cell surface death receptors. Cell 1998;94:481-90.
6. Enari M, Sakahira H, Yokoyama H, Okawa K, Iwamatsu A, Nagata S. A caspase-activated DNase that degrades DNA during apoptosis, and its inhibitor ICAD. Nature 1998;391:43-50.
7. Irmler M, Thome M, Hahne M, Schneider P, Hofmann K, Steiner V, Bodmer J-L, Schroter M, Burns K, Mattmann C, Rimoldi D, French L, Tschopp J. Inhibition of death receptor signals by cellular FLIP Nature 1997;388:190-5.
8. Hu S, Vincenz C, Ni J, Gentz R, Dixit VM. I-FLICE, a novel inhibitor of tumor necrosis factor receptor-1 and CD-95-induced apoptosis J Biol Chem 1997;272:17255-7.
9. Srinivasula SM, Ahmad M, Otilie S, Bullrich F, Banks S, Fernandes-Alnemri T, Croce CM, Litwack G, Tomaselli KJ, Armstrong RC, Alnemri ES. FLAME-1, a novel FADD-like anti-apoptotic molecules that regulates Fas/TNFR1-induced apoptosis J Biol Chem 1997;272:18542-5.
10. Refaeli Y, Van Parijs L, London CA, Tschopp J, Abbas AK. Biochemical mechanisms of IL-2-regulated Fas-mediated T cell apoptosis Immunity 1998;8:615-23.
11. Griffith TS, Brunner T, Fletcher SM, Green DR, Ferguson TA. Fas ligand-induced apoptosis as a mechanism of immune privilege Science 1995;270:1189-92.
12. Bellgrau D, Gold D, Selawry H, Moore J, Franzusoff A, Duke RC. A role of CD95 ligand in preventing graft rejection Nature 1995;377:630-2.

13. Hahne M, Rimoldi D, Schröter M, Romero P, Schreier M, French LE, Schneider P, Bornand T, Fontana A, Lienard D, Cerottini J-C, Tschopp J. Melanoma cell expression of Fas (Apo-1/CD95) ligand: Implications for tumor immune escape. Science 1996;274:1363-6.

14. Strand S, Hofman WJ, Hug H, Müller M, Otto G, Strand D, Mariani SM, Stremmel W, Krammer PH, Galle PR. Lymphocyte apoptosis induced by CD95 (APO-1/Fas) ligand expressing tumor cells-A mechanism of immune evasion? Nature Med 1996;2:1361-6.

15. Niehans GA, Brunner T, Frizelle SP, Liston JC, Salerno CT, Knapp DJ, Green DR, Kratzke RA. Human lung carcinomas express Fas ligand Cancer Res 1997;57:1007-12.

16. Springer TA. Traffic signals on endothelium for lymphocyte recirculation and leukocyte emigration Ann Rev Physiol 1995;57:827-72.

17. Luscinskas FW, Gimbrone MAJ. Endothelial-dependent mechanism in chronic inflammatory leukocyte recruitment Ann Rev Med 1996;47:413-21.

18. Ross R. The pathogenesis of atherosclerosis: a perspective for the 1990s Nature 1993;362:801-9.

19. Sata M, Walsh K. TNFα Regulation of Fas ligand expression on the vascular endothelium modulates leukocyte extravasation Nature Med 1998;4:415-20.

20. Suda T, Takahashi T, Golstein P, Nagata S. Molecular cloning and expression of the Fas ligand, a novel member of the tumor necrosis factor family. Cell 1993;75:1169-78.

21. Suda T, Okazaki T, Naito Y, Yokota T, Arai N, Ozaki S, Nakao K, Nagata S. Expression of the Fas ligand in T cell lineage J Immunol 1995;154:3806-13.

22. Richardson BC, Lalwani ND, Johnson KJ, Marks RM. Fas ligation triggers apoptosis in macrophages but not endothelial cells. Eur J Immunol 1994;24:2640-5.

23. Rodriguez I, Matsuura K, Khatib K, Reed JC, Nagata S, Vassalli P. A bcl-2 transgene expressed in hepatocytes protects mice from fulminant liver destruction but not from rapid death induced by anti-Fas antibody injection J Exp Med 1996;183:1031-6.

24. Lacronique V, Mignon A, Fabre M, Viollet B, Rouquet N, Molina T, Porteu A, Henrion A, Bouscary D, Varlet P, Joulin V, Kahn A. Bcl-2 protects from lethal hepatic apoptosis induced by an anti-Fas antibody in mice. Nature Med 1996;2:80-6.

25. Itoh N, Tsujimoto Y, Nagata S. Effect of bcl-2 on Fas antigen-mediated cell death J Immunol 1993;151:621-7.

26. Strasser A, Harris AW, Huang DCS, Krammer PH, Cory S. Bcl-2 and Fas/APO-1 regulates distinct pathways to lymphocyte apoptosis EMBO J 1995;14:6136-47.

27. Sata M, Walsh K. Endothelial cell apoptosis induced by oxidized LDL is associated with the downregulation of the cellular caspase inhibitor FLIP. J Biol Chem 1998;In press.

28. Sata M, Perlman H, Muruve DA, Silver M, Ikebe M, Libermann TA, Oettgen P, Walsh K. Fas ligand gene transfer to the vessel wall inhibits neointima formation and overrides the adenovirus-mediated T cell response. Proc Natl Acad Sci USA 1998;95:1213-7.

29. Geng Y-J, Henderson LE, Levesque EB, Muszynzki M, Libby P. Fas is expressed in human atherosclerotic intima and promotes apoptosis of cytokine-primed human vascular smooth muscle cells. Arterioscler Thromb Vasc Biol 1997;17:2200-8.

30. Tanaka M, Itai T, Adachi M, Nagata S. Downregulation of Fas ligand by shedding. Nature Med 1998;4:31-6.

31. Suda T, Hashimoto H, Tanaka M, Ochi T, Nagata S. Membrane Fas ligand kills human peripheral blood T lymphocytes, and soluble Fas ligand blocks the killing. J Exp Med 1997;186:2045-50.

32. Wick G, Schett G, Amberger R, Kleindienst R, Xu Q. Is atherosclerosis an immunologically mediated disease? Immunol Today 1995;16:27-33.

33. Jonasson L, Holm J, Skalli O, Bondjers G, Hansson GK. Regional accumulations of T cells, macrophages, and smooth muscle cells in the human atherosclerotic plaque Arteriosclerosis 1986;6:131-8.

34. Munro JM, van der Walt JD, Munro CS, Chalmers JAC, Cox E. An immunohistochemical analysis of human aortic fatty streaks Hum Path 1987;18:375-80.

35. Emeson EE, Robertson AL. T lymphocytes in aortic and coronary intimas: their potential role in atherogenesis. Am J Pathol 1988;130:369-76.

36. van der Wal AC, Das PK, van de Berg DB, van der Loos CM, Becker AE. Atherosclerotic lesions in human: in situ immunophenotypic analysis suggesting an immune mediated response Lab Invest 1989;61:166-70.

37. Tanaka H, Swanson SJ, Sukhova G, Schoen FJ, Libby P. Smooth muscle cells of the coronary arterial tunica media express tumor necrosis factor-α and proliferate during acute rejection of rabbit cardiac allografts. Am J Pathol 1995;147:617-26.

38. Libby P, Hansson GK. Involvement of the immune system in human atherogenesis: Current knowledge and unanswered questions Lab Invest 1991;64:5-15.

39. Billingham ME. Cardiac transplant atherosclerosis Transplantation Proceedings 1987;19:19-25.

40. Ross R. Genetically modified mice as models of transplant atherosclerosis Nature Med 1996;2:527-8.

41. Clausell N, Milossi S, Sett S, Rabinovitch M. In vivo blockade of tumor necrosis factor-α in cholesterol-fed rabbits after cardiac transplant inhibits acute coronary artery neointimal formation. Circulation 1994;89:2768-79.

42. Hansson GK, Holm J, Jonasson L. Detection of activated T lymphocytes in the human atherosclerotic plaque Am J Pathol 1989;135:169-75.

43. Sata M, Walsh K. The Fas/Fas ligand pathway mediates vascular endothelial cell apoptosis induced by oxidized LDL J Clin Invest 1998;(in press).

44. McBride W, Lange RA, Hillis LD. Restenosis after successful coronary angioplasty: pathophysiology and prevention. N Engl J Med 1988;318:1734-7.

45. Nobuyoshi M, Kimura T, Nosaka H, Mioka S, Ueno K, Yokoi H, Hamasaki N, Hriuchi H, Ohishi H. Restenosis after successful percutaneous transluminal coronary angioplasty: serial angiographic follow-up of 229 patients. J Am Coll Cardiol 1988;12:616-23.

46. Moreno PR, Bernardi VB, Lopez-Cuellar J, Newell JB, McMellon C, Gold HK, Palacios IF, Fuster V, Fallon JT. Macrophage infiltration predicts restenosis after coronary intervention in patients with unstable angina Circulation 1996;94:3098-102.

47. Nobuyoshi M, Kimura T, Ohishi H, Horiuchi H, Nosaka H, Hamasaki N, Yokoi H, Kim K. Restenosis after percutaneous transluminal coronary angioplasty: pathologic observations in 20 patients. J Am Coll Cardiol 1991;17:433-9.

48. Kearney M, Pieczek A, Haley L, Losordo DW, Andrés V, Schainfeld R, Rosenfield K, Isner JM. Histopathology of in-stent restenosis in patients with peripheral artery disease. Circulation 1997;95:1998-2002.

49. Kornowski R, Hong MK, Tio FO, Bramwell O, Wu H, Leon MB. In-stent restenosis: contributions of intlammatory responses and arterial injury to neointimal hyperplasia J Am Coll Cardiol 1998;31:224-30.

50. Ohno T, Gordon D, San H, Pompili VJ, Imperiale MJ, Nabel GJ, Nabel EG. Gene therapy for vascular smooth muscle cell proliferation after arterial injury. Science 1994;265:781-4.

51. Guzman RJ, Hirschowitz EA, Brody SL, Crystal RG, Epstein SE, Finkel T. In vivo suppression of injury-induced vascular smooth muscle cell accumulation using adenovirus-mediated transfer of the herpes simplex virus thymidine kinase gene. Proc Natl Acad Sci USA 1994;91:10732-6.

52. Chang MW, Barr E, Seltzer J, Jiang Y, Nabel GJ, Nabel EG, Parmacek MS, Leiden JM. Cytostatic gene therapy for vascular proliferative disorders with a constitutively active form of the retinoblastoma gene product. Science 1995;267:518-22.

53. French BA, et al. Percutaneous transluminal in vivo gene transfer by recombinant adenovirus in normal porcine coronary arteries, atherosclerotic arteries, and two models of coronary restenosis. Circulation 1994;90:2402-13.

54. Dai Y, Schwarz EM, Gu D, Zhang W-W, Sarvetnick N, Verma IM. Cellular and humoral immune responses to adenoviral vectors containing factor IX gene: Tolerization of factor IX and vector antigens allows for long-term expression. Proc Natl Acad Sci USA 1995;92:1401-5.

55. Chang MW, Barr E, Lu MM, Barton K, Leiden JM. Adenovirus-mediated over-expression of the cyclin/cyclin-dependent kinase inhibitor, p21 inhibits vascular smooth muscle cell proliferation and neointima formation in the rat carotid artery model of balloon angioplasty. J Clin Invest 1995;96:2260-8.

56. Smith RC, Branellec D, Gorski DH, Guo K, Perlman H, Dedieu J-F, Pastore C, Mahfoudi A, Denèfle P, Isner JM, Walsh K. p21^{CIP1}-mediated inhibition of cell proliferation by overexpression of the *gax* homeodomain gene. Genes Dev 1997;11:1674-89.

57. Yang Y, Nunes FA, Berencsi K, Furth EE, Gönczöl E, Wilson JM. Cellular immunity to viral antigens limits E1-deleted adenoviruses for gene therapy. Proc Natl Acad Sci USA 1994;91:4407-11.

58. Risau W. Mechanisms of angiogenesis Nature 1997;386:671-4.

59. Folkman J. Clinical-applications of research on angiogenesis N Engl J Med 1995;333:1757-63.

60. Arras M, Ito WD, Scholz D, Winkler B, Schaper J, Schaper W. Monocyte activation in angiogenesis and collateral growth in the rabbit hindlimb J Clin Invest 1998;101:40-50.

61. Freeman MR, Schneck FX, Gagnon ML, Corless C, Soker S, Niknejad K, Peoples GE, Klagsbrun M. Peripheral blood T lymphcytes and lymphocytes infiltrating human cancers express vascular endothelial growth factor: a potential role for T cells in angiogenesis Cancer Res 1995;55:4140-5.

62. Polverini PJ, Cortran RA, Gimbrone MAJ, Unanue ER. Activated macrophages induce vascular proliferation Nature 1977;269:804-6.

63. Risau W. Angiogenesis is coming of age Circ Res 1998;82:926-8.

64. Frater-Schroder MW, Risau R, Hallmann P, Gautschi P, Bohlen P. Tumor necrosis factor type alpha, a potent inhibitor of endothelial cell growth in vitro, is angiogenic in vivo Proc Natl Acad Sci USA 1987;84:5277-81.

65. Rupia E, Montrucchio G, Battaglia E, Modena V, Camussi G. Role of tumor necrosis factor-alpha and platelet-activating factor in neoangiogenesis induced by synovial fluids of patients with rheumatoid arthritis Eur J Immunol 1996;26.:1690-4.

8 MOLECULAR MECHANISMS OF PLATELET ACTIVATION AND INHIBITION

A. Koneti Rao, M. D.
Temple university School of Medicine

PLATELET ROLE IN HEMOSTASIS AND THROMBOSIS

The basic mechanisms that operate in hemostasis and thrombosis are similar although the inciting processes and the consequences are different. Both encompass a complex sequence of interrelated events involving the vessel wall, platelets, and the coagulation system. Following injury to the blood vessel, platelets adhere to exposed subendothelium by a process (adhesion) which involves the interaction of a plasma protein, von Willebrand factor (vWF), and a specific protein on the platelet surface, glycoprotein Ib (GPIb). Adhesion is followed by recruitment of additional platelets which form clumps, a process called aggregation (cohesion). This platelet-platelet interaction involves binding of fibrinogen to specific platelet surface receptors - a complex comprised of glycoproteins IIb-IIIa (GPIIb-IIIa). In the resting state, platelets do not bind fibrinogen; platelet activation induces a conformational change in the GPIIb-IIIa complexes leading to fibrinogen binding and a sequence of events resulting in aggregation. Activated platelets release contents of their granules (secretion or release reaction), such as adenosine diphosphate (ADP) and serotonin from the dense granules, which cause recruitment of additional platelets. In addition, platelets play a major role in hemostasis and thrombosis by contributing to coagulation mechanisms; several key enzymatic reactions in blood coagulation occur on the platelet membrane lipoprotein surface. Thrombin generation and formation of a clot composed of blood cells and fibrin strands leads to restoration of hemostasis or thrombosis with its attendant sequalae. Thrombin not only induces fibrin formation but is also a potent platelet agonist. Conversion of plasminogen to plasmin by activators, including tissue plasminogen activator and urokinase, leads to endogenous lysis of the clot. Therapeutic agents have been developed that modulate several of the above mentioned aspects of the thrombotic process. These include agents or approaches that modify the risk factors contributing to the vascular process, antiplatelet agents, anticoagulants and thrombolytic agents. This review will focus on the mechanisms of platelet activation and on the approaches to inhibit platelets in the general context of vascular diseases.

Platelets are anucleate cells that are produced by shedding from megakaryocytes. Platelets have an active machinery for production and utilization of ATP but they do not have the ability to synthesize proteins. Platelets have at least 3 types of granules: α granules, dense granules and acid hydrolase containing vesicles. A number of physiological agonists interact with specific receptors on platelet surface to induce responses including a change in platelet shape from discoid to spherical (shape change), aggregation, secretion, and thromboxane A_2 formation. (Fig. 1). These agonists include ADP, epinephrine, thromboxane A_2,

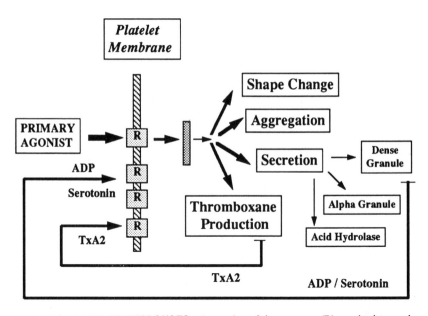

Fig 1. BASIC PLATELET RESPONSES. Interaction of the receptors (R) on platelet membrane with agonists results in several responses including shape change, aggregation, secretion and thromboxane A_2 formation. Substances released from dense granules (ADP, serotonin) and thromboxane A2 form positive feedback loops amplifying the activation process.

thrombin, platelet activating factor (PAF), collagen, vasopressin and serotonin, which vary in their relative abilities to induce various responses, their sources, and the mechanisms by which they cause different responses. Some, but not all agonists, can induce all of the responses. For example, thrombin is a strong agonist that induces all of the responses; ADP, epinephrine and PAF are weaker agonists that require thromboxane A_2 production to induce secretion. Receptors for several of these agonists share common features such as a heptahelical structure that traverses the plasma membrane and the intervention of G-proteins in mediating their effects. Thrombin induces effects in platelets that are both G-protein dependent and independent.

PLATELET ACTIVATION

Interaction of platelets with an agonist initiates the production or release of several intracellular messenger molecules including calcium ions, products of phosphoinositide hydrolysis (diacylglycerol and inositol 1,4,5-trisphosphate, $InsP_3$), thromboxane A_2 and cyclic nucleotides (cyclic adenosine monophosphate, cAMP) [1] (Fig 2)· These modulate the various discernible platelet responses of calcium mobilization, protein phosphorylation, aggregation, secretion, and the liberation of arachidonic acid. The interaction between the agonist receptors on the platelet surface and the key intracellular effector enzymes (e.g. phospholipase A_2, phospholipase C, adenylyl cyclase) are mediated by a group of GTP-binding proteins which are modulated by GTP [2]. These G-proteins function as molecular on-off switches in regulating the transduction of signals from the surface receptors to intracellular effectors and enzymes. Phosphoinositides constitute a small fraction of the total platelet membrane lipids and, on platelet stimulation, they are hydrolyzed by phospholipase C (PLC) to diacylglycerol and various inositol phosphates, including 1,4,5 $InsP_3$. Diacylglycerol is hydrolyzed by lipases to free arachidonic acid and glycerol, or is phosphorylated by a kinase to form phosphatidic acid, which then recycles to phosphatidylinositol. Platelet activation results in a rise in cytoplasmic ionized calcium concentration which is a combination of release of Ca^{2+} from intracellular stores and influx of external Ca^{2+}. $InsP_3$ functions as a messenger to mobilize Ca^{2+} from intracellular source, the dense tubular system in platelets [3]. Functional consequences of Ca^{2+} mobilization include phosphorylation of myosin light chain by a specific Ca^{2+} dependent kinase. This has been considered to play a role in shape change and secretion. Another Ca^{2+} dependent process in platelets is the release of arachidonic acid from phospholipids by the action of the Ca^{2+} dependent phospholipase A_2. The free arachidonic acid is converted by cyclooxygenase (COX) to prostaglandins G_2 and H_2, and subsequently by thromboxane synthetase to thromboxane A_2. In the presence of suitable phospholipids, diacylglycerol activates protein kinase C at basal intracellular Ca^{2+} levels and this results in the phosphorylation of a 47kD protein Pleckstrin. Protein kinase C activation is considered to play a major role in platelet secretion and in the expression of platelet surface fibrinogen binding sites (consisting of GP IIb-IIIa), which is a requisite for platelet aggregation [4, 5].

Although exposure of platelet to agents such as ADP and thrombin leads to activation of platelets, there are other agents that inhibit the platelet mechanisms. Prostacyclin (PGI_2) produced by the endothelium and PGD_2 produced by platelets stimulate adenylate cyclase to elevate platelet cyclic AMP levels. These agonists bind to specific receptors on platelets and mediate their responses via G-protein $G\alpha_s$. Elevated cAMP levels inhibit most platelet responses including

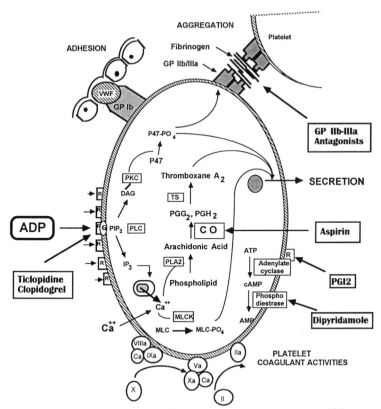

Fig 2. PLATELET ACTIVATION MECHANISMS AND ACTION OF PLATELET INHIBITORS:
cAMP = cyclic adenosine monophosphate; CO = cyclooxygenase;
DAG = diacylglycerol; G = GTP-binding protein; IP_3 = inositoltrisphosphate; MLC = myosin light chain; MLCK = myosine light chain kinase; PIP_2 = phosphatidylinositol bisphosphate; PKC = protein kinase C; PLC = phospholipase C; PLA_2 = phospholipase A_2; R = receptor; TS = thromboxane synthesis; vWD = von Willebrand Factor

phosphoinositide hydrolysis, Ca^{2+} mobilization, activation of GPIIb-IIIa, platelet aggregation and secretion. Nitric oxide inhibits platelet activation by increasing production of cyclic guanosine monophosphate (cGMP) by stimulating cytosolic guanylate cyclase. Moreover, responses to some of the stimulatory agonists, such as ADP, epinephrine, and thrombin, can be decreased by the phenomenon of receptor desensitization.

PLATELETS, INTEGRINS AND ADHESIVE PROTEINS

Fundamental to the platelet processes of adhesion and aggregation are the interactions between several glycoprotein receptors on the platelets and the multiple adhesive proteins that bind them in a relatively specific manner (Table 1). Several of the glycoprotein receptors belong to the integrin family consisting of heterodimeric molecules composed of a series of α and β subunits. The α and β subunits combine to constitute receptors that vary in their specificity to bind various ligands [6, 7] (Table 1). One integrin on platelets is the GPIIb-IIIa receptor which consists of α_{IIb} and β_3 chains and binds to fibrinogen and other adhesive ligands including , vWF, fibronectin, and vitronectin. The specific amino acid sequence that mediates the binding of these adhesive proteins to GPIIb-IIIa consists of the tripeptide Arg-Gly-Asp (RGD). Fibrinogen contains two RGD sequences in the Aα chain. There is evidence that interaction of fibrinogen with GPIIb-IIIa is also mediated by another sequence (Lys-Gln-Ala-Gly-Asp-Val) located at the carboxyl terminal of the γ chain of fibrinogen [8, 9] and that this sequence may be the predominant site for the binding of fibrinogen to GPIIb-IIIa receptors [10, 11]. The interaction of GPIIb-IIIa with vWF, fibronectin and vitronectin is also mediated by the RGD recognition sequence. Another platelet integrin is the vitronectin receptor consisting of $\alpha_v\beta_3$ which binds vitronectin, fibrinogen, fibronectin and vWF. In addition to the integrins, platelets possess non-integrin receptors; a major one is the receptor for vWF consisting of GPIb, GPIX and GPV. From a pharmacological perspective, peptides containing the RGD sequence are potent inhibitors of platelet integrin-fibrinogen interaction and thereby inhibit aggregation.

Table 1: Platelet-Membrane Glycoprotein Receptors

Receptor	Ligand	Receptor Mediated Action	Surface Copies/ Platelet
Integrins			
$\alpha_{IIb}\beta_3$ (glyco-protein IIb/IIIa)	Fibrinogen Fibronectin von Willebrand Factor Vitronectin	Aggregation	40,000-80,000
$\alpha_v\beta_3$	Vitronectin Fibrinogen Fibronectin von Willebrand Factor	Adhesion	500
$\alpha_2\beta_\square$ (glyco-protein Ia/IIa)	Collagen	Adhesion	1000
$\alpha_5\beta_1$ (glyco-protein Ic/IIa)	Fibronectin	Adhesion	1000
$\alpha_6\beta_1$	Laminin	Adhesion	1000
Non Integrins			
Glycoprotein Ib	von Willebrand Factor	Adhesion	20,000-30,000
Glycoprotein IV	Thrombospondin Collagen	Adhesion	25,000
Glycoprotein VI	Collagen	Adhesion	Unknown

INTERACTION OF PLATELETS WITH VESSEL WALL: ADHESION

Circulating platelets do not adhere to the normal endothelium; and this is related to a number of mechanisms including the endothelial production of inhibitory substances PGI_2 and nitric oxide. These compounds inhibit platelets by elevating intracellular levels of cAMP and cGMP, respectively. Endothelium has mechanisms that limit the activation process by modulating production or destruction of agonists. For example, endothelium possesses a protein thrombomodulin which induces the activation of protein C by thrombin; the activated protein C rapidly degrades activated factors V and VIII thereby limiting further thrombin generation. Heparan sulfate and other sulfated mucopolysaccharides on the endothelial surface inhibit thrombin by enhancing the interaction with its inhibitor antithrombin. Endothelial cells possess surface ADPase which degrades ADP. These mechanisms that limit platelet activation are altered in the diseased endothelium which becomes thrombogenic as a result of diverse processes such as atherosclerosis, viral injury, and hyperhomocysteinemia.

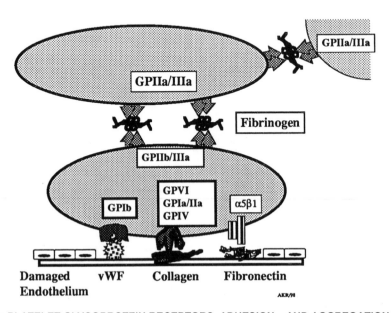

Fig 3: PLATELET GLYCOPROTEIN RECEPTORS, ADHESION , AND AGGREGATION

Injury to the endothelial barrier results in the exposure of a large number of matrix components that can directly or indirectly and readily bind platelets (Fig 3). These include different types of collagen (particularly types I, III, VI), vWF, laminins, fibronectin, and thrombospondin. The simultaneous availability of circulating plasma proteins such as vWF and fibrinogen adds to the interactions between platelets and the injured vessel wall.

vWF is present in plasma, platelet α-granules and endothelial cells, and in the subendothelium. Under appropriate stimuli both endothelial cells and platelets release vWF. Thus, at the site of platelet-vessel wall interaction the local vWF levels are elevated and consistent with a major role of vWF in platelet adhesion. vWF is a large multimeric protein that circulates in plasma bound to coagulation factor VIII and, therefore, serves to enhance local thrombin generation by virtue of transporting factor VIII. vWF binds to platelets and this is mediated by two specific receptors, GPIb and GPIIb-IIIa. In addition, vWF binds rapidly and tightly to collagen, as do platelets to collagen directly, mediated by as yet not fully delineated collagen receptors (GPIa/IIa, GPVI, GPIV). Although vWF binds to both platelet GPIb and GPIIb-IIIa receptors, it is the GPIb-vWF interaction that plays a major initial role in platelet adhesion in blood vessels with high velocity blood flow and shear rate. At high shear rates, platelets adhere to the subendothelium through the interaction of vWF with GP-Ib receptors, and this interaction is stabilized by subsequent intervention of GPIIb-IIIa-vWF binding. The binding of vWF to GP-Ib is mediated by the A1 domain of vWF; vWF binds to GPIIb-IIIa by the interaction of the RGDS sequence in its C1 domain.

PLATELET-PLATELET INTERACTION: AGGREGATION

The major mediator of platelet-platelet interaction (aggregation) is the integrin GPIIb-IIIa, a heterodimer consisting of two subunits. Platelets have ~ 40,000 - 80,000 copies of this complex on their surface, and they constitute the major binding site on platelets for fibrinogen (Fig 3). Additional GPIIb-IIIa binding sites also become available as a result of surface expression of the intracellular granule pools. In the resting state platelets do not bind fibrinogen. On platelet activation, the GPIIb-IIIa complex undergoes a conformational change leading to an enhanced affinity for the binding of fibrinogen; this is a prerequisite for aggregation. (Fig 4). Although vWF also binds to GPIIb-IIIa, also mediated by the RGD sequence, the major ligand for platelet aggregation is fibrinogen. Activation of GPIIb-IIIa complex on the platelet surface is modulated by intracellular signaling events that occur following agonist activation of platelets (inside-out signaling). In addition, there is evidence that binding of fibrinogen to the GPIIb-IIIa complex results in additional signaling events (such as activation of tyrosine kinases Syk, Src, FAK) that have been referred to as "outside-in" signaling.

Platelet aggregation is, thus, a major mechanism in thrombus formation. Antibodies directed against the GPIIb-IIIa complex, and RGD peptides and peptidomimetics, inhibit platelet aggregation and constitute an important strategy to inhibit platelets. These compounds inhibit not only fibrinogen binding but also of vWF to GPIIb-IIIa complex; many inhibit binding of ligands to the vitronectin receptor (integrin $\alpha_v\beta3$).

ROLE OF PLATELETS IN BLOOD COAGULATION

A major role of platelets in hemostasis is their contribution to several of the key enzymatic events of the coagulation cascade which occur on the platelet membrane

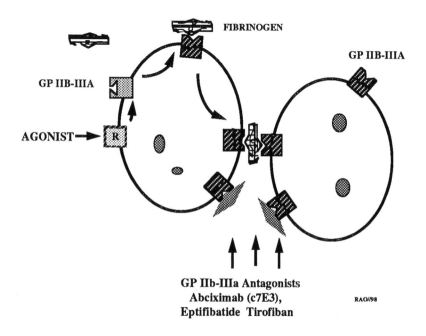

Fig 4. ACTIVATION AND INHIBITION OF PLATELET GPIIB-IIIA COMPLEX. GPIIb-IIIa complexes on resting platelets do not bind fibrinogen. Platelet activation results in intracellular signaling events leading to a conformational change in the GPIIb-IIIa complex and fibrinogen binding which is aprerequisite for aggregation. GPIIb-IIIa antagonists bind GPIIb-IIIa complex and inhibit aggregation.

surface [12]. This role of platelets has been referred to as the platelet procoagulant activity. Platelet α-granules are endowed with several coagulation factors, and platelets promote blood coagulation by various mechanisms including exposure of specific binding sites for the coagulation proteins, providing the surface for assembly of the involved coagulation proteins thereby inducing a profound acceleration of the enzymatic reactions, and by protecting the coagulation enzymes from inactivation by naturally occurring inhibitors [12]. They play a remarkable role in specific coagulation steps such as in activation of prothrombin and factor X. For example, activated platelets express activated factor V (Va) on their surface which serves as a binding site for factor Xa; thus, platelets participate in the conversion of prothrombin to thrombin (Fig 1).

The platelet role in blood coagulation is attributed to exposure of an anionic phospholipid (phosphatidylserine) on platelet surface following activation. In resting platelets, this phospholipid is located in the inner leaflet of the lipid bilayer of the plasma membrane. On platelet activation there is increased surface expression of phosphatidylserine with a concomitant inward redistribution of the neutral phospholipids present in the outer leaflet of the resting membranes. This process of "scrambling" of platelet phospholipids requires agonist-induced calcium influx and results in the exposure of docking sites on the membrane for various coagulation factors. In addition, there is budding off from the platelet membrane of small microparticles which also have the capability to support coagulation reactions on their surface. The asymmetry of platelet phospholipids in the resting state is maintained by the activity of an enzyme (aminophospholipid translocase, *scramblase*) which is inhibited by activation-induced influx of calcium leading to the reorientation of phosphatidylserine. A selective defect in the platelet procoagulant activity is associated in a bleeding diathesis (Scott Syndrome) [13].

A major recent finding is the report [14] for a role of the GPIIb-IIIa complex in blood coagulation. These studies indicate that prothrombin binds to the platelet GPIIb-IIIa complex and that this interaction accelerates prothrombin activation to thrombin. Moreover, the interaction of prothrombin with GPIIb-IIIa is inhibited by monoclonal antibodies to GPIIb-IIIa, and by fibrinogen and RGD peptides. These mechanisms provide a cogent explanation for the diminished tissue-factor stimulated thrombin generation in the presence of platelets exposed to GPIIb-IIIa antagonists [15].

MECHANISMS OF PLATELET INHIBITION

Because of the important role of platelets in the acute events of vascular diseases, antiplatelet therapy is an important strategy in the overall antithrombotic armamentarium. Reviewed here are the mechanisms by which various antiplatelet agents (Table 2) function in this role. For each drug selected clinical studies are cited. No attempt is made to cover all of the large number of clinical trials performed with various agents

ANTIPLATELET AGENTS

Aspirin (Acetylsalicylic Acid) at One Hundred Years. August 10, 1997, marked the centenary of aspirin (acetylsalicylic acid) which has been hailed as the first, and most commercially successful synthetic drug the world has seen [16]. It was registered by Bayer AG in 1899 under the name "Aspirin" with 'a' coming from acetyl and 'spir' from the first part of *Spirea ulmania*, the plant from which salicylic acid was first isolated. In the USA, about 35,000 kg of aspirin is consumed daily [16]. Its usage and sales still continue to increase with newer beneficial effects being recorded.

Table 2	Platelet Inhibiting Drugs

Aspirin
Dipyridamole
Sulfinpyrazone
Ticlopidine
Clopidogrel
GPIIb/IIIa Antagonists*
      Abciximab (c7E3 Fab)
      Epitifibatide
      Tirofiban
Other Agents:
      Thromboxane A_2 Receptor Antagonists
      Thromboxane Synthetase Inhibitors
      Prostacyclin Analogs
      Nitric Oxide Donors
      Phosphodiesterase III Inhibitors (Cilostazol)
      Serotonin Antagonists (Keranserin)

*Includes selected drugs in this group

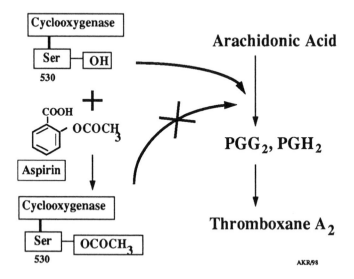

Fig 5. MECHANISM OF ACTION OF ASPIRIN. Aspirin irreversibly acelytates Ser 530 of the cyclooxygenase and inhibits its ability to catalyze the conversion of arachidonic acid to prostaglandin G_2.

The primary mechanism by which aspirin acts as an antithrombotic agent is its effect on platelet cyclooxygenase (COX) (also referred to as prostaglandin H synthase, PGHS), which catalyzes the conversion of arachidonic acid to PGG_2 and subsequently of PGG_2 to PGH_2 (Fig 2). This enzyme exists in two forms: COX-1 which is constitutively expressed in several tissues, and COX-2 which is present in low levels but can be induced rapidly by thrombin, cytokines, and growth factors in endothelial cells, monocytes and other cells [17]. Shear stress also induces COX-2 activity in endothelial cells. Platelets possess only COX-1. Aspirin irreversibly acetylates the COX and inhibits the formation of PGG_2 and PGH_2 which in platelets are converted to thromboxane A_2 by thromboxane synthase and in endothelial cells to PGI_2 by prostacyclin synthase (Fig 5).

The molecular mechanisms by which aspirin influences the catalytic action of COX have been delineated based on crystal structure of the enzyme [17, 18]. The carboxylic moiety of salicylic acid interacts reversibly with Arg residue 120 of COX and irreversibly acetylates an hydroxyl group on a serine residue in position 530. This acetylation prevents the catalytic action of COX by sterically interfering with the binding of arachidonic acid. The net result of this irreversible effect is inhibition of thromboxane A_2 production by the platelet for its entire life span because platelets, unlike endothelial cells, lack protein synthetic ability to replenish the COX stores. Moreover, the effect of aspirin on the two isozymes (COX-1 and COX-2) are not identical with a greater effect on COX-1. Because of its irreversible effect, chronic administration of even low dose aspirin have a cumulative effect on platelets leading to a very striking inhibitory effect on thromboxane A_2 production over a period of several days. In addition to the effect on COX, aspirin has been reported to have other effects [19] including acetylation of plasma proteins, especially fibrinogen with impairment in its role in platelet aggregation, and the platelet membrane proteins with an inhibitory effect on thrombin generation [20].

Pharmacokinetics. Aspirin is absorbed rapidly from the stomach and the small intestine. Peak plasma levels of aspirin occur 15-20 min after ingestion and the levels decay with half-life of 15-20 min. The major effect of aspirin on platelets occurs in the presystemic circulation [21]. In plasma the ester is hydrolyzed to salicylate which has a dose-dependent half-life ranging from 2-12 hours. It is also hydrolyzed to salicylate in the liver, lungs, and erythrocytes and excreted mainly by the kidneys.

Platelets are exquisitely sensitive to aspirin: a single 100 mg dose reduces thromboxane A_2 production in serum by 98% by 1 hour; 30 mg/day daily effectively eliminate thromboxane A_2 production. After a single oral dose of aspirin, the recovery of COX activity occurs after a lag of 48 hours which has been interpreted as evidence for an effect on megakaryocyte COX. Aspirin effect on platelets is demonstrable by an effect on platelet aggregation response ex vivo; aggregation responses in vitro to agonists such as ADP, epinephrine and PAF are decreased with a loss of the second-wave of aggregation. There is also an inhibition of dense granule secretion. In response to low dose, but not high doses of collagen or thrombin, these responses are decreased. The bleeding time is prolonged in normal subjects following repeated daily administration of aspirin as low as 20-80 mg. From the perspective of a clinical benefit, patients with a wide range of vascular   diseases   benefit   from   doses   for   long   term   therapy

Table 3 - Minimum Aspirin Dose That Has Been Shown to be Effective	
Disorder	Minimum Effective Daily Dose, mg
Stable Angina	75
Unstable angina	75
Acute myocardial infarction	160
Transient cerebral ischemia and incomplete stroke	75

as small as 75-160 mg (Table 3) and the antithrombotic effect appears not to be dose-related (Table 4) [22]. There has been considerable discussion regarding the relative impact of aspirin on platelet versus endothelial COX. In theory, an ideal antithrombotic effect would be characterized by a selective inhibition of platelet COX without impairment of the endothelial PGI_2 production which is mediated by both COX-1 and the inducible COX-2. Although it has been considered that lower aspirin doses may have limited effect on endothelial PGI_2 production, results from the clinical studies have not established this otherwise elegant concept.

Table 4 - Comparison of Aspirin Dosages Affecting Vascular Events in High-risk Trials*			
Dose (mg/day)	No of Trials	No of Patients	Odds Reduction %
Aspirin (500-1000) 30	18,471	21±4	
Aspirin (160-325) 12	23,670	28±3	
Aspirin (75) 4	5,012	29±7	
* Data from Antiplatelet Trialists' Collaboration, Reference 23			

Clinical Trials of Aspirin.
Primary Prevention of Myocardial Infarction. Aspirin has beneficial effects in the primary and secondary prevention of myocardial infarction (MI) and in the prevention of stroke [22, 23]. There have been 4 large studies of aspirin on the primary prevention of MI [24-27]. The Physicians' Health Study [24] was a double blind, placebo controlled, randomized trial involving 22,071 male U.S. physicians, age 40-80 years, who were randomly allocated to low dose aspirin (325 mg every other day) or placebo, plus beta carotene (50 mg every other day) or placebo, according to a 2 x 2 factorial design. With a follow up of 60 months, the results showed no reduction in the total cardiovascular mortality in the aspirin group, but there was striking reduction in the rates of MI with aspirin (risk reduction 44%, p < 0.00001). A statistically significant reduction was noted in fatal and nonfatal

infarction. The combined outcome of important vascular events (nonfatal MI, nonfatal stroke, and death from cardiovascular causes) was significantly reduced in aspirin group (risk reduction 18%, p = 0.01). The reduction in MI was noted only among those over the age of 50 years. The overall stroke rate was higher on aspirin (relative risk 1.22, not significant) with an increased risk of hemorrhagic stroke (relative risk 2.14, p = 0.06). The second trial, the British Doctors' Study [25] was an open, randomly allocated trial of aspirin 500 mg daily versus aspirin avoidance, involving 5139 apparently healthy male physicians followed for up to 6 years. There was no significant difference in the incidence of MI or stroke. However, there were considerably more disabling strokes in the aspirin group (relative risk 2.58, p < 0.05). The third study [26] was a large prospective cohort study in 87,678 U.S. registered nurses, aged 34-65 years, free of diagnosed coronary artery disease, stroke and cancer at baseline, who were followed for 6 years. Regular aspirin usage was documented at intervals. Among women taking one to six aspirin per week, the age adjusted relative risk of first MI was 0.68 (p = 0.005). This benefit was confined to women age 50 years or older. In those who took 7 or more aspirin per week there was no benefit. In the recently reported Thrombosis Prevention Trial [27] involving 5499 men aged 45-69 years at high risk of ischemic heart disease, aspirin 75 mg daily reduced the incidence of acute events with a 32% reduction in non-fatal MI. Based on the above trials it has been recommended [28] that aspirin be considered for primary prevention in individuals older than 50 years who have at least one additional major risk factor for coronary artery disease. The overall enthusiasm for aspirin for primary prevention has been tempered by the small increase in bleeding related strokes and by gastrointestinal hemorrhage.

Chronic Stable Angina and Unstable Angina. In the Physicians' Health Study [29] a subset of 333 patients had chronic stable angina. In these patients aspirin reduced the incidence of first MI by 87% (p < 0.001). Four randomized, double-blind, placebo-controlled trials, [28] showed that aspirin reduces the incidence of MI and death from cardiac causes by 50-70% in patients with unstable angina.

Acute Myocardial Infarction. Aspirin is efficacious in patients with acute MI when used alone or with thrombolytic therapy. In the ISIS-II trial [30], involving 17,187 patients with acute MI, aspirin (160 mg daily for one month) reduced the incidence of nonfatal re-infarction by 44% and fatal events by 21%. The mortality at 5 weeks were 13.2% with placebo, 9.4% with aspirin, 9.2% with streptokinase and 8.0% with streptokinase and aspirin, indicating that aspirin further reduced the mortality over that observed with streptokinase alone. The impact of aspirin alone in this trial was comparable to that of streptokinase alone.

Secondary Prevention of MI. Multiple trials have been conducted and no single study showed a significant reduction in mortality with aspirin use. However, meta-analysis by Antiplatelet Trialists' Collaboration [23] of 145 randomized trials of prolonged antiplatelet therapy (predominantly aspirin) showed that among high risk patients with primarily occlusive vascular disease antiplatelet therapy reduced vascular mortality (odds reduction, 18% ; < 0.00001), non-fatal MI (odds reduction, 35%, p <0.00001), non-fatal stroke (odds reduction, 31%, p < 0.00001) and vascular events, (odds reduction, 17%, p < 0.0001).

Coronary Angioplasty and Coronary Bypass Grafting. In patients undergoing angioplasty the two main issues revolve around early abrupt closure and delayed restenosis. Randomized placebo-controlled trials [28] showed that aspirin (650-990 mg daily) and dipyridamole (225 mg daily) begun at least 24 hours before angioplasty reduced the incidence of abrupt closure. Aspirin does not reduce the incidence of restenosis. A number of trials have shown that aspirin alone or combined with dipyridamole reduced the incidence of graft thrombosis in patients with saphenous-vein grafts after bypass surgery when begun 1 day before surgery, on the day of surgery, or the day after surgery [31]. Therapy must be started pre-operatively or within 48 hours after surgery. Dipyridamole does not add to the benefits from aspirin alone in the prevention of saphenous vein graft occlusion.

Cerebrovascular Disease. Several studies have established the beneficial effect of aspirin and other antiplatelet agents in reducing stroke and death in patients with stroke or transient ischemic attacks. In the meta-analysis published by the Antiplatelet Trialists' Collaboration [23], prolonged antiplatelet therapy resulted in a 22% reduction in vascular events in patients presenting with completed stroke or transient ischemic attack. This reduction was similar for patients presenting with a completed stroke (23%, p<0.001) and for those presenting with only a transient ischemic attack (22%, p < 0.001). Some earlier studies showed a lack of benefit or lesser-benefit from aspirin in women, but the Antiplatelet Trialists' meta-analysis including more recent trials does not support a gender effect [23]. Although a dose of 75 mg/day has been shown to be effective in the Swedish Aspirin Low-Dose Trial (SALT) [32] the optimum aspirin dose in patients with cerebrovascular diseases remains controversial [33].

Sulfinpyrazone. Sulfinpyrazone is a competitive cyclooxygenase inhibitor and weaker in its effect than aspirin. It normalizes shortened platelet survival in patients with prosthetic heart valves and its benefits appear to be more marked on prosthetic rather than natural surfaces. Although there are two trials [34-36] indicating benefit of sulfinpyrazone in patients with MI, the findings have been controversial [37] and there are no clear cut advantages of this drug over aspirin.

Dipyridamole. Dipyridamole acts as an antiplatelet agent by raising the platelet cyclic AMP which inhibits platelet responses. There is little good evidence that dipyridamole is an effective antithrombotic agent when used alone [38]. It prolongs the survival of platelets in patients with prosthetic valves [39], and in combination with warfarin is more effective than warfarin alone in preventing systemic embolism in prosthetic valves [40]. In most other situations the benefit of added dipyridamole over that of aspirin alone has not been shown convincingly [38].

Ticlopidine and Clopidogrel. ADP plays an important role in platelet function. It causes platelets to change shape from disk to spheres, activates the GPIIb-IIIa complex, and induces aggregation and secretion. ADP is present in platelet dense granules and is secreted on platelet activation; the released ADP further amplifies the activation process [Fig 2]. In addition, in vitro ADP inhibits the elevated cAMP levels induced by platelet inhibiting agents such as PGI_2. These responses are mediated by specific ADP receptors on platelets and current evidence indicates that platelets possess at least three types of ADP receptors [41] which mediate distinct responses. Ticlopidine and the newer analog clopidogrel inhibit platelet function by inhibiting the binding of ADP to platelet receptors, particularly those involved in the inhibition of adenylate cyclase [42]. However, our understanding of the specific ADP receptors involved is incomplete. Both drugs inhibit ADP-induced platelet aggregation, but not shape change, or thromboxane A_2 synthesis. They inhibit aggregation induced by collagen and thrombin but these inhibitory effects are agonist-concentration dependent; high concentrations of collagen and thrombin over-ride the inhibition. The inhibitory effect on collagen and thrombin induced aggregation reflect the potentiating effect of ADP released from the dense granules on the response to other agonists.

Ticlopidine and clopidogrel are thienopyridine derivatives and differ from each other by the addition of a carboxymethyl side group in clopidogrel. Neither of these agents inhibits platelet aggregation in vitro indicating in vivo conversion to as yet unidentified active metabolites in the liver. These metabolites are excreted primarily by the kidneys. Both drugs are rapidly absorbed by oral route but the maximal platelet inhibitory effect is delayed by several days. Maximal inhibition following recommended doses of ticlopidine (500 mg/day) or clopidogrel (75 mg/day) is noted at 4-7 days of therapy although inhibition of platelet aggregation is demonstrable at 2 to 3 days. Once discontinued, the inhibitory effect of ticlopidine persists for 7-10 days. Both these agents prolong the bleeding time with a maximal effect after 5-6 days of administration.

Ticlopidine. Ticlopidine has been established as an effective antiplatelet agent in a number of arterial diseases. In the double-blind Canadian American Ticlopidine Study (CATS), ticlopidine (250 mg twice daily) reduced the combined end-point of stroke, myocardial infarction, or vascular death in patients with recent thromboembolic stroke by 23.3% at 2 years of follow up [43]. In the subsequent Ticlopidine Aspirin Stroke Study (TASS) [44] comparing ticlopidine, 250 mg twice daily, with aspirin, 625 mg twice daily, the ticlopidine group had a 12% reduction in the primary end point of non-fatal stroke or death compared to aspirin (17% compared to 19%, p=0.048). There was a significant reduction in all strokes (10% versus 13%, p=0.024) as well as recurrent transient ischemic attacks (30% versus 43%; p = 0.007) [45]. More recently, ticlopidine was found to be superior to a nonsteroidal anti-inflammatory agent indobufen in reducing the primary end point of death, stroke or myocardial infarction in patients with recent transient ischemic attack, amaurosis fugax, or minor strokes (2.9% with ticlopidine versus 5.8% with indobufen; p=0.004) [46]. Ticlopidine has a number of side effects, particularly neutropenia, and these have limited its use which is currently FDA approved for treatment of patients with cerebrovascular disease who cannot tolerate or fail on aspirin therapy.

Ticlopidine has been studied in the context of unstable angina [47]. Patients were randomized to receive conventional therapy (β-blockers, calcium channel blockers, nitrates but no aspirin) alone or in combination with ticlopidine (250 mg twice daily). At 6 months follow up, ticlopidine decreased the combined end point of vascular death and non-fatal MI by 46% (7.3% compared with 13.6%, p=0.009). More recently, several studies have assessed the role of ticlopidine in the prevention of coronary artery stent thrombosis and have reported impressive results.

Thrombosis and excessive hemorrhage related to vigorous anithrombotic regiments have been two problems encountered with cardiac stents. Following impressive results in initial non-randomized trials, two randomized trials have defined the optimum regimens associated with antithrombotic efficacy as well as low incidence of bleeding. In the Intracoronary Stenting and Antithrombotic Regimen (ISAR) trial [48] 517 patients were randomized after successful stent placement to receive antiplatelet therapy (aspirin 100 mg twice daily, and ticlopidine 250 mg twice daily for four weeks) or anticoagulant therapy (initial intravenous heparin for 5-10 days; phenprocoumon and aspirin 100 mg twice daily for 4 weeks). The primary cardiac endpoint was a composite measuring death from cardiac causes or the occurrence of MI, coronary bypass surgery or repeated angioplasty. At 30 days, the primary end point was reached in 1.6% of patients in antiplatelet therapy group compared to 6.2% in the anticoagulant group (p<0.001). The incidence of stent thrombosis was also strikingly lower in the antiplatelet therapy group. Moreover, the superiority of the antiplatelet therapy group on the cardiac end points persisted at 6 and 12 months [49].

In a second randomized trial (The Stent Antithrombotic Regimen Study, STARS) [50], 1653 patients were randomly assigned to receive aspirin 325 mg once daily, plus warfarin (INR 2.0-2.5); aspirin plus ticlopidine, 250 mg twice daily; or aspirin alone for 1 month. The combined end point of death, Q-wave MI, emergency surgery, target vessel revascularization, and angiographic thrombosis was reduced by 80% at 30 days in the ticlopidine-aspirin group (0.5%) compared with aspirin plus warfarin group (2.7%, p=0.007) and the aspirin alone group (3.6, p<0.001). Based on these studies, the role of ticlopidine in patients undergoing stent placement is well established. Several other trials have examined the use of ticlopidine in relation to stents and in maintaining patency of saphenous vein grafts and these are reviewed elsewhere [51]. Two trials have examined the effect of ticlopidine in patients with peripheral arterial disease with beneficial effects on vascular events [52, 53]

Clopidogrel. Acute myocardial infarction, cerebrovascular disease and peripheral arterial disease all represent different facets of the common underlying atherosclerotic process. While the majority of studies of antiplatelet agents have focused separately on patients with the above vascular disorders, the CAPRIE trial (Clopidogrel vs. Aspirin in Patients at Risk for Ischemic Events) [54] studied patients with symptomatic atherosclerosis including patients with recent ischemic stroke (within one week to six months), myocardial infarction (within 35 days) or documented peripheral arterial disease. 19,000 patients were randomly assigned to receive either clopidogrel 75 mg once daily, or aspirin, 325 mg once daily. There was an 8.7% reduction in the primary end point of ischemic stroke, myocardial infarction or vascular death in the clopidogrel group (5.32% compared with 5.83%; p=0.03). Subgroup analysis showed that there was a greater benefit in patients with peripheral arterial disease and that patients with myocardial infarction group had an increase in events which was not significant (5.03% per year compared with 4.84%; p>0.2). However, in a secondary post-hoc analysis including all patients with previous myocardial infarction (even though they were entered into the trial on the basis of either stroke or peripheral arterial disease) clopidogrel was associated with a 7.4% decrease in the combined end point. Further analysis of the data also showed that clopidogrel had a greater benefit in preventing MI than stroke or vascular death [55]. Clopidogrel has been recently approved by the FDA for the secondary prevention for vascular events in patients with symptomatic atherosclerosis.

As indicated earlier, clopidogrel functions as an antiplatelet agent by virtue of inhibiting the interaction of ADP with platelets. It does not have an impact on thromboxane production in platelets. Thus a cogent rationale can be presented for evaluating the effect of combination of clopidogrel and aspirin, which both function by separate mechanisms. In future studies, the efficacy of such a combination needs to be compared with the individual agents.

Side Effects of Ticlopidine and Clopidogrel. Aside from the potential side effects of bleeding due to platelet inhibition, Ticlopidine has a number of side effects including diarrhea, dyspepsia, nausea, skin rash and neutropenia [51]. In the TASS Study [44] neutropenia (<1200 cells/mm^3) was observed in 2.4% of patients; severe neutropenia (<450 cells/mm^3) occurred in 0.9%. However, in the trials of patients undergoing coronary stenting [48, 50-51] the neutropenia has been observed less frequently, possibly due to the shorter duration of therapy. Because of this potential side effect, patients on ticlopidine therapy have required monitoring of blood counts, particularly in the initial months of therapy. Clopidigrel appears not to be associated with this troublesome neutropenia [54]. Ticlopidine has also been associated with an increase in cholesterol levels [44], not noted with clopidogrel [54].

Attention has been recently focused on the association of ticlopidine with thrombotic thrombocytopenia purpura (TTP) [56], a serious complication characterized by thrombocytopenia, angiopathic hemolytic anemia, neurologic manifestations and renal failure. In a review of 60 such cases of TTP [56] 80% of patients had been on the drug for less than a month; 12 patients had received ticlopidine for 3 weeks or less after placement of cardiac stents. The frequency of TTP associated with cardiac stents has been estimated to be 1 in 1600 patients [57]. Given the structural similarity between ticlopidine and clopidogrel, there is a need for awareness regarding this potential life-threatening complication with the use of either drug.

Glycoprotein IIB-IIIA Antagonists. In the pathogenesis of thrombus formation on a ruptured atherosclerotic plaque, adhesion of an initial layer of platelets (mediated predominantly by GPIb and vWF) is followed by accretion of platelets by aggregation (platelet-platelet interaction) mediated largely by GPIIb-IIIa and its ligand fibrinogen (Fig 3). Thus, interruption of the platelet-platelet interaction is a powerful antithrombotic strategy in occlusive vascular disease. A second important rationale for the development of GPIIb-IIIa antagonists hinges on the role of GPIIb-IIIa-fibrinogen interaction as the final common pathway leading to aggregation in response almost all agonists including thrombin, collagen, ADP and thromboxane A_2. To this end, inhibition of aggregation has been accomplished by blocking the GPIIb-IIIa receptor with monoclonal antibodies and with peptide or peptidomimetics based on the RGD recognition sequence [58, 59] (Fig 4).

In the quest to develop GPIIb-IIIa antagonists based on the RGD sequence, studies in snake venoms have played a major role [60, 61]. Numerous products from snake venoms with activity against GPIIb-IIIa receptor have been isolated and studied; the first of these being Trigramin, isolated from the venom of viper *Trimeresurus gramineus* [62]. These compounds inhibit platelet aggregation by virtue of their RGD sequence and they have been collectively referred to as disintegrins [60, 61].

A number of GPIIb-IIIa antagonists have gone on to clinical trials and some have now become available commercially including the monoclonal antibody c7E3 (abciximab, ReoPro™), eptifibatide (Integrilin™), and tirofiban (MK-383, Aggrastat™). Several other compounds including lamifiban, fradafiban, roxifiban, orbofiban, and xemilofiban are at various stages of clinical development. Common to all of the GPIIb-IIIa antagonists is their ability to inhibit platelet aggregation in vitro and ex vivo in response to all of the usually used agonists. In addition, they prolong the bleeding time. In general, GPIIb-IIIa antagonists are more potent platelet inhibitors than aspirin and likely to be associated with somewhat more bleeding symptoms. Patients with Glanzmann thrombasthenia, whose platelets are devoid of GPIIb-IIIa complexes have severe mucocutaneous bleeding manifestations [63].

c7E3 monoclonal antibody is the Fab fragment of the mouse/human chimeric constructed to reduce immunogenicity from the variable region of the mouse antibody and constant region of the human immunoglobulin. This compound has undergone extensive clinical evaluation. Following intravenous bolus administration, free plasma c7E3 concentrations decrease rapidly with an initial half life of less than 10 min with a second phase half life of about 30 min. c7E3 is avidly bound to platelets and is detectable in the circulation for 15 days or more in platelet-bound state. c7E3 can be demonstrated on circulating platelets for longer periods than predicted based on the life span of platelets. This suggests the possibilities of transfer of the c7E3 molecule between platelets or that the inhibitor binds to megakaryocytes with subsequent release into circulation [64]. More than 80% of platelet GPIIb-IIa receptors were blocked after bolus administration of 0.25 mg/kg to patients with ischemic heart disease and reduce platelet aggregation induced by 20 μM ADP to less than 20% of baseline [65]. The median bleeding times were prolonged over 30 min. The peak effects were observed at two hours, the first sampling time. Administration of continuous infusion at 10 μg/min maintained the profound effect on platelet aggregation with recovery of platelet function gradually over 48 hours after discontinuation. The bleeding times returned to normal by 12 hours [65].

In the EPIC (Evaluation of c7E3 to Prevent Ischemic Complications) trial 2099 patients undergoing percutaneous transluminal coronary angioplasty (PTCA) or atherectomy were randomly assigned to receive c7E3 bolus (0.25 mg/kg) followed by a 12 hour infusion, c7E3 bolus followed by placebo infusion or placebo bolus and infusion [66, 67]. The composite end point of death, myocardial infarction, or need for urgent intervention was significantly reduced at 30 days in patients receiving the c7E3 bolus and infusion and the benefit was sustained at 6 months [67]. Of particular interest, c7E3 bolus plus 12 hour infusion improved outcomes as long as 3 years after the procedure [68]. The results at 6 months and 3 years are landmark findings because they indicate that pharmacologic intervention impacts on clinical restenosis. In the EPIC trial the rate of major bleeding was higher in the c7E3 groups than in the placebo group [66]. It is relevant to note that all patients received concomitant heparin therapy. In the subsequent EPILOG (Evaluation of PTCA to Improve Long-Term Outcome by c7E3 GPIIb-IIIa Receptor Blockade) [69] the dose of heparin was decreased and weight-adjusted, and there was no increase in major bleeding with c7E3. In this trial, a broad group of patients undergoing percutaneous coronary intervention (PCI) were enrolled. Administration of c7E3 reduced the end point consisting of death, MI or urgent intervention at 48 hours, 30 days and 6 months follow-up [69]. Careful modification of clinical management issues, such as intensity of heparin anticoagulation, have resulted in an acceptable bleeding rates with this and other GPIIb-IIIa antagonists.

While patients enrolled in the EPIC and EPILOG were studied essentially in the setting of PCI, the CAPTURE (Chimeric Anti-platelet Therapy in Unstable Angina Refractory to standard medical therapy) trial [70] studied patients with refractory angina in whom PCI was planned to be performed within 24 hours. Administration of c7E3 for 18 to 24 hours prior to PCI significantly reduced the composite primary end point of death, MI and urgent intervention at 30 days. There was also a reduction in the incidence of MI occurring prior to and after angioplasty.

Eptifibatide (Integrilin™) is a synthetic cyclic peptide GPIIb-IIIa antagonist that has been modeled after the snake venom disintegrin barbourin [71] and contains the KGD instead of the RGD sequence present in other GPIIb-IIIa antagonists. Eptifibatide has a rapid onset of action and short half-life of 50-60 min. Following discontinuation of infusion in human volunteers, inhibition of platelet aggregation and the bleeding time prolongation were reversible within 30 min with normalization of the bleeding time and platelet aggregation at 2-4 hours. In the IMPACT-II trial (Integrilin to Minimise Platelet Aggregation and Coronary Thrombosis-II trial) [72], 4010 patients undergoing elective, urgent or emergency coronary intervention were assigned to placebo or two dosage regimens of eptifibatide administered as a bolus followed by an infusion. Eptifibatide reduced the early abrupt closure and ischemic events at 30 days. This drug has been approved recently by the FDA for the treatment of patients with acute coronary syndromes, including patients who are to be managed medically, and those undergoing PCI.

Tirofiban (Aggrastat™) is a highly selective, short-acting (terminal half-life ~1.5 hours) small non-peptide GPIIb-IIIa antagonist. In the RESTORE trial (Randomized Efficacy Study of Tirofiban for Outcomes and Restenosis) [73], 2212 patients with an acute coronary syndrome and undergoing PCI were administered bolus and 36-hour infusion of tirofiban or placebo. There were significant reductions in the adverse cardiac events at 2 days and 7 days post-angioplasty but not at 30 days [73]. Two large trials of tirofiban have been recently reported involving patients with unstable angina or non-Q-wave MI. The PRISM trial (Platelet Receptor Inhibition in Ischemic Syndrome Management) [74] involved 3232 patients who were randomly assigned to receive intravenous tirofiban or heparin for 48 hours, with all patients receiving aspirin. In the tirofiban treated patients, there was a reduction in the primary end point, a composite of death, MI, or refractory ischemia at 48 hours (3.8 percent versus 5.6 percent, p = 0.01). Although the rates of refractory ischemia and MI at 30 days were not significantly reduced with tirofiban, there was a significant reduction in mortality (2.3 percent versus 3.6 percent in the group, p = 0.02).

In the PRISM-PLUS (Platelet Receptor Inhibition in Ischemic Syndrome Management in Patients Limited by Unstable Signs and Symptoms) trial [75], 1915 patients were randomly assigned to receive infusion of heparin, tirofiban plus heparin, or tirofiban alone; all patients received aspirin. The primary end point was a composite of death, MI, or refractory ischemia at 7 days. At 7 days there was excess mortality in the tirofiban alone group compared to the other two groups (4.6 percent versus 1.1 percent with heparin alone and 1.5 percent with the combination). The composite primary end point at 7 days was lower in the tirofiban plus heparin group compared to heparin alone group, (12.9 percent versus 17.9 percent, p = 0.004), and the beneficial effect persisted at 30 days and 6 months. Tirofiban has been recently approved by the FDA for treatment of patients with acute coronary syndrome.

Lamifiban is a non-peptide, selective GPIIb-IIIa antagonist that has gone on to clinical trials in patients with unstable angina. The Canadian Lamifiban Study showed a decrease in severe ischemic events during a 3-5 day infusion and reduced the incidence of death and MI at 1 month [76].

Bleeding in the face of intense antithrombotic therapy is a feared complication. In general, the large trials with c7E3 and the synthetic GPIIb-IIIa antagonists have demonstrated that efficacy can be attained with acceptable bleeding risk. Thrombocytopenia has been observed with several of the GPIIb-IIIa antagonists. In one study [77] 0.5% of 744 patients treated with c7E3 developed acute profound thrombocytopenia (<20,000/μl within 24 hours of bolus). Thrombocytopenia has been noted with use of other GPIIb-IIIa antagonists as well. Of particular interest is the report documenting pre-existing antibodies to a conformational epitope induced in GPIIb-IIIa in two primates administered non-antibody GPIIb-IIIa antagonists [78]. More importantly, drug-dependent antibodies against GPIIb-IIIa where noted in 1% of over 1000 human plasma samples from subjects not exposed to GPIIb-IIIa antagonists. This study indicates the presence of pre-existing antibodies in some individuals; they may be of clinical significance in inducing thrombocytopenia on drug administration. Thrombocytopenia has been reported after the first dose in one patient and on day 7 in another following administering of an oral agent (RPR 10891 [79]. Mild transient thrombocytopenia has also been reported in two of 20 patients treated with Xemilofiban [80], another oral antagonist. The mechanisms and frequency of thrombocytopenia with GPIIb-IIIa antagonists need to be defined.

Impact of Platelet GPIIb-IIIa Antagonists on Thrombin Generation. Platelet function and blood coagulation have traditionally been viewed as distinct prongs of the hemostatic system. Incontrovertible evidence supports that the two mechanisms are closely intertwined and platelets play a major role in thrombin generation [12]. Further proof for this is provided by the studies demonstrating an effect of GPIIb-IIIa antagonists on thrombin generation. In the EPIC study the activated clotting times were more prolonged in patients receiving c7E3 compared to controls [81]. In vitro, c7E3 decreases thrombin generation triggered by tissue factor [15]. In the baboon model, tirofiban reduces thrombin generation during cardiopulmonary bypass and this effect is discernible on top of the effect of heparin [82]. There is also evidence from in vitro and in vivo studies [15] that other antiplatelet agents such as aspirin, indomethacin, PGE_1, and PGI_2, also impact on thrombin generation.

The impact of antiplatelet agents on thrombin generation, hitherto unrecognized, may be an important aspect of the antithrombotic effects of some of these agents. Of particular significance in this context are the observations that thrombin has a mitogenic effect on smooth muscle cells. Inhibition of thrombin generation may contribute to the effect on restenosis noted following percutaneous coronary intervention.

Other Issues With GPIIb-IIIa Antagonist. The issue of relative integrin specificity of the various GPIIb-IIIa antagonists and its impact on clinical efficacy needs to be defined. Compared to other synthetic GPIIb-IIIa antagonists, c7E3 has the distinction of being relatively non-specific and is the only one to inhibit the vitronectin receptor (integrin $\alpha_v\beta_3$) in addition to the GPIIb-IIIa ($\alpha_{IIb}\beta_3$) [83]. The $\alpha_v\beta_3$ integrin is widely distributed on several cell types (platelets, endothelial, smooth muscle, osteoclasts) and also binds to fibrinogen, vWF and other RGD-containing ligands. It has been implicated in intimal hyperplasia and inhibition of $\alpha_v\beta_3$ receptors shown to decrease the extent of intimal hyperplasia in animal models [84, 85]. In addition this receptor may contribute to the thrombin generation [15]. Thus, the contribution of $\alpha_v\beta_3$ inhibition to the overall effect of c7E3 in decreasing the restenosis in patients undergoing percutaneous coronary intervention is currently unknown and needs to be clarified. The findings may impact on drug-design approaches in developing newer agents.

Several compounds are currently being developed as oral GPIIb-IIIa antagonists. Aside from issues they share with intravenous agents (such as the intensity of GPIIb-IIIa inhibition, half life, cost, etc.), the requirement of safety (bleeding, thrombocytopenia) may be different for chronic long-term administration in ambulatory patients compared to their use in the acute setting of ischemic heart disease. Moreover, the need and methods for laboratory monitoring require to be defined.

Other Antiplatelet Agents. Several other groups of compounds have antiplatelet effects (Table 2) and have been tested as potential antithrombotic agents. A number of compounds that inhibit thromboxane synthase, the enzyme that converts PGH_2 to thromboxane A_2, or inhibit the platelet thromboxane A_2 receptor have been developed but have not been proven to be effective or provide an advantage over aspirin. Prostanoids such as PGI_2 and PGE_1, and their analogs (iloprost, beraprost, cicaprost, ciprostene) inhibit platelet responses by elevating cAMP levels. Both PGI_2 and PGE_1 have a short half-life, and cause vasodilation and hypotension which has limited their development. Iloprost also shares these effects. Phosphodiesterase inhibitors also elevate platelet cAMP levels (Fig 1). Cilostazol is a phosphodiesterase III inhibitor that has gone on to clinical trials particularly in the context of peripheral arterial disease. Several compounds function as platelet inhibitors by virtue of elevating cGMP levels. These include nitric oxide (NO) and agents that generate NO (NO donors). Langford et al [86] have reported inhibition of platelet function in patients with acute MI and unstable angina by infusion of NO donor (glyceryl trinitrate or S-nitrosoglutathione). Serotonin is a weak platelet agonist which is also released from platelet dense granules on activation. Ketanserine is a serotonin antagonist that has been of interest for some time and has been evaluated in patients with peripheral arterial disease [87]. Inhibition of vWF interaction with GPIb presents an attractive strategy for inhibiting platelet adhesion in thrombosis. This strategy has been approached using antibodies that block vWF binding to GPIbα [88], recombinant fragment of vWF (A1 domain) [89-91], aurintricarboxylic acid [92], and heparins designed to specifically inhibit platelet interaction with vWF [93]. As of this writing, none of these agents are approved in the US for clinical use although some are approved in other countries.

REFERENCES:

1. Schafer AI: Biochemical mechanisms of platelet activation. Blood 1989; 74: 1181-1195.
2. Brass LF, Hoxie JA, Manning DR: Signaling through G Proteins and G Protein-coupled Receptors during Platelet Activation. Thromb and Haemostas 1993; 70: 217-223.
3. Berridge MJ: Inositol triphosphate and calcium signaling. Nature 1993; 361: 315-325.
4. Shattil SJ, Brass LF: Induction of the fibrinogen receptor on human platelets by intracellular mediators. J Biol Chem 1987; 262: 992-1000.
5. van Willigen G, Akkerman JWN: Protein kinase C and cAMP regulate reversible exposure of binding sites for fibrinogen on glycoprotein IIb-IIIa complex of human platelets. Biochemical Journal 1991; 273: 115-120.
6. Hynes RO: Integrins: a family of cell surface receptors. Cell 1987; 48: 549-54.
7. Smyth SS, Joneckis CC, Parise LV: Regulation of vascular integrins. Blood 1993; 81: 2827-43.
8. Kloczewiak M, Timmons S, Hawiger J: Recognition site for the platelet receptor is present on the 15-residue carboxy-terminal fragment of the gamma chain of human fibrinogen and is not involved in the fibrin polymerization reaction. Thromb Res 1983; 29: 249-55.
9. Kloczewiak M, Timmons S, Lukas TJ, Hawiger J: Platelet receptor recognition site on human fibrinogen. Synthesis and structure-function relationship of peptides corresponding to the carboxy-terminal segment of the gamma chain. Biochemistry 1984; 23: 1767-74.
10. Farrell DH, Thiagarajan P, Chung DW, Davie EW: Role of fibrinogen alpha and gamma chain sites in platelet aggregation. Proc Natl Acad Sci USA 1992; 89: 10729-32.
11. Weisel JW, Nagaswami C, Vilaire G, Bennett JS: Examination of the platelet membrane glycoprotein IIb-IIIa complex and its interaction with fibrinogen and other ligands by electron microscopy. J Biol Chem 1992; 267: 16637-43.
12. Walsh PN: Platelet-coagulant protein interactions. In: Colman RW, Hirsh J, Marder VJ, eds. Hemostasis and Thrombosis. Basic Principles and Clinical Practice. Philadelphia: J.B.Lippincott, 1994; 629-651.
13. Weiss HJ: Scott syndrome: a disorder of platelet coagulant activity. Semin Hematol 1994; 31: 312-9.
14. Byzova TV, Plow EF: Networking in the hemostatic system. Integrin alphaIIb beta3 binds prothrombin and influences its activation. J Biol Chem 1997; 272: 27183-8.
15. Reverter JC, Beguin S, Kessels H, Kumar R, Hemker HC, Coller BS: Inhibition of platelet-mediated, tissue factor-induced thrombin generation by the mouse/human chimeric 7E3 antibody. Potential implications for the effect of c7E3 Fab treatment on acute thrombosis and "clinical restenosis". J Clin Invest 1996; 98: 863-74.
16. Jack DB: One hundred years of aspirin. Lancet 1997; 350: 437-9.
17. Smith WL, Garavito RM, DeWitt DL: Prostaglandin endoperoxide H synthases (cyclooxygenases)-1 and -2. J Biol Chem 1996; 271: 33157-60.
18. Loll PJ, Picot D, Garavito RM: The structural basis of aspirin activity inferred from the crystal structure of inactivated prostaglandin H2 synthase. Nat Struct Biol 1995; 2: 637-43.
19. Patrono C: Aspirin as an antiplatelet drug. N Engl J Med 1994; 330: 1287-94.
20. Szczeklik A, Krzanowski M, Gora P, Radwan J: Antiplatelet drugs and generation of thrombin in clotting blood. Blood 1992; 80: 2006-11.
21. Pedersen AK, Fitzgerald GA: Dose-related kinetics of aspirin. Presystemic acetylation of platelet cyclooxygenase. N Engl J Med 1984; 311: 1206-1211.
22. Hirsh J, Dalen JE, Fuster V, Harker LB, Salzman EW: Aspirin and other platelet-active drugs; the relationship between dose, effectiveness, and side effects. Chest 1995; 102: 327S-336S.

23.Antiplatelet Trialists' Collaboration: Collaborative overview of randomised trials of antiplatelet therapy--I: Prevention of death, myocardial infarction, and stroke by prolonged antiplatelet therapy in various categories of patients. Antiplatelet Trialists' Collaboration. Br Med J 1994; 308: 81-106.

24.The Steering Committee of the Physician's Health Study Research Group: Final report on the aspirin component of the ongoing Physicians' Health Study. Steering Committee of the Physicians' Health Study Research Group. N Engl J Med 1989; 321: 129-35.

25.Peto R, Gray R, Collins R, et al: Randomised trial of prophylactic daily aspirin in British male doctors. Br Med J 1988; 296: 313-316.

26.Manson JE, Stampfer MJ, Colditz GA, et al: A prospective study of aspirin use and primary prevention of cardiovascular diseases in women. JAMA 1991; 266: 521-527.

27. The Medical Research Council's General Practice Framework: Thrombosis prevention trial: randomised trial of low-intensity oral anticoauglation with warfarin and low-dose aspirin in the primary prevention of ischaemic heart disease in men at increased risk. Lancet 1998; 351: 233-241.

28.Cairns JA, Lewis HD Meade TW, Sutton GC, Theroux P: Antithrombotic agents in coronary artery disease. Chest 1995; 108: 380S-400S.

29.Ridker PM, Manson JE, Gaziano M, Buring JE, Hennekens CH: Low-dose aspirin therapy for chronic stable angina: a randomized, placebo-controlled clinical trial. Ann Intern Med 1991; 114: 835-839.

30.ISIS-2 (Second International Study of Infarct Survivial) Collaborative Group: Randomised trial of intravenous streptokinase, oral aspirin, both, or neither among 17,187 cases of suspected acute myocardial infarction: ISIS-2. Lancet 1988; 2: 349-60.

31. Stein PD, Dalen JE, Goldman S, Schwartz L, Theroux P, Turpie AG: Antithrombotic therapy in patients with saphenous vein and internal mammary artery bypass grafts. Chest 1995; 108: 424S-430S.

32. The SALT Collaborative Group: Swedish aspirin low-dose trial (SALT) of 75 mg aspirin as secondary prophylaxis after cerebrovascular ischemic events. Lancet 1991; 338: 1345-1349.

33. Sherman DG, Dyken ML, Jr., Gent M, Harrison MJG, Hart RG, Mohr JP: Antithrombotic therapy for cerebrovascualr disorders. An update. Chest 1995; 108: 444S-456S.

34.The Anturane Reinfarction Trial Research Group: Sulfinpyrazone in the prevention of cardiac death after myocardial infarction. The Anturane Reinfarction Trial. N Engl J Med 1978; 298(6): 289-95.

35.The Anturane Reinfarction Trial Research Group: Sulfinpyrazone in the prevention of sudden death after myocardial infarction. N Engl J Med 1980; 302(5): 250-6.

36.Report from the Anturane Re-Infarction Italian Study: Sulfinpyrazone in postmyocardial infarction. Lancet 1989; 1: 1215-1220.

37.Temple R, Pledger GW: The FDA's critique of the anturane reinfarction trial. N Engl J Med 1980; 303: 1488-92.

38. Fitzgerald GA: Dipyridamole. N Engl J Med 1987; 316: 1247-1257.

39.Harker LA, Slichter SJ: Studies of platelets and fibrinogen kinetics in patients with prothetic heart valves. N Engl J Med 1970; 299: 53-59.

40. Chesebro JH, Fuster V, Elveback LR, et al: Trial of combined warfarin plus dipyridamole or aspirin therapy in prosthetic heart valve replacement: danger of aspirin compared with dipyridamole. Am J Card 1983; 51: 1537-1541.

41. Daniel JL, Dangelmaier C, Jin J, Ashby B, Smith JB, Kunapuli SP: Molecular basis for ADP-induced platelet activation. I. Evidence for three distinct ADP receptors on human platelets. J Biol Chem 1998; 273: 2024-9.

42. Mills DC, Puri R, Hu CJ, Minniti C, Grana G, Freeman MD: Clopidogrel inhibits the binding of ADP analogues to the receptor mediating inhibition of platelet adenylate cyclase. Arterioscler Thromb 1992; 12: 430-436.

43.Gent M, Blakely JA, Easton JD, et al: The Canadian American Ticlopidine Study (CATS) in thromboembolic stroke. Lancet 1989; 2: 1215-1220.

44. Hass WK, Easton JD, Adams HP, et al: A randomized trial comparing ticlopidine hydrochloride with aspirin for the prevention of stroke in high-risk patients. N Engl J Med 1989; 321: 501-507.

45. Bellavance A: Efficacy of ticlopidine and aspirin for prevention of reversible cerebrovascular ischemic events. The Ticlopidine Aspirin Stroke Study. Stroke 1993; 24: 1452-7.

46. Bergamasco B, Benna P, Carolei A, Rasura M, Rudelli G, Fieschi C: A randomized trial comparing ticlopidine hydrochloride with indobufen for the prevention of stroke in high-risk patients (TISS Study). Ticlopidine Indobufen Stroke Study. Funct Neurol 1997; 12: 33-43.

47. Balsano F, Rizzon P, Violi F, et al: Antiplatelet treatment with ticlopidine in unstable angina: a controlled multicenter trial. Circulation 1990; 82: 17-26.

48. Schomig A, Neumann FJ, Kastrati A, et al.: A randomized comparison of antiplatelet and anticoagulant therapy after the placement of coronary-artery stents. N Engl J Med 1996; 334: 1084-9.

49. Dirschinger J, Schuhlen H, Walter H, Hadmitzky M, Zitzmann EM: Intracoronary stenting and antithrombotic regimen trial: one-year clinical follow-up (abstract). Circulation 1997; 94: I-257.

50. Leon MD, Faim DS, Gordon P, et al: Clinical and angiographic results from the Stent Anticoagulation Regimen Study (STARS). Circulation 1996;94:I-685.

51. Sharis PJ, Cannon CP, Loscalzo J: The antiplatelet effects of ticlopidine and clopidogrel. Ann Intern Med 1998; 129: 394-405.

52. Janzon L, Bergqvist D, Boberg J, et al.: Prevention of myocardial infarction and stroke in patients with intermittent claudication; effects of ticlopidine. Results from STIMS, the Swedish Ticlopidine Multicentre Study. J Intern Med 1990; 227: 301-8.

53. Arcan JC, Blanchard J, Boissel JP, Destors JM, Panak E: Multicenter double-blind study of ticlopidine in the treatment of intermittent claudication and the prevention of its complications. Angiology 1988; 39: 802-11.

54. CAPRIE Steering Committee: A randomised, blinded, trial of clopidogrel versus aspirin in patients at risk of ischaemic events (CAPRIE). Lancet 1996; 348: 1329-1339.

55. Gent M: Benefit of clopidorel in patients with coronary artery disease (abstract). Circulation 1997; 96: I-467.

56. Bennett CL, Weinberg P, Rozenberg-Ben-Dror K, Yarnold P, Kwaan U, Green D: Thrombotic thrombocytopenia purpura associated with ticlopidine. Ann Intern Med 1998; 128: 541-544.

57. Bennett C, Kiss J, Weinberg P, et al.: Thrombotic thrombocytopenic purpura after stenting and ticlopidine. Lancet 1998; 352: 1036-1037.

58. Lefkovits J, Plow EF, Topol EJ: Platelet glycoprotein IIb/IIIa receptors in cardiovascular medicine. N Engl J Med 1995; 332: 1553-9.

59. Coller BS: Platelet GPIIb/IIIa antagonists: the first anti-integrin receptor therapeutics. J Clin Invest 1997; 100: S57-60.

60. Gould RJ, Polokoff MA, Friedman PA, et al.: Disintegrins: a family of integrin inhibitory proteins from viper venoms. Proc Soc Exp Biol Med 1990; 195: 168-71.

61. Niewiarowski S, McLane MA, Kloczewiak M, Stewart GJ: Disintegrins and othe rnaturally occurring anatoginists of platelet fibrinogen receptors. Sem Hematol 1994; 31: 289-3000.

62. Huang TF, Holt JC, Kirby EP, Niewiarowski S: Trigramin: primary structure and its inhibition of von Willebrand factor binding to glycoprotein IIb/IIIa complex on human platelets. Biochem 1989; 28: 661-6.

63. Rao AK: Congenital disorders of platelet function: disorders of signal transduction and secretion. Am J Med Sci 1998; 316: 69-76.

64. Christopoulos C, Mackie I, Lahiri A: Flow cytometric observations on the in vivo use of Fab gragments of a chimeric monoclonal antibody to platelet glycoprotein IIb-IIIa. Blood Coagul Fibrinol 1993; 4: 729.

65. Tcheng JE, Ellis SG, George BS, et al.: Pharmacodynamics of chimeric glycoprotein IIb/IIIa integrin antiplatelet antibody Fab 7E3 in high-risk coronary angioplasty. Circulation 1994; 90: 1757-64.

66. The EPIC Investigators: Use of a monoclonal antibody directed against the platelet glycoprotein IIb/IIIa receptor in high-risk coronary angioplasty. N Engl J Med 1994; 330: 956-61.

67. Topol EJ, Califf RM, Weisman HF, et al.: Randomised trial of coronary intervention with antibody against platelet IIb/IIIa integrin for reduction of clinical restenosis: results at six months. The EPIC Investigators. Lancet 1994; 343: 881-6.

68. Topol EJ, Ferguson JJ, Weisman HF, et al.: Long-term protection from myocardial ischemic events in a randomized trial of brief integrin beta3 blockade with percutaneous coronary intervention. EPIC Investigator Group. JAMA 1997; 278: 479-84.

69. The EPILOG Investigators: Platelet glycoprotein IIb/IIIa receptor blockade and low-dose heparin during percutaneous coronary revascularization. N Engl J Med 1997; 336: 1689-96.

70. The CAPTURE Investigators: Randomised placebo-controlled trial of abciximab before and during coronary intervention in refractory unstable angina: the CAPTURE Study. Lancet 1997; 349: 1429-35.

71. Scarborough RM, Naughton MA, Teng W, et al.: Design of potent and specific integrin antagonists. Peptide antagonists with high specificity for glycoprotein IIb-IIIa. J Biol Chem 1993; 268: 1066-73.

72. The IMPACT-II Investigators: Randomised placebo-controlled trial of effect of eptifibatide on complications of percutaneous coronary intervention: IMPACT-II. Lancet 1997; 349: 1422-8.

73. The RESTORE Investigators: Effects of platelet glycoprotein IIb/IIIa blockade with tirofiban on adverse cardiac events in patients with unstable angina or acute myocardial infarction undergoing coronary angioplasty. Circulation 1997; 96: 1445-53.

74. THE Platelet Receptor Inhibition in Ischemic Syndrome Management (PRISM) Study Investigators. A comparison of aspirin plus tirofiban with aspirin plus heparin for unstable angina. N Engl J Med 1998; 338: 1498-505.

75. Platelet Receptor Inhibition in Ischemic Syndrome Management in Patients Limited by Unstable Signs and Symptoms (PRISM-PLUS) Study Investigators. Inhibition of the platelet glycoprotein IIb/IIIa receptor with tirofiban in unstable angina and non-Q-wave myocardial infarction. N Engl J Med 1998; 338: 1488-97.

76.Theroux P, Kouz S, Roy L, et al.: Platelet membrane receptor glycoprotein IIb/IIIa antagonism in unstable angina. The Canadian Lamifiban Study. Circulation 1996; 94: 899-905.

77. Berkowitz SD, Harrington RA, Rund MM, Tcheng JE: Acute profound thrombocytopenia after C7E3 Fab (abciximab) therapy. Circulation 1997; 95: 809-13.

78. Bednar B, Bednar RA, Cook JJ, et al.: Drug-dependent antibodies against GPIIb/IIIa induce thrombocytopenia (abstract). Circulation 1996; 94: I-99.

79.Catella-Lawson F, Kapoor S, Skammer W, Fitzgerald DJ, Rocca B, Tamby JF: Chronic inhibition of the plateletl glycoprotein IIb/IIIa by a new oral agent: dose escalation study in patients with coronary artery disease (CAD) (abstract). Thrombos Haemost 1997; 77: 393.

80. Simpfendorfer C, Kottke-Marchant K, Lowrie M, et al.: First chronic platelet glycoprotein IIb/IIIa integrin blockade. A randomized, placebo-controlled pilot study of xemilofiban in unstable angina with percutaneous coronary interventions. Circulation 1997; 96: 76-81.

81. Moliterno DJ, Califf RM, Aguirre FV, et al.: Effect of platelet glycoprotein IIb/IIIa integrin blockade on activated clotting time during percutaneous transluminal coronary angioplasty or directional atherectomy (the EPIC trial). Evaluation of c7E3 Fab in the Prevention of Ischemic Complications trial. JACC 1995; 75: 559-62.

82.Rao AK, Sun L, Hiramatsu Y, Gikakis N, Anderson HL, Gorman JH, Edmunds LH, Jr. Glycoprotein IIb/IIIa receptor antagonist Tirofiban (Aggrastat(inhibits thrombin generationduring cardiopulmonary bypass in baboons.

83.Charo IF, Bekeart LS, Phillips DR: Platelet glycoprotein IIb-IIIa-like proteins mediate endothelial cell attachment to adhesive proteins and the extracellular matrix. J Biol Chem 1987; 262: 9935-8.

84.Matsuno H, Stassen JM, Vermylen J, Deckmyn H: Inhibition of integrin function by a cyclic RGD-containing peptide prevents neointima formation. Circulation 1994; 90(5): 2203-6.

85. van der Zee RJ, Passeri JJ, Barry DA, Cheresh, Isner JM: A neutralizing antibody to the alpha v beta 3 integrin reduces neointimal thickening in a balloon-injured rabbit iliac artery. Circulation 1996; 98: I-257a.

86. Langford EJ, Wainwright RJ, Martin JF: Platelet activation in acute myocardial infarction and unstable angina is inhibited by nitric oxide donors. Arterioscler Thromb Vasc Biol 1996; 16: 51-5.

87.PACK Trial Group: Prevention of atherosclerotic complications: controlled trial of ketanserin. Br Med J 1989; 298: 424-430.

88. Bellinger DA, Nichols TC, Read MS, et al.: Prevention of occlusive coronary artery thrombosis by a murine monoclonal antibody to porcine von Willebrand factor. Proc Natl Acad Sci U S A 1987; 84: 8100-4.

89. Sixma JJ, Ijsseldijk MJ, Hindriks G, et al.: Adhesion of blood platelets is inhibited by VCL, a recombinant fragment (leucine504 to lysine728) of von Willebrand factor. Arterioscler Thromb Vasc Biol 1996; 16: 64-71.

90. Yao SK, Ober JC, Garfinkel LI, et al.: Blockade of platelet membrane glycoprotein Ib receptors delays intracoronary thrombogenesis, enhances thrombolysis, and delays coronary artery reocclusion in dogs. Circulation 1994; 89: 2822-8.

91. Zahger D, Fishbein MC, Garfinkel LI, et al.: VCL, an antagonist of the platelet GP1b receptor, markedly inhibits platelet adhesion and intimal thickening after balloon injury in the rat. Circulation 1995; 92: 1269-73.

92. Golino P, Ragni M, Cirillo P, et al.: Aurintricarboxylic acid reduces platelet deposition in stenosed and endothelially injured rabbit carotid arteries more effectively than other antiplatelet interventions. Thromb Haemost 1995; 74: 974-9.

93. Sobel M, Bird KE, Tyler-Cross R, et al.: Heparins designed to specifically inhibit platelet interactions with von Willebrand factor. Circulation 1996; 93: 992-9.

9 MOLECULAR DETERMINANTS OF THE T WAVE

Michael R. Rosen, M. D.
College of Physicians and Surgeons of Columbia University

The last two decades have seen an impressive increment in our understanding of the determinants of cardiac electrical activity, as molecular and genetic techniques applied initially to bacteria, yeast and drosophila have been used to explore the structure - function relationships of mammalian ion channels. A major asset in these studies has been the pattern of conservation that characterizes so many processes in nature; i.e., the ion channels studied molecularly and biophysically in less complex life forms have a good deal of homology with channels in mammalian heart. These points of similarity have facilitated our understanding of the physiology and the structure of the channels and - as a result - are providing new directions for exploring pathophysiology and developing therapy.

The goal of this paper is to consider how an understanding of the molecular biology of the heart facilitates our understanding of the electrocardiographic T wave. The complexity of the repolarization processes that underlie the T wave can be appreciated in light of transmural and regional electrical gradients, and these shall be reviewed below. However, the electrical signals that determine the ST segment and T wave are, themselves, the result of molecular and biochemical processes that determine electrical activity.[1,2] Making the situation even more complex is the fact that electrical activity, in turn, influences the molecular and biochemical processes importantly.[3]

In the following pages I shall first review the molecular determinants of the T wave. I shall then demonstrate how alterations in these determinants cause long-lasting and pathological changes in the T wave that are harbingers of lethal arrhythmias. Here I shall use the congenital long QT syndrome as an example. Finally, the effect of the environment on molecular function in the heart will be demonstrated using "cardiac memory"[4,5] in which changes in ventricular activation pathways modify cellular repolarization[6,7] and the T wave.[6,8]

MOLECULAR DETERMINANTS OF THE T WAVE

Ventricular resting and action potentials.   Figure 1A demonstrates a typical myocardial action potential. Salient points regarding this action potential is that it has a high (i.e. negative) level of resting potential determined by an imbalance of charge maintained across the cell membrane. This imbalance is in part the result of the permanent charges residing on the lipids that constitute the cell membrane (with negative charge on the intracellular side), as well as the high conductance of a specific K channel, referred to as I_{K1} (see below) and the operation of biochemical pumps, such as the Na/K ATPase, that drive Na^+ out of the cell in excess of the K^+ brought into the cell.[9]

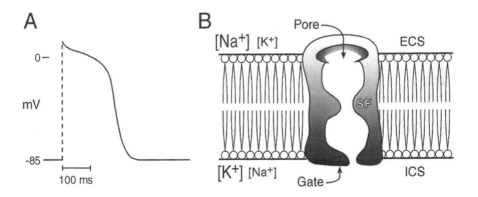

FIGURE 1: Panel A: A typical myocardial action potential. See text for description. Panel B: The lipid bilayer of the cell membrane is depicted schematically. Shown as well is a channel spanning the bilayer, whose pore links the aqueous solutions of the extracellular (ECS) and extracellular (ICS) spaces. Critical to the ability of the channel to determine the passage of ions are a selectivity filter (SF) and gate (see text for description of both). Also depicted are the disparate concentrations of Na^+ and K^+ ions in the ECS and ICS.

To generate an action potential, a cell requires the presence of a good conducting medium (i.e., the aqueous solutions of the cytosol and of the extracellular space) as well as the presence of an insulating membrane (the lipid bilayer of the membrane) (Figure 1B). The separation of ions across the membrane is such that the inside of the cell has a high K^+ concentration (about 135 mM) and a low Na^+ concentration (about 15 mM). This is in contrast to the extracellular space, in which the Na^+ concentration is about 135 mM, and K^+, about 4 mM.[9]

Generation of an action potential requires a mechanism to carry charge across the membrane. This mechanism is provided by ion channels, which are protein pores that traverse the lipid bilayer of the membrane (Figure 1B). Structures critical to the function of the channels are:

1: The selectivity filter, which is a narrowing near the outer surface of the channel. The selectivity filter has a particular configuration, size and charge that determine which ion is most likely to transverse the channel to the relative exclusion of other ions.[9]

2: Gates are protein structures on the inner margin of the channel: these can be in open or closed positions.[9-11] The Na^+ channel, which is responsible for carrying the inward current that induces the upstroke of the ventricular action potential and the QRS complex is depicted schematically. The Na channel has two gates, referred to as "m" and "h" in Figure 2. In the resting state, the "m" gate is closed and the "h" is open. When the channel is activated the m gate opens and Na ion enters the cell, traveling down both concentration and voltage gradients. As membrane voltage becomes more positive, the h gate, which is voltage-dependent closes. At this time Na can no longer enter the cell, and the channel is said to be inactivated. As membrane potential moves back towards its resting level, the m gate closes and the h reopens.

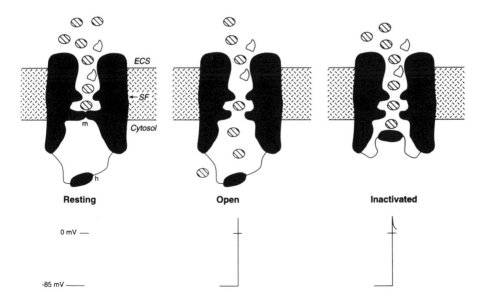

FIGURE 2: Depiction of Na^+ channel in resting, open and inactivated states. In the resting state the m gate is closed and h is open. At this time only a resting membrane potential is recorded from the myocyte. In the open state, both gates are open, Na^+ enters, carrying positive charge into the cell, and the phase 0 upstroke of the action potential is recorded. In the inactivated state, the h gate now closes and the cell begins to repolarize. See text for further description.

The inward current that depolarizes ventricular muscle cells is carried in the main by Na^+ ion. With respect to repolarization, the situation is far more complex. Figure 3, modified from the Sicilian Gambit publications,[12] approximates the temporal relationship between a ventricular myocardial action potential, and the ion channels that determine repolarization. Both inward and outward currents are

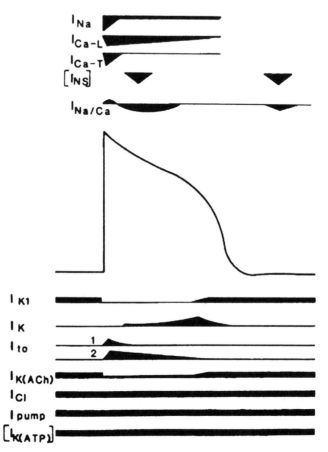

FIGURE 3: Depiction of a ventricular myocyte action potential. Above it are the various inward currents that would maintain a depolarized state during the plateau, as well as the Na/Ca exchanger, which can carry net inward or outward current. Below are various outward, repolarizing currents. The temporal relationships indicated here are all approximate and no depiction of current amplitude is provided. See text for description. (Reprinted by permission of the American Heart Association from reference 12).

involved. The inward currents depolarize the cell and tend to maintain it at a positive level of membrane potential; the outward currents repolarize it and return it to its resting potential. Two major inward, depolarizing currents contribute to repolarization: a slow inward current carried by calcium, referred to as the L-type calcium current,[13] and a persistent inward current carried by Na.[14] The major

outward, repolarizing currents are carried by potassium. The first of these to occur is the transient outward current (I_{to}) responsible for phase 1 repolarization.[15] The delayed rectifier current, I_k, has three components: one is ultra-rapidly activating (I_{Kur}),[16] one is rapidly activating (I_{Kr}), and one is slowly activating (I_{Ks}).[17] These are responsible for the termination of the phase 2 plateau and the early portion of phase
3 repolarization. The remainder of repolarization is determined by an inwardly rectifying potassium current, I_{K1}, which not only returns the membrane to its resting potential, but contributes to the negative potential achieved during electrical diastole (phase 4).[12]

Many of these channels have been studied molecularly and have been cloned, although their three-dimensional structures have not yet been identified. Each can be understood not only as a functional entity, but one for which we are steadily acquiring information about structure-function relationships. The latter are deduced from experiments in which specific amino acids or sequences of amino acids are replaced or deleted and the effects of this process on channel function are noted.

Heterogeneity of repolarization. In the neonatal heart there tends to be great homogeneity of action potential duration. However, with growth and development there is increasing heterogeneity across the ventricular wall. Single myocytes or slabs of tissue isolated from the epicardium, midmyocardium or endocardium show significant differences in the voltage-time course of repolarization (figure 4).[18-21] The epicardial action potential has a large phase 1 notch and a relatively short duration. That in the myocardium (the so- called M cell region[18,19]) has a large notch as well, and a long action potential duration. The endocardial action potential is short, and there is a minimal notch. These differences in action potential duration and configuration have important underlying ionic determinants. The phase 1 notch of the action potential is induced to a great extent by the transient outward K current, I_{to}. This current is prominent in epicardial and M cells but is minimal in endocardium.[22] The rapidly activating delayed rectifier current I_{kr} is of approximately equal magnitude in epi-, mid- and endocardium, but the slowly activating delayed rectifier, I_{Ks}, is reportedly of lesser magnitude in midmyocardium.[23] This property plus the presence of a larger inward (depolarizing) Na current in the midmyocardial cells than in epi- and endocardial is presumed responsible for the longer midmyocardial potential duration.[2]

Despite these differences in cellular electrophysiologic properties, there is a relatively smooth gradient for repolarization transmurally in the ventricle. Different studies of the intact ventricle have shown that gradients of less than 30 msec and approaching 0 msec occur across the myocardial wall at cycle lengths of about 1.5 sec.[21,24-26] Electrotonic coupling among myocytes in the ventricular wall is believed to account for the reduction in heterogeneity across the myocardial wall in situ.[27] Nonetheless, some heterogeneity persists in the intact heart, such that at physiologic rates epicardial action potentials tend to be longer than endocardial, and apical shorter than basal.

There are important determinants of transmural heterogeneity: one is growth and development; for example in the neonatal canine heart there is no I_{to} or phase 1 notch in the action potential until about 2 months of age,[28] and the action potentials are far more homogeneous than in the adult. Gender is another determinant of repolarization; i.e. women have significantly longer electrocardiographic QT intervals than men.[29] Moreover, women are at greater risk than men of death from administration of drugs that prolong repolarization, such as certain antiarrhythmics (e.g., d-sotalol[30]) and non-sedating antihistamines (e.g., terfenadine), either alone or in combination with macrolide antibiotics or ketoconazole antifungals.[31] All these drugs share the common property of blocking I_{Kr}.

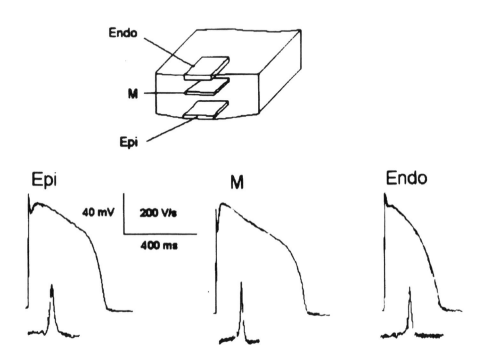

FIGURE 4: Left ventricular epicardial (epi), midmyocardial (M) and endocardial (endo) myocyte action potentials. The upper traces are the action potentials and the lower, the electronically differentiated maximal upstroke velocity of phase 0, reflecting rapid Na entry that contributes to the upstroke. The schematic indicates a transmural section of LV myocardium and the site from which each tissue sample is obtained. See text for further description. (Modified from reference 27 by permission).

GENETICALLY-DETERMINED ALTERATIONS IN MOLECULAR DETERMINANTS AND THEIR EFFECTS ON THE ECG

Experiments of nature provide an important window into the workings of specific biological processes. One such experiment, unfortunate as it has been for those individuals afflicted, is the congenital long QT syndrome (LQTS). This rare disorder is characterized by a long QT interval on ECG and a propensity to torsades de pointes, syncope and sudden death.[2,32] The inheritance pattern is autosomal recessive, yet interestingly, there is a greater predilection for syncope and death in female than in male patients, perhaps determined by the gender-associated differences in repolarization described above.

Major anomalies contributing to LQTS have been linked to chromosomes 3, 4, 7, 11 and 21.[33-41] Mutated genes have thus far been identified at four of the chromosomal loci.[2,32] Mutations in KvLQT1 which is responsible for LQT1, are localized to chromosome 11; mutations in HERG, responsible for LQT2, are localized to chromosome 7; mutations in SCN5A are responsible for LQT3 and are localized to chromosome 3; and mutations in KcNE1 are responsible for LQT5 and are localized to chromosome 21. Examples of the HERG and SCN5A abnormalities are shown respectively in Figures 5 and 6.

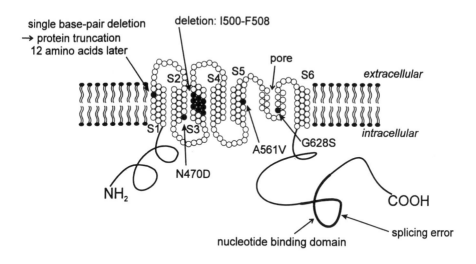

FIGURE 5: Molecular organization of HERG. The topology of this protein resembles one domain of the sodium channel, and it is thought that four proteins co-assemble to form functional channels. The locations of identified mutations are shown. Those in S1 and S3 are not likely to form functional channels, whereas the single amino acid changes indicated in S2, S5, and the pore might. HERG contains a cyclic nucleotide-binding domain in its intracytoplasmic C-terminal, and a sixth mutation has been identified there. (Reprinted from Roden et al., J Cardiovasc Electrophysiol 1995;6:1023-1031, by permission.)

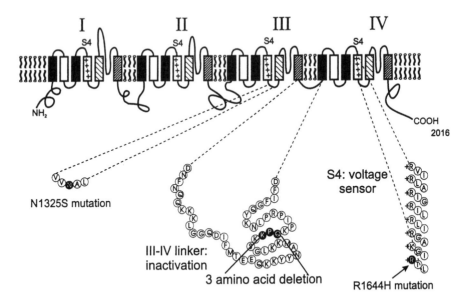

FIGURE 6: Molecular organization of the human cardiac sodium channel (hH1). The SCN5A gene encodes the sodium channel _-subunit, a protein 2016 amino acids long. The protein consists of four roughly homologous domains (I-IV) each containing six transmembrane spanning segments (S1-S6). The 52 amino acids linking domains III and IV are shown by their single letter codes; this region is known to be important for normal sodium channel inactivation. Three different mutations causing LQTS have been identified in SCN5A. One is a deletion of three amino acids (KPQ) in the III-IV linker, and the other two are point mutations. (Reprinted from Roden et al., J Cardiovasc Electrophysiol 1995;6:1023-1031, by permission.)

LQT1, LQT2 and LQT5 all are associated with abnormal K currents (respectively I_{Ks}, I_{Kr} and I_{Ks}) whereas LQT3 involves the channel responsible for inward Na current during the plateau of the action potential. With respect to the two I_{Ks} abnormalities that are involved, it should be noted that LQT1 is associated with mutations in $KvLQT_1$, whose protein product is an important component of I_{Ks}; whereas LQT5 is associated with mutations in KcNE1 whose protein product, minK, coassembles with $KvLQT_1$ to produce I_{Ks}.[33] Hence, in three instances (i.e. the K channel abnormalities) there is a reduction of outward, repolarizing current during the action potential and in the fourth (i.e., the Na channel abnormality) there is an increase in inward, depolarizing, Na current. The result in all four instances is similar on the ECG; i.e., an increase in the QT interval. Of particular note in reviewing figures 5-8 should be the multiple amino acid deletions and point mutations that occur. It is these diverse lesions in the genes determining channel structure that result in the malfunction of the Na or K channel, and prolongation of the QT interval.

Even though all the lesions described prolong the QT interval, there are clinical differences in the syndromes associated with each channel abnormality. For example, SCN5A patients tend to have torsades de pointes that occurs at rest; the torsades de pointes of KvLQT1 tends to occur during activity.[32] Important from a therapeutic viewpoint is that SCN5A patients respond to the Na channel blocking drug, mexiletine, with greater shortening of the QT interval than KvLQT1 patients, while the latter tend to show a greater shortening of the QT in response to elevations of extracellular potassium.[42,43] This observation of mexiletine effect in SCN5A patients may explain the earlier clinical observation made prior to genotyping that some patients with LQTS have a favorable clinical response to mexiletine whereas many do not.[2] Presumably this heterogeneous response reflects the unknowing inclusion of patients with SCN5A (who would tend to respond favorably) and those with K channel abnormalities (who would not).

Whether the QT shortening induced by mexiletine in SCN5A patients is also associated with a reduction in torsades de pointes, syncope and death is not yet known. While it might be logical to expect that shortening of the QT interval would reduce the incidence of lethal arrhythmias, it should be noted that some subsets of LQTS patients have a long QT interval and no arrhythmias and others have a normal QT interval yet experience arrhythmias.[32] Hence, the factors contributing to arrhythmogenesis in these patients are more complex than was initially believed.

We can hypothesize that the complexity of arrhythmogenesis is LQTS patients might be understood via the contribution of two factors to the overt expression of LQTS, arrhythmias and death. These are the substrate (i.e. the K or Na channel involved) and a trigger mechanism.[44] The trigger would be the autonomic nervous system, specifically its beta-adrenergic limb. Supporting this view is that beta-adrenergic blockade remains the most effective single therapy for the prevention of arrhythmias in LQTS, regardless of the channel involved.[32] Moreover, left sympathectomy has been an effective adjunct in those cases where beta-blockade alone has not sufficed.[32] The mechanism for the efficacy of beta-adrenergic blockade is thought to be as follows: beta-adrenergic stimulation increases inward L-type Ca current would tends to prolong the action potential plateau further (especially in the face of persistent inward Na current or reduced outward K current) to the point where oscillations referred to as early afterdepolarizations occur (Figure 7). The latter induce triggered arrhythmias having the characteristics of torsades de pointes. Trigger-directed therapy such as beta-adrenergic blockade would be expected to show efficacy regardless of the substrate, although the expression of the arrhythmia would vary further, depending on the magnitude of the substrate abnormality. In contrast, administration of specific therapy targeted at the substrate is anticipated to be most effective when the substrate is correctly identified (i.e., mexiletine would be anticipated to show greater effectiveness in shortening the QT interval in SCN5A than KvLQT$_1$). However, even if there is a salutary effect on the appropriate ion channel, presence of a large amount of catecholamine might provide a sufficient trigger to override this.

Given the associations among lesions in channel structure, the currents that determine repolarization, and clinical syndromes with a high potential for lethality, we can begin to understand, using LQTS as a paradigm, the inconsistent success of some prior clinical therapies (e.g., mexiletine) and the more consistent success of

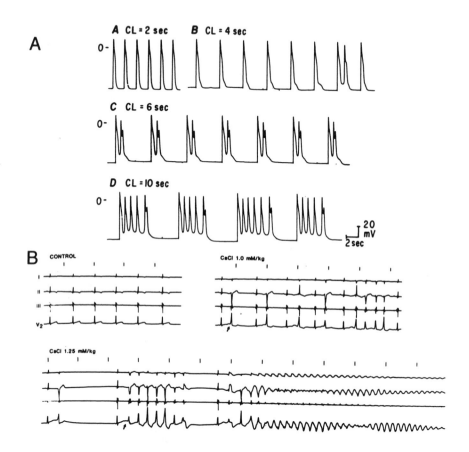

FIGURE 7: A: The initiation of early afterdepolarizations (EAD) and triggered activity by cesium in isolated canine Purkinje fibers. In the presence of Cs at a CL of 2 sec no EAD are seen. However as CL is increased to 4 sec, EAD appear as a "shoulder" during phase 3, one of which attains threshold, resulting in a triggered action potential (next to last cycle). At a CL of 6 sec, single triggered action potentials occur with each cycle and at 10 sec there are bursts of triggered activity. This sequence highlights the bradycardia-dependence of triggered activity induced by EAD. (Reprinted by permission of the American Heart Association, from Daminao and Rosen, Circulation 69:1013-1025, 1984). B: Cesium-induced triggered activity in an intact, anesthetized dog. As cesium is administered note the occurrence of single premature depolarizations, long pauses, and in the lower panel, bursts of pleomorphic ventricular tachycardia having some resemblance to torsade de pointes, and degenerating into fibrillation (Reprinted by permission of the American Heart Association from Brachmann et al., Circulation 1983;68:846-856.)

others (e.g., beta blockade). We also can begin to consider new approaches for other conditions; examples that come to mind are: those patients who develop long QT intervals on administration of certain antiarrhythmic, antibiotic or antihistaminic drugs;[31] or the approximately 25% of patients with myocardial infarction who develop potentially lethal arrhythmias.[44] The implication of work to date is that genetic determinants of the function of specific channels are such that a substrate favoring arrhythmias is present in these patients. The widespread role of genetic predisposition to abnormal function was given further credence recently by the discovery of three additional abnormalities in the SCN5A channel (Figure 8).[45] However, instead of resulting in a long QT interval and persistent inward Na current, these anomalies induced an abnormally rapid recovery from inexcitability of the Na channel. As a result, the effective refractory period was excessively short and ventricular tachycardias (presumably reentrant) in the absence of QT prolongation occurred. In summary, it is clear that unraveling the mysteries surrounding LQTS has let us to visualize more imaginative approaches to other arrhythmias. It is believed that further understanding of LQTS and these other clinical conditions will lead to evolution and application of more rational approaches to therapy.

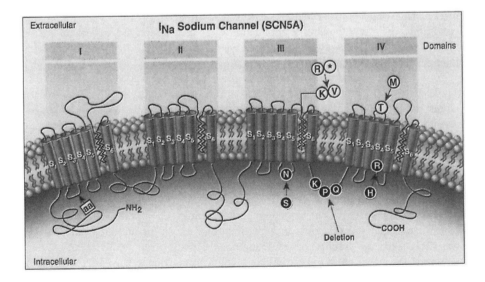

FIGURE 8: Predicted secondary structure of the cardiac Na channel, including these mutations causing idiopathic ventricular fibrillation (in white symbols) and chromosome 3 linked LQTS (in black circles). The channel incorporates four transmembrane domains (DI-DIV) each of which houses six transmembrane segments (S1-S6). (Reprinted by permission from reference 45.)

ALTERED PATHWAYS OF ACTIVATION INFLUENCE THE MOLECULAR DETERMINANTS OF THE T WAVE

Thus far I have discussed the contrasting situations seen in normal hearts and hearts in which molecular lesions are present. Each has a clear pattern of molecular determinism and clinical expression. Far more subtle and in some ways elusive are the interfaces between normal and disease states.[44] Similarly, the effects on cardiac electrophysiologic function of transient stresses that may not be pathological can be difficult to identify. To illustrate how transient interventions may imprint the heart with changes of varying magnitude and duration, I shall discuss the changes in the T wave that occur as the result of varying periods (from minutes to weeks) of cardiac rhythm change associated with an altered activation pathway. Chatterjee et al[5] and, subsequently Rosenbaum et al[6] described these changes in some detail, noting the relationship between the abnormal QRS vector of altered ventricular activation (as appears with either pacemaker therapy or an intermittent ventricular arrhythmia) and the occurrence of an abnormal T wave whose vector mirrors that of the paced QRS complex and that persists long after the heart had returned to normal sinus rhythm and a normal QRS complex. This phenomenon was referred to as "cardiac memory" by Rosenbaum et al.[6]

Cardiac memory is defined as a specific change in the T wave vector that (1) is induced by, yet long outlasts, a change in ventricular activation pathway, and (2) is cumulative, increasing with the extent of abnormal activation.[6] This phenomenon created a dilemma for those who described it: if, as was originally thought, the T wave change results entirely from an electrotonic influence on repolarization,[6] why does it last so long after the return to a normal activation pathway?[1,6,8] The answer appears to lie in the extraordinary sensitivity of the mechanisms that control functional expression of ion channels to environmental conditions, including the simple application of a ventricular pacing protocol and an altered activation pathway. In the remainder of this section, I shall illustrate the linkages that occur here.

Figure 9 shows the events that follow pacing the ventricle for a period of 21 days. Note that the T wave vector moves to approximate the QRS vector. Under these conditions there is no myocardial ischemia, no cardiac failure, and no cardiac hypertrophy.[6] Once this altered T wave occurs, anywhere from 1 week to well over 1 month is required for resolution. As shown in Figure 10, pharmacological inhibition of new protein synthesis markedly attenuates the accumulation of the T wave change.[6] Hence, it can be suggested that the altered activation pattern associated with pacing in turn alters the synthesis of protein structures that control repolarization.

That a very real change occurs in the cardiac action potential in this setting of cardiac memory was shown in experiments in which the action potential notch was decreased, the duration of the action potential was prolonged, and the gradient between epicardial, midmyocardial and endocardial fibers was altered as well (Figure 11). All this is consistent with altered ion channel function.

Given the loss of the action potential notch in epicardial myocytes, we studied I_{to}, the transient outward current responsible for phase 1 repolarization. The activation of the channel was moved positively from about -20 to -5 mV, and the recovery from inactivation was increased almost twenty-fold, from about 35 to 690 msec. Moreover, the density of the current was reduced by about $1/3$.[3] Of particular interest is that the message level for Kv4.3, the gene responsible for I_{to}, is also reduced by about $1/3$.[3]

VECTOROCARDIOGRAPHIC VIEW OF CM
frontal plane

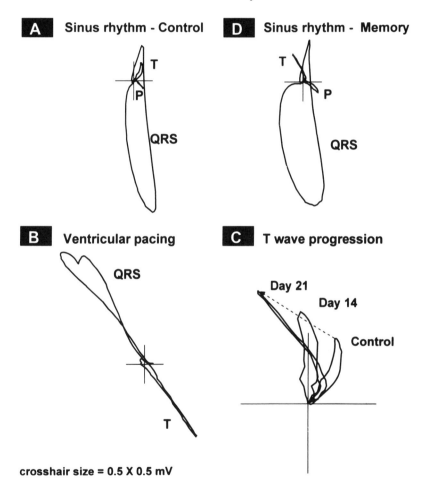

crosshair size = 0.5 X 0.5 mV

FIGURE 9: Frontal plane vectorcardiographic depiction of cardiac memory in a dog. Panel A shows P, QRS and T wave vectors in control, prior to the onset of pacing. Panel B depicts the QRS and T vectors during ventricular pacing. Panel C is the T wave vector alone (note enlarged scale as well as dotted line indicating the change in vector) during sinus rhythm in control (identical to panel A) and on days 14 and 21. Note the increase in amplitude of the vector as well as the shift in vector angle from that in control to one which approximates the QRS vector during pacing (panel B). In panel D is a record made within one hour of returning to sinus rhythm on day 21. (Reprinted by permission of the American Heart Association from reference 6).

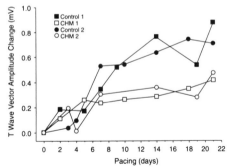

FIGURE 10: Effects of administration of cycloheximide (CHM) on evolution of cardiac memory in one dog. T wave vector amplitude change is used as the form of measurement here. Four consecutive experiments were done. The sequence was control 1-CHM 1-control 2-CHM 2. For control 1 a standard protocol was used to induce memory. Note the evolution of a steady state in T wave amplitude by about day 14. Complete resolution of the memory was then permitted, after which the animal was administered CHM and pacing was reinstituted. The result was only partial induction of memory, as seen in a curve that was displaced downward and to the right of control. Resolution of the memory process was permitted, after which a second control experiment was done. The results were nearly identical to the initial control. After resolution of the memory, a second course of CHM was given, and the pacing protocol again was repeated. In this case, the result was essentially identical to that of the initial CHM experiment. (Reprinted by permission of the American Heart Association from reference 6).

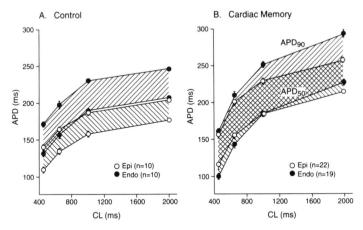

FIGURE 11: Action potential duration to 50% (APD_{50}) and 90% (APD_{90}) of repolarization measured from epicardium and endocardium of left ventricle in a control dog (panel A) and a dog with cardiac memory (panel B). Preparations were paced over a range of cycle lengths (horizontal axis) from 2000 to 400 msec. Three to 5 minutes were required for equilibration at each cycle length. Recordings were made at 10 minutes. Three sets of preparations were used per heart and multiple impalements were made per preparation. The shaded areas are those inscribed between APD_{50} and APD_{90} of the epicardial and the endocardial preparations. In panel A at almost all cycle lengths almost all values for endocardium differ from those at corresponding cycle lengths in epicardium (P<.05 for all). In panel B statistical significance (P<.05) was seen only for APD_{90} at the two longest cycle lengths. (Reprinted by permission of the American Heart Association from reference 6).

Hence it is clear that long-term pacing (and, by implication, cardiac arrhythmias) can induce T wave changes that reflect only the altered pattern of activation and no other pathological condition. If the same type of pacing protocol is applied for brief periods of time (i.e. 20-120 min) then the same pattern of T wave change occurs, but is of a duration that last minutes to hours, at most.[8] This short term memory has been studied from the point of view of its molecular signal transduction. Altering the pathway of activation of myocytes in tissue culture for brief periods, increases cellular synthesis of angiotensin II.[46] If we hypothesize that angiotensin II synthesis might be increased as a result of pacing the intact ventricle, then we would expect that interventions that either prevent angiotensin II synthesis (e.g. infusion of an ACE inhibitor or a tissue chymase inhibitor) or block at the level of the angiotensin II receptor will suppress the occurrence of this memory process. This, in fact, does occur, with either captopril or saralasin literally abolishing the expression and accumulation of the memory induced by short-term pacing.[47] Moreover, voltage clamp studies have shown that incubation with angiotensin II for a period of hours changes the threshold of activation of I_{to} in otherwise normal cardiac myocytes from around -22 to -5 mV and increases the time required for recovery from inactivation from about 25 to 490 msec[3] - precisely mirroring the changes shown above in I_{to} in the setting of cardiac memory.

Putting this information together, it would appear that pacing the ventricle and altering its pathway of activation triggers a signaling cascade (angiotensin II) that alters the function of I_{to} and also alters the synthesis of the I_{to} channel such that the memory process can accumulate and persist.[48] Therefore, it should be clear that the electrical events set into motion by pacing operate via complex pathways such that the modulation of ion channels is altered as is the expression of electrical activity.

There is an important interface between these findings and those that occur in pathological conditions. Angiotensin II is known to induce cardiac hypertrophy,[49] and one might hypothesize that long-term exposure to the stimuli that induce memory might result in the occurrence of hypertrophy as well. Moreover, in the setting of cardiac failure, in which there is myocyte hypertrophy, I_{to} function is altered significantly in a pattern not unlike that seen with memory.[50] Similarly, in myocardial infarction the peri-infarct zone of the heart is hypertrophied and changes in I_{to} are seen.[51] The point to be emphasized is that in a variety of settings that range from the physiological to the pathological, but in all of which there is an alteration of activation and/or alteration in a hypertrophic hormone, the ion channel used as an example, I_{to}, changes in a consistent direction. Using this information as a guideline, it is reasonable to test whether the electrocardiographic changes associated with memory are also indicators of likelihood, or at least risk, of imminent expression of cardiac pathology.

CONCLUSIONS

In the preceding pages, I have attempted to demonstrate that repolarization and the T wave must be thought of as much more than the result of electrical events. While the signals themselves are electrical their occurrence and the changes seen in them are the result of profound interactions that are molecular and biochemical. If we consider the etiology and the expression of these T wave changes in an electrical sense only, we will comprehend neither the mechanisms responsible for their occurrence nor the myriad possibilities that exist to return abnormal to normal function. Hence, the study of this important interface permits us not only to understand the elegant control mechanisms that exist but the very practical approaches to therapy and prevention that are afforded us.

REFERENCES

1. Katz AM: T Wave "Memory": Possible causal relationship to stress-induced changes in cardiac ion channels? *J Cardiovasc Electrophysiol.* 1992;3:150-159.
2. Roden DM, Lazzara R, Rosen M, Schwartz P, Towbin J, Vincent GM. Multiple mechanisms in the long-QT syndrome: Current knowledge, gaps, and future directions. *Circulation.* 1996;94:1996- 2012.
3. Yu H, McKinnon D, Dixon JE, Gao J, Wymore R, Cohen IS, Danilo P Jr, Shvilkin A, Anyukhovsky EP, Sosunov EA, Hara M, Rosen MR. The transient outward current, I_{to1}, is altered in cardiac memory. *Circulation. , in press.*
4. Rosenbaum MB, Blanco HH, Elizari MV, Lazzari JO, Davidenko JM. Electrotonic modulation of the T wave and cardiac memory. *Am J Cardiol.* 1982;50:213-222.
5. Chatterjee K, Harris AM, Davies JG, Leatham A. Electrocardiographic changes subsequent to artificial ventricular depolarization. *Br Heart J.* 1969;31:770-779.
6. Shvilkin A, Danilo P, Jr, Wang J, Burkhoff D, Anyukhovsky EP, Sosunov EA, Hara M, Rosen MR. The evolution and resolution of long-term cardiac memory. *Circulation.* 1998; 97:1810-1817.
7. Geller JC Rosen MR. Persistent T-wave changes after alteration of the ventricular activation sequence. New insights into cellular mechanisms of 'cardiac memory'. *Circulation.* 1993;88:1811- 1819.
8. del Balzo U, Rosen MR. T wave changes persisting after ventricular pacing in canine heart are altered by 4-aminopyridine but not by lidocaine. Implications with respect to phenomenon of cardiac 'memory'. *Circulation.* 1992;85:1464-1472.
9. Hille, B. *Ionic Channels of Excitable Membranes. 2nd Edition* Massachusetts: Sinauer Associates; 1992.
10. Hodgkin AL and Huxley AF. Currents carried by sodium and potassium ions through the membrane of the giant axon of *Loligo. J Physiol. (Lond.)* 1952a; 116:449-472.
11. Hodgkin AL and Huxley AF. The components of membrane conductance in the giant axon of *Loligo. J Physiol. (Lond.)* 1952b; 116:473-496.
12. Task Force of the Working Group on Arrhythmias of the European Society of Cardiology: The Sicilian Gambit. A New Approach to the Classification of Antiarrhythmic Drugs Based on Their Actions on Arrhythmogenic Mechanisms. *Circulation.* 1991;84:1831-1851.
13. Pelzer D, Pelzer S, MacDonald TF. Properties and regulation of calcium channels in muscle cells. *Rev Physiol Biochem Pharmacol.* 1990;114:107-207.
14. Hagiwara N, Irisawa H, Kasanuki H, Hosoda S. Background current in sinoatrial node cells of rabbit heart. *J Physiol. (Lond.)*;1992;448:53-72.
15. Coraboeuf E, Carmeliet E. Existence of two transient outward currents in sheep cardiac Purkinje fibers. *Pflügers Arch.* 1982;392:352-359.
16. Backx PH, Marban E. Background potassium current active during the plateau of the action potential in guinea pig ventricular myocytes. *Circ Res.* 1993;72:890-900.
17. Sanguinetti MC, Jurkiewicz NK. Role of external Ca^{2+} and K^+ in gating of cardiac delayed rectifier K^+ currents. *Pflügers Arch.* 1992;420:180-186.
18. Sicouri S, Antzelevitch C. A subpopulation of cells with unique electrophysiological properties in the deep subepicadium of the canine ventricle. The M cell. *Circ Res.* 1991;68:1729-1741.
19. Liu D-W, Antzelevitch C. Characteristics of the delayed rectifier current (I_{Kr} and I_{Ks}) in a canine epicardial, midmyocardial and endocardial myocytes. *Circ Res.* 1995;76:351-365.
20. Drouin E, Charpentier F, Gauthier C, et al: Electrophysiological characteristics of cells spanning the left ventricular wall of human heart. *J Am Coll Cardiol.* 1995;26:185-192.
21. Anyukhovsky EP, Sosunov EA, and Rosen MR. Regional differences in electrophysiological properties of epicardium, midmyocardium, and endocardium: in vitro and in vivo correlations. *Circulation.* 1996;94:1981-1988.

22. Litovsky SH, Antzelevitch C. Transient outward current prominent in canine ventricular epicardium but not in endocardium. *Circ Res.* 1988;62:116-125.

23. Liu DW, Gintant GA, Antzelevitch C. Ionic bases for electrophysiological distinctions among epicardial, midmyocardial and endocardial myocytes from the free wall of the canine left ventricle. *Circ Res.* 1993;72:671-687.

24. Weissenburger J, Nesterenko VV, Antzelevitch C. Intramural monophasic action potentials (MAP) display steeper APD-rate relations and higher sensitivity to class III agents than epicardial and endocardial MAPs: Characteristics of M cells in vivo. *Circulation.* 1995;92:I-300. (Abstract)

25. El-Sherif N, Caref E, Yin H, et al. The electrophysiological mechanism of ventricular arrhythmias in the long QT syndrome: Tridimensional mapping of activation and recovery patterns. *Circ Res.* 1996;79:474-492.

26. Anyukhovsky EP, Sosunov EA, Feinmark SJ, Rosen MR: Effects of quinidine on repolarization in canine epicardium, midmyocardium, and endocardium: II. In vivo study. *Circulation.* 1997;96:4019-4026.

27. Anyukhovsky EP, Sosunov EA, Gainullin RZ, Rosen MR. The controversial M cell. *J Cardiovasc Electrophysiol, in press.*

28. Jeck CD. Boyden PA. Age-related appearance of outward currents may contribute to developmental differences in ventricular repolarization. *Circ Res.* 1992;71:1390-1403.

29. Peter W. MacFarlane and T. D. Veitch Lawrie (eds.). Comprehensive Electrocardiology, Theory and Practice in Health and Disease, University of Glasgow, UK; Pergamon Press, Elmsford, N.Y., 1989.

30. Waldo AL, Camm AJ, Deruyter H, Friedman PL, Macneil DJ, Pauls JF, et al. Effect of d-sotalol on mortality in patients with left ventricular dysfunction after recent and remote myocardial infarction. *Lancet* 1996;348:7-12

31. Rosen MR. Of Oocytes and Runny Noses. *Circulation.* 1996;94:607-609.

32. Schwartz PJ. The *Long QT Syndrome-Clinical Approaches to Tachyarrhythmias series* - Camm AJ, editor. Armonk: Futura, 1997: 1-108.

33. Splawski I, Tristani-Firouzi M, Lehmann M, Sanguinetti M, Keating M. Mutations in the hminK gene cause long QT syndrome and suppress I_{Ks} function. *Nature Genetics.* 1997;17:338-340.

34. Curran ME, Splawski I, Timothy KW, Vincent GM, Green ED, Keating MT. A molecular basis for cardiac arrhythmia: *HERG* mutations cause long QT syndrome. *Cell.* 1995;80:795-80.

35. Sanguinetti MC, Jiang C, Curran ME, Keating MT. A mechanistic link between an inherited and an acquired cardiac arrhythmia: *HERG* encodes the I_{Kr} potassium channel. *Cell.* 1995;81:299-307.

36. Sanguinetti MC, Curran ME, Spector PS, Keating MT. Spectrum of HERG K^+ channel dysfunction in an inherited cardiac arrhythmia. *Proc Natl Acad Sci.* 1996a;93:2208-2212.

37. Sanguinetti MC, Curran ME, Zou A, Shen J, Spector PS, Atkinson DL, et al. Coassembly of $KvLQT_1$ and *minK* (IsK) proteins to form cardiac I_{Ks} potassium channel. *Nature.* 1996;384:80-83.

38. Wang Q, Shen J, Li Z, Timothy K, Vincent GM, Priori SG, et al. Cardiac sodium channel mutations in patients with long QT syndrome, an inherited cardiac arrhythmia. *Hum Molec Gen.* 1995;4:1603-1607.

39. Wang Q, Shen J, Splawski I, Atkinson D, Li Z. SCN5A mutations associated with an Inherited cardiac arrhythmia, long QT syndrome. *Cell.* 1995;80: 805-811.

40. Wang Q, Curran ME, Splawski I, Burn TC, Millholland JM, Vanraay TJ, et al. Positional cloning of a novel potassium channel gene: *KVLQT₁* mutations cause cardiac arrhythmias. *Nature Genetics.* 1996;12:17-23.

41. Schott JJ, Charpentier F, Peltier S, Foley P, Drouin E, Bouhour JB, et al. Mapping of a gene for long QT syndrome to chromosome 4q25-27. *Am J Hum Genet.* 1995;57:1114-1122.

42. Schwartz PJ, Priori SG, Locati EH, Napolitano C, Stramba-Badiale M, Diehl L, et al. QT_c responses to mexiletine and to heart rate changes differentiate LQT1 from LQT3 but not from LQT2 patients. *Circulation.* 1996;94:I-204. (Abstract).

43. Compton SJ, Lux RL, Ramsey MR, Strelich KR, Sanguinetti MC, Green LS, et al. Genetically defined therapy of inherited long-QT syndrome. Correction of abnormal repolarization by potassium. *Circulation.* 1996;94:1018-1022.

44. Members of the Sicilian Gambit. The search for novel antiarrhythmic strategies. *Eur Heart J.* 1998; 19:1178-1196.

45. Chen Q, Kirsch GE, Zhang D, Brugada R, Brugada J, Brugada P, et al. Genetic basis and molecular mechanism for idiopathic ventricular fibrillation. *Nature.*1998;392:293-296.

46. Sadoshima J-I, Izumo S. Mechanical stretch activates multiple signal transduction pathways in cardiac myocytes: Potential involvement of an autocrine/paracrine mechanism. *EMBO J.* 1993;12:1681-1692.

47. Ricard P, Yu H, Danilo P Jr, Gao J, Wymore R, Cohen IS, Rosen MR. The role of the renin-angiotensin II system in cardiac T-wave memory. *Circulation.* 1996;94:I-6. (Abstract)
48. Rosen MR, Cohen IS, Danilo P Jr, Steinberg SF. The heart remembers. *Cardiovascular Res., in press.*
49. Sadoshima J-I, Izumo S: Molecular characterization of angiotensin II-induced hypertrophy of cardiac myocytes and hyperplasia of cardiac fibroblasts. *Circ Res.* 1993;73:413-423.
50. Tomaselli GF, Beuckelmann DJ, Calkins HG, Berger RD, Kessler PD, Lawrence JH, Kass D, Feldman AM, Marban E. Sudden cardiac death in heart failure: The role of abnormal repolarization. *Circulation* . 1994;90:2534-2539.
51. Jeck C, Pinto JMB, Boyden PA. Transient outward currents in subendocardial Purkinje myocytes surviving in the 24 and 48 hr infarcted heart. *Circulation.* 1995;92:465-473.

10 SEXUAL DIMORPHISM IN CARDIOVASCULAR DISEASE

Stephen Bakir, M.D.
Suzanne Oparil, M.D.
University of Alabama at Birmingham

INTRODUCTION: EPIDEMIOLOGY OF CORONARY ARTERY DISEASE IN WOMEN

The United States has experienced an overall decline in mortality from cardiovascular disease during the past twenty years, but this rate of decline has been slower in women than men.[1] Although there has been an increasing awareness of cardiovascular disease in women over the past decade, this has not resulted in a decline in their rate of cardiovascular death. On the contrary, as the population ages, the percentage of women increases along with the absolute number of cardiovascular deaths in women (Figure 1).[1,2]

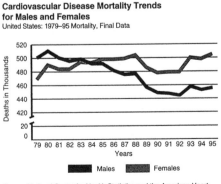

Cardiovascular Disease Mortality Trends for Males and Females
United States: 1979–95 Mortality, Final Data

Source: National Center for Health Statistics and the American Heart Association.

Figure 1. From reference 2 with permission

Cardiovascular disease is responsible for more than 500,000 female deaths each year, which accounts for 45.2% of all deaths in women - more than stroke and lung and breast cancers combined.[1,2] In 1997 alone, cardiovascular disease cost more than $250 billion and was the most common reason for hospital admission in both sexes.[1] Despite these sobering statistics, there is evidence that coronary disease may be underdiagnosed and undertreated in women in the United States.[3,4] This is true notwithstanding the long-recognized cardioprotective effects of estrogen in women.

Cardioprotective Effects of Estrogen

The gender differences in cardiovascular disease have largely been ascribed to the biologic effects of sex hormones. All sex hormones, androgens in men and estrogens in women, are steroids synthesized from the common precursor androstenedione, a cholesterol derivative. In premenopausal women, the major effector sex hormone is 17β-estradiol synthesized in the ovaries. Following menopause however, estrone, produced in fat tissue by the aromatization of testosterone, becomes the predominant estrogen[5]. Estrogens produce their biologic effect by binding to ligand specific soluble receptor molecules located inside the cell's nucleus, referred to as the *estrogen receptor*. Estrogen receptor-α is coded for by a gene of 140,000 base-pairs which is split into eight exons[6]. Its cDNA has an open reading frame of 1,785 nucleotides which is translated into a peptide of 595 amino acids with a molecular weight of 66,200 daltons[7,8]. This nuclear receptor molecule is not only expressed in reproductive tissues, but also found widely in other sites, including importantly the cardiovascular system. Both the estrogen receptor–α, as well as the more recently discovered 54,200 dalton estrogen receptor-β, have been found in vascular smooth muscle cells, including the coronary arteries and aorta, cardiac fibroblasts and cardiomyocytes. Moreover, estradiol itself is produced locally in both coronary arteries and cardiomyocytes by the aromatization of androgens; although it induces the expression of estrogen receptor only in females[9-11]. Although expressed in diverse tissues, the individual biologic consequence of estrogen receptor activation is controlled by the presence of other tissue specific co-activators[5].

Estrogens are lipid soluble molecules which pass through cell membranes and migrate to the nucleus where they bind to a hydrophobic ligand binding pocket in the estrogen receptor[12]. This appears to cause the dissociation of a molecule of heat shock protein-90 (Hsp-90), which in turn allows the homodimerization of two estrogen receptor molecules and their activation by conformational alteration[13,14]. Once activated, the estrogen:estrogen receptor complex, along with tissue-specific co-activators[15,16]attach to specific non-coding enhancer sequences upstream of estrogen responsive genes. These *estrogen responsive elements* (ERE's) are fifteen nucleotide long sequences composed of two 6 base-pair palindromic half-sites separated by a 3 base-pair spacer[13,14,17]. Site-specific recognition and attachment occurs through the tertiary structure of the estrogen receptor DNA-binding domain. This sixty-six amino acid sequence forms two *zinc fingers*, specialized DNA binding structures, which bind to the two palindromic half-sites in the ERE[18].

Transactivation of estrogen responsive genes, that is genes with an ERE in their enhancer region, is followed by transcription of the specified proteins, in our case proteins related to cardiovascular biology. (See discussion in Chapter One).

The main biologic response to estrogen responsible for sexual dimorphism in cardiovascular disease has classically been thought to relate to the differences in lipid profiles of women and men. Estrogens have been seen as cardioprotective as a consequence of premenopausal women's lower LDL and higher HDL[19,20]. Strong supportive evidence comes from the loss of this protective lipid pattern following menopause and its continuation with estrogen replacement therapy. However, there have been recent observations suggesting important alternative estrogen effects in the cardiovascular system, as will be detailed throughout this chapter. For example, as already noted, estrogens can induce the expression of estrogen receptor in the coronary arteries of women, but not of men.

Sudden Cardiac Death

Sudden cardiac death, natural death from cardiovascular causes within one hour of onset of symptoms, is responsible for over 300,000 deaths in the US each year, with an incidence of 0.1 - 0.2 % per year. CHD is the etiology of 80% of these, and up to one half of all coronary artery deaths are unexpected and sudden[21,22]. In the 26-year follow up of the Framingham study, 320 men and 146 women died of CHD. There were 146 male and 50 female sudden, unexpected deaths. Of these, 1/2 of the male compared to 2/3 of the female sudden deaths occurred in patients without previously diagnosed CHD.[23] Several other epidemiologic studies and autopsy series have observed this interesting paradox: while the overall incidence of sudden cardiac death is much greater in men than in women, women are more likely to experience sudden death as the first manifestation of their CHD.

The disparity in the prevalence of sudden death with respect to gender is most notable in younger age groups, and trends towards "equalization" as age progresses.[21] The excess of sudden, unexpected cardiac deaths as the first manifestation of CHD in younger women is likely due to a different pathophysiological mechanism from that seen in men. Younger women who experience sudden cardiac death have different risk factors than either older women or men. Further, the dogma that the initial acute event in unstable coronary syndromes is rupture of the lipid laden atherosclerotic plaque does not seem to apply to women - particularly young women with sudden cardiac death. While this process indeed occurs in the majority of acute coronary events in men, recent data point to more heterogeneity in this process in women. In two recent autopsy series of women and men who died suddenly, a substantial percentage (44%) of the lesions involved a thrombus overlying an *eroded* but not *ruptured* plaque (Figure 2).[24,25]

In the recent series of sudden deaths in women reported by Burke et al, there was a notable difference in plaque morphology in younger (presumably premenopausal) as compared to older (presumably postmenopausal) women. Thirty-five percent of the series exhibited eroded (but not ruptured) plaques with an overlying thrombus. Fifty nine percent of the women in this series were under 50 years of age. There were also some notable differences in risk factor profile between younger and older women. In cases of plaque erosion in younger women, the only major atherosclerotic risk factor identified was smoking. For the most part, these women were previously young and healthy without hypercholesterolemia, obesity or diabetes.[25] In older women, more traditional *ruptured* plaques were observed in combination with healed areas of myocardial infarction. The traditional risk factors of elevated total cholesterol, diabetes and hypertension were more common in this group.[25] This would seem to suggest differing strategies of risk factor reduction in different age groups.

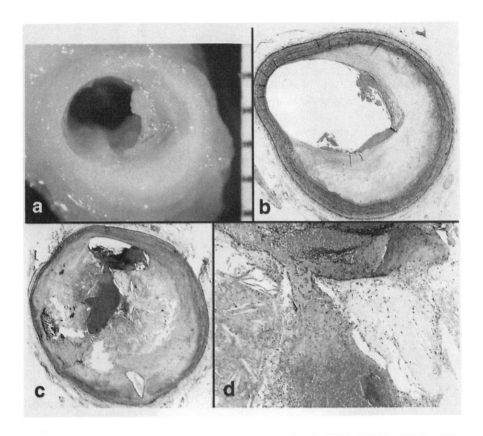

Figure 2. Substrates of acute coronary thrombosis. A. Plaque erosion: eccentric plaque with overlying subocclusive thrombosis. The narrowing is not critical, and disruption of the cap is absent. B. Microscopic illustration of plaque demonstrates thrombus overlying intact plaque. The patient was a 58 year-old smoker with a history of emphysema but no heart disease. She recently complained of chest pain but was not extensively evaluated. She had an apparent seizure and developed cardiac arrest from which she could not be resuscitated. C. Plaque rupture: critical narrowing of this section of the left anterior descending artery by atheroma rich in cholesterol crystals. Central hemorrhage into plaque is continuous with the small residual lumen above. Black reflects the postmortem injection of contrast material D. Higher magnification of C demonstrates rupture site. From reference 25 with permission.

In addition to the differences is plaque morphology, there are distinct electrophysiologic gender differences promoting arrhythmia and sudden death in women. As noted by Rosen in the previous Chapter, there is a gender difference in the inward rectifying potassium current in ventricular myocardium leading to an increased heterogeneity of repolarization. This makes women more susceptible to the fatal arrhythmias associated with the long QT syndrome as well as drugs which increase   repolarization, such as certain antihistamines (pages 173-175). Furthermore, estrogen receptor has been shown to regulate the density of the slow L-type calcium channels such that decreased estrogen may lead to an increase in their number with a concomitant increase in excitability and risk of arrhythmia[26]. On the other hand, estrogen may decrease the susceptibility to lethal arrhythmias by reducing the expression of the sodium/calcium exchanger associated with ischemia and reperfusion injury[27].

Perhaps the most striking barrier to reducing sudden death in women is the absence of premonitory signs and symptoms. In the Burke series, only 22 % of the sudden deaths that were witnessed were preceded by chest pain.   Thirty-three percent of sudden death victims complained of symptoms other than chest pain, such as back pain, dizziness, fever, shortness of breath or malaise.   Forty-five percent of the coronary deaths were preceded by no symptoms whatsoever. Moreover, only 18% of the women had a history of diagnosed heart disease. The absence of accurate predictors of sudden death combined with the hazard to the individual and to the public (e.g. when an affected individual is driving) makes sudden death - particularly sudden death in women - a challenging area in need of investigation.

ACUTE MYOCARDIAL INFARCTION

Outcome data from numerous studies appear to indicate that women have a higher mortality rate than men after myocardial infarction, likely because women are generally older and have more comorbid conditions when they are diagnosed with coronary disease.   In 1995, Vaccarino et al. reviewed the literature on gender differences in mortality after myocardial infarction and found that most of the increased female mortality after myocardial infarction was attributable to age. After adjustment for age and other factors predictive of mortality - such as previous coronary disease, hypertension, diabetes, and a history of congestive heart failure - mortality in women was comparable to that in men.[28]   More recent studies have reported similar results.   In a retrospective analysis of the Thrombolysis in Myocardial Infarction III B (TIMI IIIB) population, women experienced similar rates of death, reinfarction, and recurrent ischemia as men. Women tended to have less severe coronary disease, and it could be argued that their incidence of events should have been lower.   However, age was a significant factor in that elderly patients (including a higher percentage of women) had higher rates of the endpoints mentioned.[29]   The Myocardial Infarction Triage and Intervention Registry (MITI) study did not show a significant difference in total mortality between the sexes.

Women did tend to have more recurrent angina and bleeding complications, but there were no differences in the incidence of congestive heart failure, need for temporary pacemaker, stroke or recurrent infarction.[3] In the Global Utilization of Streptokinase and Tissue Plasminogen Activator for Occluded Coronary Arteries (GUSTO) trial, despite the higher stroke rates in women, there was no mortality difference between men and women.[30]

Although there are data suggestive of differing practices of diagnosis and treatment of coronary heart disease (CHD) in women, there are regional variations, and a considerable amount of equally convincing data shows no bias against women. The outcome data are difficult to evaluate because of the many confounding variables, but if age is taken into account, there are no striking differences between the sexes with respect to survival post myocardial infarction.

In the following pages, we will further explore some of the issues dealing with the sexual dimorphism of CHD, including gender differences in prevalence, diagnosis, and treatment. We will restrict our discussion to CHD and some of the factors that contribute to the sexual dimorphism in its prevalence and clinical manifestations. We will not address other forms of cardiovascular disease such as stroke, peripheral vascular disease, and end stage renal disease, which are also common in women and are consequences of the same set of risk factors.

TRADITIONAL RISK FACTORS FOR CORONARY HEART DISEASE

The major risk factors for CHD are similar in both sexes, but some gender differences have been described. The major modifiable cardiovascular risk factors are cigarette smoking, diabetes mellitus, dyslipidemia, systolic and diastolic hypertension, obesity, and sedentary lifestyle. Some relative newcomers to this list are hyperhomocysteinemia, fibrinogen, plasminogen activator inhibitor-1 (PAI-1), and other clotting factors. Though we will not discuss each of these risk factors in depth, we will address the major areas of discrepancies between men and women. Following each section are suggestions for optimal risk reduction in women as modified from an AHA/ACC consensus statement on risk factors for CHD in women.[31]

Cigarette Smoking. Cigarette smoking is the leading *preventable* cause of death for men and women in the United States; more than 50% of myocardial infarctions in middle aged women can be attributed to tobacco.[32] The risk of cardiovascular disease is increased with minimal exposure to cigarettes (1 to 4 per day), and is incremental with the number of cigarettes smoked per day (Figure 3).[32,33] Observational studies have consistently shown that smoking increases mortality from CHD by up to 70%.[32] Passive exposure to cigarette smoke has also been associated with a threefold increase in relative risk of CHD mortality in individuals who lived with current or former smokers compared to people who had never smoked.[22]

It is uncertain whether smoking affects the sexes differentially, but smoking is synergistic with other risk factors associated with CHD – especially the use of oral contraceptives.[22,34] The excess cardiovascular risk associated with smoking is reversible, with the risk of CHD declining within months of smoking cessation. However, smoking rates are declining more slowly in women than men in the United States, and some sources report increasing smoking rates in younger women.[1,22,32] This is troublesome when considering the future prevalence of CHD in women.

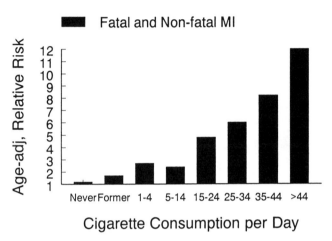

Figure 3. Smoking and CHD risk (from reference 33 with permission)

Goals:
- **Complete cessation**
- **Avoid passive smoke**

Diabetes. Diabetes mellitus is the cardiovascular risk factor with the most pronounced gender difference in its effect on atherosclerosis and cardiovascular events. It is a more powerful predictor of CHD in women than in men, and provides more prognostic information about female patients than any other traditional cardiovascular risk factor.[32,34] In the Nurses' Health Study, maturity onset diabetes was associated with a three to sevenfold increase in cardiovascular events.[35] In most studies, the increase in relative risk for cardiovascular disease in diabetic vs. nondiabetic women is twice that seen in diabetic vs. nondiabetic men.[36] Diabetes also increases mortality after myocardial infarction more in women than in men.[22]

The mechanism(s) of the association between diabetes and atherosclerotic vascular disease are incompletely defined, but candidates include hyperglycemia, hyperinsulinemia, dyslipidemia, and hypertension. Control of hyperglycemia will reduce the progression of the microvascular complications of diabetes (retinopathy and proteinuria), but the link between hyperglycemia and macrovascular complications is less clear. Epidemiologic evidence has shown that elevated plasma fasting glucose concentrations and increased glycosylated hemoglobin percentages are associated with an increased risk of cardiovascular events. However, the University Group Diabetes Program (UGDP) found that improved glycemic control, by any therapy, did not reduce the risk of cardiovascular endpoints. Two additional studies from the United Kingdom Prospective Diabetes Study Group (UKPDS) confirmed this finding.[37,38]

Hyperinsulinemia (endogenous or exogenous) has been implicated in atheroma formation. Prospective studies in both men and women have found a weak and inconclusive association between plasma insulin levels and coronary heart disease. The "metabolic syndrome" of elevated insulin, triglyceride, and PAI-1 levels, hypertension, and low HDL levels has been called the "metabolic syndrome X". It is associated with a stronger predisposition toward atherosclerosis in women than in men[22,39] However, much more investigation is needed to clarify the role of each of these factors in the pathogenesis of CHD in women.

Current evidence suggests that the best strategy for reducing CHD in women with diabetes involves controlling the concomitant risk factors. Along with vigilant control of hypertension and reasonable glucose control (maintenance of HbA1c < 7%), a recent AHA/ACC consensus panel recommended keeping the low density lipoprotein cholesterol (LDL-C) value below 130mg/dL in diabetic women without known CHD.[31] For those women with known CHD, LDL-C should be <100mg/dL. Of note, however, is the growing opinion that the LDL value should be < 100mg/dL in *all* men and women with diabetes[40] It is also recommended that triglyceride levels be kept <150mg/dL in diabetic patients.

Goals:
- **Maintain reasonable glucose control with HbA1c <7%; post prandial blood glucose 80 - 120mg/dL; and bedtime blood glucose 100 - 140mg/Dl.**
- **LDL-C < 100 mg/dL**
- **Triglycerides < 150 mg/dL**
- **Tight blood pressure control (BP< 130/85)[41]**

Dyslipidemia. Premenopausal women have long been recognized as being at relatively lower risk for coronary heart disease due to the association of estrogen with lower LDL-C and higher high density lipoprotein cholesterol (HDL-C). Recent evidence suggests that this phenomenon may operate via LDL receptor (LDL-R) independent pathways. For example, estrogen can reduce cholesterol by inducing the expression of hepatic cholesterol-7-α-hydroxylase, the rate limiting enzyme in the liver's conversion of cholesterol to bile acid without a change in LDL-R[42]. In fact, cholesterol-fed mice in which LDL-R has been genetically removed have reduced atherosclerosis when treated with 17β-estradiol[43]. We have already discussed how cardiovascular sexual dimorphism is not entirely estrogen receptor dependent, in that this molecule is estrogen inducible only in the coronary arteries of women. On the other hand, mutation of the estrogen receptor gene in men might be a cryptic risk factor for coronary disease[44]. One must also be aware of the effect on coronary risk of the anti-estrogen drugs currently being used for the treatment and prevention of breast cancer[45,46].

An elevated level of HDL-C is strongly associated with a lower risk of CHD in women.[39] In the Lipid Research Clinics Follow-up Study, HDL-C was second only to age as a predictor of CHD risk in women.[32] The association between HDL-C and coronary heart disease is stronger in women than men,[21] and elevated triglycerides are also more predictive of coronary disease in women than in men. This is particularly true in older women.[32,34]

The end of the 20th century has been marked by many well conceived and well-conducted prospective placebo controlled lipid reduction trials in different patient populations. Most of the recent trials have involved the 3-hydroxy-3-methylglutaryl coenzyme A (HMG-CoA) reductase inhibitors (statins). These trials have shown that treatment with statins can reduce coronary events in patients with elevated or even average cholesterol levels. While the number of women studied was limited in earlier investigations, data for women have markedly increased since 1994.

The Scandinavian Simvastatin Survival Study (4S) was a trial of secondary prevention for CHD, and women comprised approximately 20% of 4444 patients in the study. The women that received simvastatin had a decrease in major coronary events similar to that seen in men. While there was not a significant mortality reduction in women on simvastatin, there were only 52 deaths in women, and showing survival benefit would, therefore, be difficult.[47] The Cholesterol and Recurrent Events (CARE) trial was another secondary prevention study in patients (14% women) with average cholesterol levels. The decrease in major coronary events (defined as CHD death, nonfatal MI, or revascularization) for women who received pravastatin was double that seen in men, and the benefits were seen earlier in women than men (Figure 4).[48,49]

The AFCAPS/TexCAPS trial (Air Force/Texas Coronary Atherosclerosis Prevention Study) enrolled generally healthy, middle-aged and older men and women (17%) with no previous coronary events and average cholesterol levels. The entry criteria included LDL-C between 130-190mg/dL, and HDL-C ≤ 45 mg/dL for men and 47mg/dL for women. Therefore, these patients were not eligible for drug therapy under the current National Cholesterol Education Program (NCEP) guidelines. The study demonstrated a reduction in coronary events in the treatment group that was greater (but not statistically different) in women than in men.[50]

Despite ample knowledge of the benefits of lowering cholesterol with respect to CHD, physicians (as a whole) do a poor job of applying this to patient care - particularly in women. The Heart and Estrogen/Progestin Replacement Study (HERS) was a secondary prevention study of hormone replacement in postmenopausal women with known coronary disease.[51] A subgroup analysis of cholesterol levels in the women enrolled in the study revealed that 91% of the participants exceeded the 1993 LDL-C treatment goal of 100mg/dL. This was despite the fact that 47% of the study participants were taking lipid-lowering medication.[52]

Data from the AFCAPS/TexCAPS trial and current perspectives on gender differences regarding HDL-C, triglycerides and CHD risk will likely be

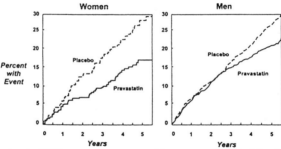

Figure 4. Reduction in CHD events in women with average cholesterol levels using pravastatin (reproduced from reference 49 with permission)

incorporated into future recommendations for the treatment of dyslipidemia in women. Current evidence supports the goals below.

Goals:
- **Low risk (< 2 risk factors) LDL < 160mg/dL (optimal <130mg/dL)**
- **Intermediate risk (≥ 2 risk factors) LDL-C <100mg/dL**
- **Established CHD LDL-C < 100mg/dL**

Obesity and Sedentary Lifestyle. America is becoming a nation of obese individuals, and this is true for both sexes. The Nurses' Health Study found that the risk of CHD was three times higher in women with a body-mass index of 29 or higher (BMI = weight in kilograms / height in square meters). Central, visceral, or "android" obesity is particularly concerning, with the risk of coronary disease rising steeply in women with a waist-to-hip ratio of 0.8 or greater. Visceral obesity is associated with dyslipidemia, insulin resistance, diabetes and CHD in women and men.[39,40]

The benefits of physical activity are well documented in men. The few studies that gave gender specific information showed a 50% reduction in CHD risk in active vs inactive women. Despite this, most women in the United States are sedentary. The level of activity does not need to be intensive to reduce cardiovascular risk: 30 to 45 minutes of walking three times per week reduces risk by up to 50%.[22]

Goals (weight):
- **Achieve and maintain desirable weight**
- **Target BMI between 18.5 - 24.9 kg/m^2**
- **Desirable waist circumference < 88cm or < 35in**

Goals (physical activity):
- **Accumulate at least 30 minutes of moderate intensity physical activity on most, and preferably all days**

Women with recent cardiovascular events or procedures should participate in a cardiac rehabilitation program, a physician-guided home exercise program, or a comprehensive secondary prevention program

Hypertension. There is a sexually dimorphic pattern of hypertension development in humans.[1,53] (Figure 5). Gender differences in blood pressure emerge during adolescence and persist through adulthood. Men tend to have higher mean systolic and diastolic blood pressure than women (by 6-7 mm Hg and 3-5 mm Hg, respectively), and through middle age, hypertension is more prevalent among men than among women. However, hypertension, particularly systolic hypertension, is more prevalent among women than among men after age 59.

Prevalence of Hypertension by Gender and Age

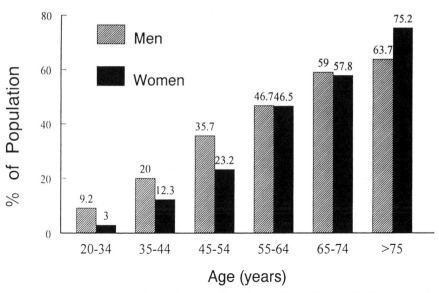

Figure 5. Sexual dimorphism in the development of hypertension (from reference 65 with permission)

The influence of menopause on blood pressure in women is controversial. Longitudinal studies from Framingham, Allegheny County, and the Netherlands did not document a rise in blood pressure with menopause. In contrast, cross-sectional studies from Belgium and the U.S. found significantly higher systolic blood pressure and diastolic blood pressure in postmenopausal compared to premenopausal women[54] The Belgian study reported a fourfold higher prevalence of hypertension in postmenopausal women than in premenopausal women (40% vs. 10%, P < 001). After adjusting for age and BMI, postmenopausal women were still more than twice as likely to have hypertension as premenopausal women. Enhanced stress-induced cardiovascular responses and higher ambulatory blood pressures have also been documented in normotensive postmenopausal compared to premenopausal women.[55] A menopause-related increase in blood pressure has been attributed to a variety of factors, including estrogen withdrawal, overproduction of pituitary hormones, weight gain, or a combination of these and other, yet undefined, neurohumoral influences. Further research is needed to elucidate the effects of the sex hormones and their withdrawal on blood pressure. Elderly (postmenopausal) women appear to be more NaCl-sensitive than men.[56] NaCl sensitivity has been shown to correlate inversely with levels of circulating ovarian hormones in postmenopausal Japanese women. Circulating levels of prolactin, estrogen, and progesterone were significantly lower in the hypertensives compared to the normotensives, suggesting that decreases in sex hormones and increased sensitivity to dietary NaCl may contribute to the pathogenesis of postmenopausal hypertension.[57]

Certain conflicting biologic effects have been reported for estrogens. Estrogens have been reported to both increase[58,59] and decrease[60] cardiac fibroblast proliferation, suggesting an important potential effect on cardiac remodeling in response to increased blood pressure. Estradiol both downregulates the expression of the angiotensin-II receptor AT-1R[61] (see Chapter 6), while estrogen receptor binds to the angiotensinogen gene promotor inducing its expression[62]. Nevertheless, estrogens have consistently been shown to have a arteriodilatory effect. This may operate via angiotensin-II, endothelin-1 or perhaps through a direct membrane effect[63,64].

AWARENESS, TREATMENT, AND CONTROL OF HIGH BLOOD PRESSURE IN WOMEN

Women are more likely than men to be aware that they are hypertensive, to be receiving antihypertensive treatment, and to have their blood pressure controlled (Figure 6).[53,65] In NHANES III, approximately 75% of non-Hispanic black and white women were aware of their high BP, while only 65% of men in these groups were so informed. Similarly, 61% of hypertensive women, but only 44% of men, were being treated with antihypertensive medication. Finally, 28% of women overall and 19% of men had their blood pressure controlled (<140/90 mm Hg). Further, in developed countries worldwide, hypertensive women are 1.33 fold (95% CI = 1.32-1.34) more likely to be treated with antihypertensive drugs than are hypertensive men.[66] On average, 66% of hypertensive women but only 48% of hypertensive men were receiving antihypertensive drugs according to this review. The higher antihypertensive treatment rates in women have been attributed to increased numbers of physician contacts because of visits for reproductive health and child care, as well as a lower probability of employment outside the home. It is encouraging that women are attentive to their own health needs in the area of hypertension and blood pressure control. This finding bodes well for the future cardiovascular health of women in the aging population.

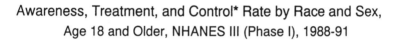

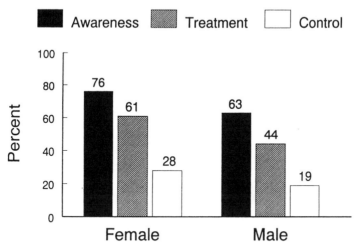

*Proportion of persons with hypertension who are controlled to < 140/90 mmHg

Figure 6. From reference 65 with permission

ORAL CONTRACEPTIVES AND BLOOD PRESSURE

The entire population of women taking oral contraceptives, most of whom are normotensive, experience a small but detectable increase in blood pressure; a small percentage experience the onset of frank hypertension, which resolves with withdrawal of oral contraceptive therapy.[67] This is true even with modern preparations that contain only 30 µg estrogen.[68] This observation has recently been validated with ambulatory blood pressure recording, the most accurate means of assessing blood pressure over time in free living individuals (Figure 7).[69]

The Nurses' Health Study found that current users of oral contraceptives had a significantly increased [Relative Risk (RR) = 1.8; 95% Confidence Interval (CI) = 1.5-2.3] risk of hypertension compared with never users.[55] Of note, absolute risk was small: only 41.5 cases of hypertension/10,000 person-years could be attributed to oral contraceptive use. Risk decreased quickly with cessation of contraceptive use: past users had only a slightly increased risk (RR= 1.2; 95% CI=1.0-1.4) compared to never users. Blood pressure generally returns to pretreatment levels within 3 months of discontinuing oral contraceptives, indicating that their blood pressure effect is relatively acute and readily reversible. Nevertheless, oral contraceptives occasionally cause accelerated, or malignant, hypertension.[67] Genetic characteristics, such as family history of hypertension, as well as environmental characteristics, including pre-existing pregnancy-induced hypertension, occult renal disease, obesity, middle age (>35 years), and duration of

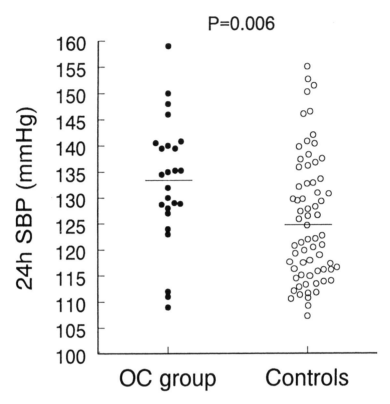

Figure 7. Blood pressure and oral contraceptive use (from reference 69 with permission)
oral contraceptive use, increase susceptibility to oral contraceptive-induced
hypertension.[67]

A family history of hypertension and a personal history of renal disease, or of
pregnancy-induced hypertension, are relative contraindications to oral contraceptive
use. Women over 35 years of age, particularly if obese, should be cautioned about
the risk of developing hypertension while taking oral contraceptives and should be
followed closely and their blood pressures measured on several occasions during
the first year of treatment and annually thereafter. Contraceptive-induced
hypertension can be diagnosed by documenting the onset of hypertension de novo
during contraceptive therapy, along with resolution of the hypertension on drug
withdrawal. The mechanism of the hypertension is unclear, but appears to be
related to the progestational potency, not the estrogenic potency, of the
preparation[68] The risk of hypertension is greater among users of monophasic
combination oral contraceptives than among users of biphasic or triphasic
combinations, perhaps because the total dose of progestin delivered is greater with
the monophasic preparation.

Women suffer from cardiovascular complications of hypertension, and their lives are shortened if blood pressure is not adequately controlled. The ultimate goal of antihypertensive treatment in women is the prevention of cardiovascular morbidity and mortality. Most of the large multicenter trials of antihypertensive therapy with "hard" end points have included slightly larger numbers of women than men, but none included enough women to analyze data from gender subgroups convincingly. Subgroup analyses from individual trials have yielded variable results regarding the risk/benefit ratio of pharmacological treatment of hypertension in women. These findings have led some to conclude that women derive less benefit than men from antihypertensive treatment. A subgroup meta-analysis of individual patient data according to sex based on seven trials from the INDANA (INdividual Data ANalysis of Antihypertensive intervention trials) database was recently carried out in order to assess treatment effect by sex and determine whether there are gender differences.[70] These trials included 20,802 women and 19,975 men recruited between 1972 and 1990 and treated with thiazide diuretics and/or beta blockers. In women, significant treatment benefits included reductions in strokes (total and fatal) and major cardiovascular events (Figure 8). In men, treatment benefits were significant for all seven outcomes considered. Expressed as relative risk, treatment benefits did not differ between the sexes. Absolute risk reduction, in contrast, is dependent on untreated risk. Untreated risk for stroke was similar in the two sexes, and for coronary events, was greater in men. Accordingly, absolute risk reduction for stroke attributed to treatment was similar in men and women, and for coronary events, was greater in men.

These results cannot be extrapolated to the newer classes of antihypertensive drugs without further research. Ongoing prospective clinical trials are examining this question, and the INDANA Group plans to review these trials. In the interim, since a major benefit of antihypertensive treatment is prevention of stroke, and the risk of stroke is similar in both sexes, it is reasonable to conclude that, in general, the sex of the patient should not play a role in decisions about whether or not to treat high blood pressure.[70] Whether the threshold for pharmacologic treatment of hypertension should be higher for young women (minor contributors to the INDANA study population) than for older women and men because of their low cardiovascular risk is currently being debated.[71]

GENERAL CONSIDERATIONS IN CHOICE OF ANTIHYPERTENSIVE DRUGS

The blood pressure lowering effect of antihypertensive drugs is generally similar in the two sexes, but some special considerations may dictate treatment choices for women. Beta-adrenergic blockers tend to be less effective than in men.[72] Diuretics are particularly useful in women, particularly elderly women, because their use may be associated with decreased bone loss and reduced risk of hip fracture.[73] Diuretics are the favorite antihypertensive drug class for the treatment of women throughout the world, while beta blockers, angiotensin converting enzyme (ACE) inhibitors

EFFECTS OF ANTIHYPERTENSIVE TREATMENT BY SEX

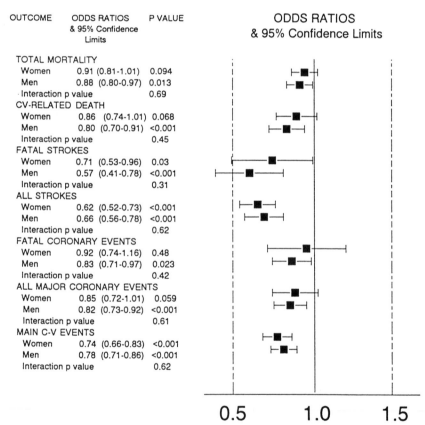

OUTCOME	ODDS RATIOS & 95% Confidence Limits	P VALUE
TOTAL MORTALITY		
Women	0.91 (0.81-1.01)	0.094
Men	0.88 (0.80-0.97)	0.013
Interaction p value		0.69
CV-RELATED DEATH		
Women	0.86 (0.74-1.01)	0.068
Men	0.80 (0.70-0.91)	<0.001
Interaction p value		0.45
FATAL STROKES		
Women	0.71 (0.53-0.96)	0.03
Men	0.57 (0.41-0.78)	<0.001
Interaction p value		0.31
ALL STROKES		
Women	0.62 (0.52-0.73)	<0.001
Men	0.66 (0.56-0.78)	<0.001
Interaction p value		0.62
FATAL CORONARY EVENTS		
Women	0.92 (0.74-1.16)	0.48
Men	0.83 (0.71-0.97)	0.023
Interaction p value		0.42
ALL MAJOR CORONARY EVENTS		
Women	0.85 (0.72-1.01)	0.059
Men	0.82 (0.73-0.92)	<0.001
Interaction p value		0.61
MAIN C-V EVENTS		
Women	0.74 (0.66-0.83)	<0.001
Men	0.78 (0.71-0.86)	<0.001
Interaction p value		0.62

ODDS RATIOS
& 95% Confidence Limits

0.5   1.0   1.5

CV=Cardiovascular
Interaction p value=significance of difference in odds ratios
between women and men

Figure 8. Gender differences in the effects of antihypertensive treatment (from reference 70 with permission)

and calcium channel blockers are more often prescribed for men.[66] Women tend to report more symptoms related to both their hypertension and their antihypertensive drugs, so treatment choices may depend more on adverse effect profile than on efficacy of a particular agent. Women are particularly vulnerable to ACE-inhibitor-induced cough,[74] calcium channel blocker-induced edema, and minoxidil-induced hirsutism. Further, ACE inhibitors and angiotensin II type 1 (AT_1) receptor blockers are contraindicated for women who are or intend to become pregnant because of the risk of fetal developmental abnormalities.

Goals:

- Achieve and maintain blood pressure (BP) <140/90mmHg and lower if tolerated
- Optimal pressure is <120/80 (note lower treatment goals in women with diabetes and renal disease with proteinuria)
- Begin therapy with lifestyle modification (weight loss, physical activity, moderation in alcohol intake, and moderate sodium restriction)
- If BP remains ≥ 140/90 or if initial level is >160mmHg systolic or 100mmHg diastolic, initiate or individualize pharmacotherapy
- In pregnant women, reduce diastolic pressure to 90 to 100mmHg if possible; attempt to minimize short term risk of elevated BP to mother while avoiding therapy that would compromise the health of the fetus

NEWER RISK FACTORS

Newer risk factors, including hyperhomocysteinemia, C-reactive protein (CRP) and clotting factors such as plasminogen activator inhibitor (PAI-1), lipoprotein [a], fibrinogen, and von Willebrand factor, have been identified for CHD. Few gender specific data (for women) concerning these risk factors are available. However, as our understanding of the pathogenesis of atherosclerosis and acute ischemic events progresses, these factors may emerge as having predictive value. Finding accurate predictors of individuals at risk for CHD and sudden death is particularly important in younger women, given their propensity to present in a catastrophic fashion.

Homocysteine. Hyperhomocysteinemia has recently been recognized as an independent risk factor for arterial occlusive disease. Homocysteine is an amino acid formed as an intermediate during methionine metabolism. It is metabolized by transsulfuration to glutathione or remythelation in a salvage pathway (Figure 9).[75] While severe hyperhomocysteinemia is rare, mildly elevated homocysteine levels are present in 5% to 7% of the general population. These individuals are typically asymptomatic until the third or fourth decades of life, when they are at risk for coronary artery disease and arterial and venous thromboses.

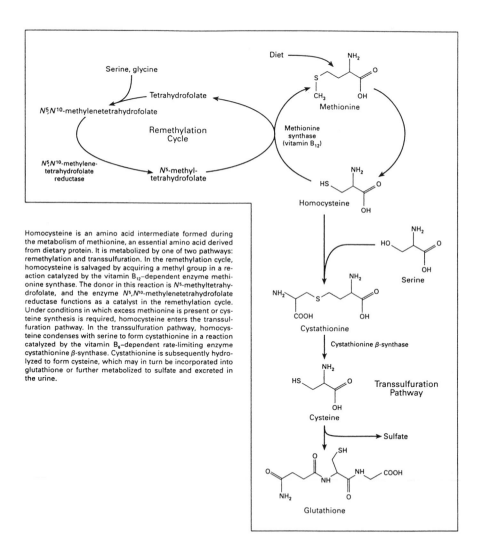

Homocysteine is an amino acid intermediate formed during the metabolism of methionine, an essential amino acid derived from dietary protein. It is metabolized by one of two pathways: remethylation and transsulfuration. In the remethylation cycle, homocysteine is salvaged by acquiring a methyl group in a reaction catalyzed by the vitamin B_{12}–dependent enzyme methionine synthase. The donor in this reaction is N^5-methyltetrahydrofolate, and the enzyme N^5,N^{10}-methylenetetrahydrofolate reductase functions as a catalyst in the remethylation cycle. Under conditions in which excess methionine is present or cysteine synthesis is required, homocysteine enters the transsulfuration pathway. In the transsulfuration pathway, homocysteine condenses with serine to form cystathionine in a reaction catalyzed by the vitamin B_6–dependent rate-limiting enzyme cystathionine β-synthase. Cystathionine is subsequently hydrolyzed to form cysteine, which may in turn be incorporated into glutathione or further metabolized to sulfate and excreted in the urine.

Figure 9. Homocysteine metabolism (from reference 75 with permission)

Elevated plasma homocysteine concentrations are most commonly caused by nutritional deficiencies or by genetic defects in the enzymes involved in homocysteine metabolism. Homozygous mutations in the cystathionine - synthase and the N^5,N^{10}-Methylene-tetrahydrofolate reductase genes cause severe hyperhomocysteinemia with resulting skeletal deformities, mental retardation, thromboembolism, and severe, premature atherosclerosis.[75] Heterozygous mutations, however, are relatively common in the general population, and cause milder elevations in plasma homocysteine levels with milder clinical manifestations. Nutritional deficiencies of one or more of the vitamin cofactors involved in homocysteine breakdown (folate, vitamin B12, and vitamin B6) are also common in the general population, and are postulated to cause between one half to two thirds of all cases of hyperhomocysteinemia.

Much effort has focused on folate intake and supplementation because of its ease of administration and its effect on lowering plasma homocysteine. Folate is easily absorbed orally and readily lowers plasma homocysteine levels by stimulating the remethylation cycle. Plasma homocysteine concentrations rise predictably with low plasma folate levels and can be readily normalized by as little as 400 µg of oral folate daily.[46] Folate deficiency is rare in individuals who do take multivitamins, but common in those who do not. In the Framingham cohort, 90% of patients who did not take multivitamins had elevated homocysteine levels.[76]

Current evidence suggests that elevated plasma homocysteine concentrations cause endothelial dysfunction by promoting oxidative damage. This may happen through direct effects on the endothelium as well as through oxidative modification of LDL molecules and formation of foam cells which produce reactive oxygen species (Figure 10).[75] Although controlled studies have not yet been performed, observational data from the Nurses' Health and other studies have correlated lower plasma homocysteine concentrations with a lower risk for vascular disease. Therefore, given the known benefits of folate in preventing neural tube defects, combined with the current observational data on homocysteine and its influence on vascular disease, dietary supplementation with 400mcg. of folate daily is prudent.

Recommendation:
- **400mcg folate daily via multivitamin or fortified cereal**

C-Reactive Protein (CRP). The role of inflammation in coronary events has been examined recently. CRP is a marker for systemic inflammation that has also been shown to be a significant predictor of cardiovascular events in men.[77] This is true for men who are healthy, at high risk for vascular events (coronary or peripheral), and with known CHD. Recently, Ridker et al showed that CRP is a powerful risk factor in women as well. Data from the Women's Health Study, showed that women with high baseline levels of CRP (>7.3 mg/L) had a 5 fold increase in risk of any vascular event and a 7 fold increase in risk of myocardial infarction or stroke.[78] These data further bolster the hypothesis that inflammation is related to coronary events. This may be particularly important for women, in whom

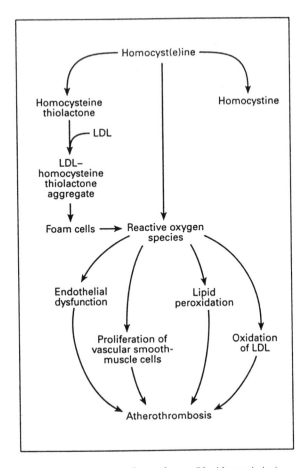

Figure 10. Mechanisms of vascular damage (from reference 75 with permission)

our suspicions of CHD are often aroused too late, and where the consequences of a first ischemic event are deadly.

ESTROGEN AND CARDIOVASCULAR DISEASE IN WOMEN

There is a strong link between menopause and an increased incidence of cardiovascular disease. Observational studies suggest that postmenopausal hormone replacement therapy, including various estrogen preparations with or without progestin (most commonly synthetic progestin), reduces cardiovascular disease risk by about half.[1,79,80] Studies also suggest that estrogen may slow the progression of existing coronary artery disease in postmenopausal women and limit the proliferation of vascular smooth muscle cells after vascular injury.[81] For example, 6-month results of the Coronary Angioplasty Versus Excisional Atherectomy Trial (CAVEAT I) showed that women undergoing atherectomy who received hormone replacement therapy (estrogen $\pm$ progestin) had significantly less late loss in minimal lumen diameter, larger lumen diameter and lower restenosis rates (27% vs. 57%, p= 0.038 for > 50% stenosis) than those not receiving estrogen.[82] In contrast, estrogen had a minimal effect on restenosis after balloon angioplasty in this trial. Two retrospective studies of women undergoing elective percutaneous transluminal coronary angioplasty (PTCA) showed improved survival and reduced cardiovascular event rates (death, nonfatal myocardial infarction or nonfatal stroke) in women treated with hormone replacement; there was no difference between treatment groups in need for subsequent revascularization, suggesting no reduction in restenosis. These device-specific results are consistent with an inhibitory effect of estrogen on neointima formation, which is thought to play a greater role in restenosis after atherectomy than after balloon angioplasty, where later recoil is a major contributor.

These studies, while provocative, suffer from the limitations of small patient numbers and noncomparability of the two treatment groups: women who take estrogen are on average better educated, have higher incomes and better access to health care and are healthier even before starting therapy.[83] This deficiency in available data concerning the cardiovascular benefits of hormone replacement therapy, combined with the known increased risk of breast and endometrial cancer and venous thromboembolism in long-term users of estrogen, have created controversy in the health care arena about the general advisability of hormone replacement.[84]

The recently published results from the Heart Estrogen-Progestin Replacement Study (HERS) have added to the controversy.[51] HERS was the first large scale randomized clinical trial to test the efficacy and safety of hormone replacement on clinical cardiovascular disease outcomes in postmenopausal women. The study population included 2,763 women with established CHD randomized to combined hormone replacement therapy or placebo who were followed for an average of 4 years. Overall, there was no significant difference between groups for the primary outcome, nonfatal myocardial infarction or CHD death, or for several secondary cardiovascular endpoints. There was a statistically significant time trend, with more CHD events in the treatment group than in the placebo group in year 1 and fewer in years 3 and beyond (Figure 11).

These results do not support instituting hormone replacement therapy in women with established CHD for the sole purpose of avoiding secondary events. HERS did not address the question of benefit (and risk) from estrogen alone or from combined hormone replacement in primary prevention, nor did it elucidate the mechanism of the apparently biphasic effect (early detriment, later benefit) of combined hormone replacement in women with atherosclerotic disease. Answers to the first questions will come from the Women's Health Initiative (WHI), a randomized trial of estrogen and combined hormone replacement therapy for primary prevention, which includes 10 times as many treated women as HERS and a longer (9 years) period of treatment, completing in 2005.[85] The last question can be answered only by further research in both human subjects and animal models on fundamental mechanisms of vasoprotection (or lack thereof) by hormones.

Outcome and Period	Estrogen-Progestin		Placebo		RH (95% CI)	P Value‡
	No.	Rate†	No.	Rate†		
Primary CHD event§						
Year 1	57	42.5	38	28.0	1.52 (1.01-2.29)	
Year 2	47	37.0	48	37.1	1.00 (0.67-1.49)	.009
Year 3	35	28.8	41	33.1	0.87 (0.55-1.37)	
Years 4 and 5	33	23.0	49	34.4	0.67 (0.43-1.04)	
Nonfatal myocardial infarction						
Year 1	42	31.3	29	21.4	1.47 (0.91-2.36)	
Year 2	34	26.8	37	28.6	0.94 (0.59-1.49)	.01
Year 3	20	16.5	29	23.4	0.70 (0.40-1.24)	
Years 4 and 5	20	13.9	34	23.9	0.58 (0.34-1.02)	
CHD death						
Year 1	17	12.5	11	8.0	1.56 (0.73-3.32)	
Year 2	19	14.4	13	9.7	1.48 (0.73-2.99)	.34
Year 3	18	14.0	16	12.3	1.14 (0.58-2.24)	
Years 4 and 5	17	11.0	18	11.6	0.95 (0.49-1.84)	
Unstable angina or coronary revascularization¶						
Year 1	101	77.1	94	71.1	1.08 (0.82-1.44)	
Year 2	52	43.3	85	70.6	0.61 (0.43-0.87)	.42
Year 3	69	61.9	56	50.5	1.22 (0.86-1.74)	
Years 4 and 5	47	36.6	67	54.2	0.67 (0.46-0.98)	
Venous thromboembolic event						
Year 1	13	9.6	4	2.9	3.29 (1.07-10.08)	
Year 2	8	6.1	2	1.5	4.09 (0.87-19.27)	.28
Year 3	7	5.5	3	2.3	2.40 (0.62-9.28)	
Years 4 and 5	6	4.0	3	2.0	2.05 (0.15-8.18)	

*RH indicates relative hazard; CI, confidence interval; and CHD, coronary heart disease.
†Event rates per 1000 women-years in the estrogen plus progestin or placebo group.
‡P values for tests of continuous trend in log-relative hazard.
§Primary CHD events include nonfatal myocardial infarction and CHD death.
¶Coronary revascularization includes coronary artery bypass graft surgery and percutaneous coronary revascularization.

Figure 11. Outcome by Treatment Group and Year Since Randomization of Women in the HERS trial (reproduced with permission)

Effects of Progestin on Estrogen-Mediated Vasoprotection.

Addition of a progestin, while needed to prevent the hyperplastic/neoplastic effects of unopposed estrogen on the endometrium, may reduce the beneficial effects of estrogen replacement therapy on the risk of cardiovascular disease.[86-89] For example, in the Postmenopausal Estrogen/Progestin Interventions (PEPI) trial, women randomized to conjugated equine estrogen and continuous or cyclical medroxyprogesterone acetate (MPA) had smaller increases from baseline in HDL cholesterol levels than women randomized to unopposed estrogen.[86] Such an effect could compromise the cardioprotective effect of estrogen, given the inverse relationship between HDL-C levels and cardiovascular disease in women. In the Framingham Offspring Study, postmenopausal women taking a combination of estrogen and progestin had higher levels of plasminogen activator inhibitor (PAI-1) than women on unopposed estrogen when adjustments were made for age, risk factors, and other covariants, suggesting that they might be more vulnerable to the development of intravascular thrombi and, therefore, cardiovascular events.[87]

Ovariectomized rhesus monkeys   treated chronically with a combination of MPA plus 17β–estradiol manifested coronary vasospasm in response to infusion of serotonin plus a thromboxane A_2 mimetic, while those treated with native progesterone plus 17β-estradiol did not.[88] This study gives evidence that different progestins have different effects on vascular function, perhaps depending on their potency, androgenicity, and other, yet to be evaluated properties.[89]

Whether these putative adverse effects of progestins are clinically important is uncertain, particularly in light of the recent report from the Nurses' Health Study which found a decrease in the risk of major coronary heart disease among women who took estrogen with progestin, compared to women who took estrogen alone or did not use hormones.[80] The recent demonstration of dose-dependent inhibition of DNA synthesis, expression of cyclin A and E mRNA levels and proliferation in human and rat aortic smooth muscle cells in culture by native progesterone is consistent with the interpretation that some progestins can be vasoprotective. Whether native progesterone has effects similar to MPA on the response to vascular injury and whether interactions between progesterone and estrogen on the vasculature are mediated at the estrogen receptor level are unanswered questions of both scientific and clinical importance.

Postmenopausal Hormone Replacement Therapy and Blood Pressure.
The conjugated and natural estrogen preparations used for postmenopausal replacement therapy are administered at doses which result in "physiologic" levels of circulating estrogen. Unlike oral contraceptives, there is no evidence that these hormones cause hypertension, or even a tendency for blood pressure elevation, when administered to normotensive women. Prospective studies have shown that administration of conjugated and natural estrogens, alone or in combination with a progestin, to normotensive postmenopausal women generally has no effect on blood pressure or tends to reduce it. The finding of significant increases in blood pressure in a small proportion (<2%) of postmenopausal women when starting treatment with oral estrogens does not alter this conclusion, since the infrequent pressor response might have been due to chance. The presence of hypertension is not a contraindication to postmenopausal hormone replacement therapy, particularly since postmenopausal hormones appear from observational studies to have a beneficial effect on overall cardiovascular risk. However, interventional studies of hormonal replacement therapy in hypertensive menopausal women have been either retrospective, short-term, small in number of participants or open in design, and caution should be exercised when treating these patients with hormones. It is recommended that all hypertensive women treated with postmenopausal hormone replacement have their blood pressure monitored at 3-6 month intervals.[53]

DIAGNOSIS AND TREATMENT OF CORONARY HEART DISEASE

Diagnosis of coronary artery disease in women presents a unique set of problems. Every diagnostic modality in current use is limited by a selection disadvantage against women. Because of the difference in age demographics, there is less coronary disease in women than in men until the seventh or eighth decade of life. The risk of death from CHD in women is similar to that of men 10 years younger. Women first develop angina on average 10 years later than men, and they infarct an average of 20 years later.[1,90] Bayes' theorem would therefore predict a lower positive predictive value of any test in women, as compared to age matched men.[14,60] Even the most basic evaluations - assessment of chest pain characteristics and the clinical history - are much more difficult to interpret in female patients. In women with typical angina, the prevalence of angiographically proven CHD is 60 - 72%. However, in women with more "atypical" chest pain syndromes, the prevalence of CHD may be as low as 2 - 7%.[91]

Stress Electrocardiographic (ECG) Testing. The diagnostic value of exercise ECG is well documented in men, but its use in diagnosing myocardial ischemia in women is problematic.[32,92] In addition to the issue of decreased prevalence of coronary disease in younger women, females without obvious heart disease have a higher incidence of repolarization abnormalities on the resting ECG. Women are more likely to be taking medications that alter the ST segment, and there is evidence that estrogen may affect the ST segment in a manner similar to digitalis. Women are also more likely to be older at the time of testing, and therefore have more difficulty reaching their target heart rate due to lack of conditioning and concomitant medical problems.[90,93] These factors limit the clinical use of exercise ECG in women. However, in women with a normal resting ECG, adequate exercise tolerance, and no ischemic changes on the stress ECG, the risk of significant CHD is low.[34] Therefore, false positive exercise ECG examinations are likely more problematic than false negatives.

Radionuclide Imaging. The addition of radionuclide imaging has enhanced the sensitivity and specificity of physiologic and pharmacologic stress testing in diagnosing CHD. This is true for both men and women, but significant limitations still exist in examining women. In addition to the issues of lower age-matched disease prevalence in women mentioned previously, myocardial perfusion imaging is limited by the female anatomy. Breast tissue attenuation can be a significant problem, especially in obese individuals. Despite this, the use of planar thallium-201 (Tl-201) imaging increased the sensitivity for detecting CHD over ECG testing in women from 61 - 73% to 70 - 84%. The specificity increased correspondingly from 59 - 78% to 85 - 93%.[34,90] This is true for both exercise and pharmacologic stress. Further improvements in imaging techniques, such as the use of single-photon emission computed tomography (SPECT), have improved the diagnostic accuracy of imaging in men, but very few data are available in women.[34,90] The problem with breast attenuation in females is particularly troublesome with Tl-201, given its lower energy (69-83 kev).[32]

The recent introduction and subsequent widespread use of technetium-99 sestamibi (Tc-99m) has improved image quality and, therefore, the accuracy of the results. With a higher energy (140kev) and a higher administered dose (five-fold more counts), breast attenuation may diminish in severity.[32] Indeed, one recent study by Taillefer et al. compared Tl-201 and Tc-99min in detecting coronary disease in women using both exercise and pharmacological stress.[4] The sensitivities were similar: 84.3% (Tl-201) vs. 80.4% (Tc-99m) for lesions ≥ to 70%. However, the specificity data favored Tc-99m over Tl-201, with values of 84.4% vs. 67.2%. The Tc-99m images are of such quality that ECG gating of the images and, therefore, evaluation of global and regional wall motion and thickening is possible. This additional information further increased the specificity of Tc-99m to 92.2%.[4] The use of Tc-99m and ECG gated images should improve accuracy in discrimination between soft tissue artifact, scar, and actual perfusion defects in women.

Echocardiography. Stress echocardiography is another technique for examining changes in global ejection fraction as well as regional contractility changes with either exercise or pharmacological stress.[32,34,90] There are inherent limitations in using echocardiography for ischemic evaluation. It is highly dependent on the technical prowess of the operator, and anatomic limitations are more problematic than with ECG or radionuclide imaging techniques. Particularly in women, breast tissue attenuation may result in inadequate image quality. Despite these mitigating factors, current studies show that stress echocardiography has a sensitivity and specificity superior to exercise ECG testing, and similar to that of Tc-99m perfusion imaging.[32,90] To date, there are only limited data on gender differences in stress echocardiography, and the results are mixed.[34] However, the cost savings, as well as the additional ancillary information obtained have led some investigators to propose that stress echocardiography be considered as the initial diagnostic evaluation in patients who are not suitable for exercise ECG testing.[22,34] This approach is promising and empirically appealing but is not currently supported by the literature - especially for women.

TREATMENT OF CORONARY HEART DISEASE

The technical aspects of coronary angiography have not been studied extensively from a gender perspective, but a variety of factors may differentially affect the outcomes of the procedure in the sexes. Women have smaller body sizes and smaller coronary artery diameters, so angiography may be more technically difficult in women as compared to men. Women are also more likely to experience renal and vascular complications such as contrast nephropathy and pseudoaneurysms or arterio-venous fistulas a result of the procedure.[22]

Gender differences in patterns of coronary angiography have stimulated a great deal of controversy. In 1987, Jonathan Tobin observed that 40% of men but only 4% of women with abnormal radionuclide scans went on to catheterization and coronary angiography.[94] Ayanian and Epstein analyzed 1987 discharge diagnoses and procedures performed during hospital admission on patients in Massachusetts and Maryland. They found that among patients hospitalized for myocardial infarction, chest pain, or chronic ischemic heart disease, approximately 28% of men vs. 17% of women underwent coronary angiography. This disparity was still present after correcting for age, the presence of congestive heart failure, and diabetes.[95] Furthermore, revascularization (angioplasty or coronary bypass surgery) was more frequent in men (15% compared with 7% in women). This study did not look at procedures done prior to admission or after discharge, and no outcome data were provided. In a study of patients from the SAVE (Survival and Ventricular Enlargement) registry, women were noted to have a prevalence of angina similar to men, but reported greater disability as a result of their symptoms prior to the infarction that placed them in the registry. Despite this, women were less likely than men to have been referred for prior cardiac catheterization (15.4 vs. 27.3 percent). Women were also less likely to have undergone previous coronary artery bypass surgery (5.9 vs. 12.7 percent). However, this difference was not statistically significant after adjusting for covariates such as age, diabetes, and previous infarction.[96]

In 1992, Krumholz et al. performed a retrospective analysis of patients admitted to the Boston Beth Israel Hospital for myocardial infarction. The rate of catheterization for women was less than that for men (odds ratio, 0.91; CI, 0.75 to 1.12), but this difference was not significant after adjusting for age. Among patients who did undergo catheterization, women exhibited a lower rate of severe (>50% left main stenosis, three vessel disease, or two-vessel disease with a proximal left anterior descending stenosis of > 70%) coronary disease than men (odds ratio of 0.67; CI; 0.48 to 0.93). There was no clear difference with respect to gender in overall numbers undergoing angioplasty or coronary bypass surgery. Overall in-hospital mortality rates were also not different in men compared to women, and this was true after controlling for age.[97] In another retrospective study, Bickell et al. examined patients catheterized at Duke University from 1969 to 1984. Overall, 46% of men and 44% of women were referred for coronary bypass surgery. When the patients were assessed for disease severity, women with advanced coronary disease - who would benefit the most from surgery - were at least as likely to be referred for surgery as men. In patients with less severe disease where surgery offered little or no benefit, men were more likely to be referred for coronary bypass.[98]

More recent studies have done little to clarify this issue. A 1994 retrospective analysis found that women were less likely to undergo arteriography after an abnormal exercise stress test or an intravenous dipyridamole thallium imaging study (33.8% in women vs. 45.0% in men). Furthermore, in those patients with an initial abnormal noninvasive test, the annual rate of cardiac death or myocardial infarction was 14.3% for women and 6.0% for men.[99] The Myocardial Infarction Triage and Intervention Registry (MITI) showed that women with acute myocardial infarction were less likely than men to receive an acute cardiac procedure (catheterization, angioplasty, coronary bypass surgery, or thrombolytic therapy) with an odds ratio of 0.5 (CI; 0.3 - 0.7). Women had twice the in hospital mortality rate as their male counterparts.[3] The Atherosclerosis Risk in Communities (ARIC) study also found that women admitted to both teaching and community hospitals for acute myocardial infarction were less likely to undergo angiography, coronary bypass surgery, and less likely to have received thrombolytic therapy. No outcome measures were examined.[100] Bernstein et al., however, were unable to a find a difference in the patterns of angiography, bypass surgery, or angioplasty in thirty New York State hospitals.[101]   A review of Emory University's angiographic and revascularization practices indicated that angiographic severity of coronary disease was the major factor in referrals to coronary bypass surgery. Gender played a significant but smaller role in referral to surgery, but only a marginal role in referral to angioplasty.[102]   Finally, a recent comparison of coronary bypass surgery in New York State and Ontario, Canada revealed that the rate of surgery in New York was 1.79 times (CI; 1.74 to 1.85) that in Canada. In all age ranges, more women underwent surgery in New York compared with Ontario.[103]

The current data on gender bias in angiography and revascularization are inconsistent at best. Several of these studies were done at a single institution, but many were multi-center and spanned several states. The heterogeneity of the results points to the difficulty in determining optimum patterns of invasive and surgical treatment of coronary disease in women and in men. This issue is further confounded by the results of the recently published Veteran's Administration Non-Q-wave Myocardial Infarction (VANQWISH)[104] trial where veterans (men) with elevated creatine kinase MB isoenzymes were randomized to "invasive" vs. "conservative" management. There was increased mortality in the hospital, at one month, and after on year in those patients assigned to the "aggressive" treatment strategy. This finding, together with previous studies showing similar increases in adverse events in patients managed aggressively,[105-107] calls into question the current practice of increasing use of invasive treatment strategies in men and women. If women are being evaluated and revascularized at rates equal to men, then it is possible that are both genders are being exposed to risk with questionable chances for benefit.[104]

REFERENCES

1. Mosca L, Manson JE, Sutherland SE, Langer RD, Manolio T, Barrett-Connor E. Cardiovascular Disease in Women: A statement for healthcare professionals from the American Heart Association. Circulation. 1997;96:2468-2482.
2. American Heart Association. *1998 Heart and Stroke Statistical Update*. Dallas, TX:American Heart Association,1997.
3. Kudenchuk PJ, Maynard C, Martin JS, Wirkus M, Weaver WD. Comparison of presentation, treatment, and outcome of acute myocardial infarction in men versus women (The Myocardial Infarction Triage and Intervention Registry). *Am J Cardiol.* 1996;78:9-14.
4. Taillefer R, DePuey G, Udleson JE, Beller GA, Latour Y, Reeves F. Comparative Diagnostic Accuracy of TI-201 and Tc-99m sestamibi SPECTimaging (perfusion and ECG-gated SPECT) in detecting coronary disease in women. *J Am Coll Cardiol.* 1997;29:69-77.
5. Gallo MA, Kaufman D. Antagonistic and agonistic effects of tamoxifen: significance in human cancer. *Semin Oncol.* 1997;24:S1-71-S1-80.
6. Ponglikitmongkol M, Green S, Chambon P. Genomic organization of the human oestrogen receptor gene. *Embo J.* 1988;7:3385-8.
7. Green S, Walter P, Kumar V, Krust A, Bornert JM, Argos P, Chambon P. Human oestrogen receptor cDNA: sequence, expression and homology to v- erb-A. *Nature.* 1986;320:134-9.
8. Greene GL, Gilna P, Waterfield M, Baker A, Hort Y, Shine J. Sequence and expression of human estrogen receptor complementary DNA. *Science.* 1986;231:1150-4.
9. Grohe C, Kahlert S, Lobbert K, Vetter H. Expression of oestrogen receptor alpha and beta in rat heart: role of local oestrogen synthesis. *J Endocrinol.* 1998;156:R1-7.

10. Register TC, Adams MR. Coronary artery and cultured aortic smooth muscle cells express mRNA for both the classical estrogen receptor and the newly described estrogen receptor beta. *J Steroid Biochem Mol Biol.* 1998;64:187-91.

11.Diano S, Horvath TL, Mor G, Register T, Adams M, Harada N, Naftolin F. Aromatase and estrogen receptor immunoreactivity in the coronary arteries of monkeys and human subjects [In Process Citation]. *Menopause.* 1999;6:21-8.

12. Maalouf GJ, Xu W, Smith TF, Mohr SC. Homology model for the ligand binding domain of the human estrogen receptor. *J Biomol Struct Dyn.* 1998;15:841-51.

13. Green S, Chambon P. Nuclear receptors enhance our understanding of transcription regulation. *Trends Genet.* 1988;4:309-14.

14. Brzozowski AM, Pike AC, Dauter Z, Hubbard RE, Bonn T, Engstrom O, Ohman L, Greene GL, Gustafsson JA, Carlquist M. Molecular basis of agonism and antagonism in the oestrogen receptor. *Nature.* 1997;389:753-8

15. Fraser RA, Heard DJ, Adam S, Lavigne AC, Le Douarin B, Tora L, Losson R, Rochette-Egly C, Chambon P. The putative cofactor TIF1alpha is a protein kinase that is hyperphosphorylated upon interaction with liganded nuclear receptors. *J Biol Chem.* 1998;273:16199-204.

16. Shiau AK, Barstad D, Loria PM, Cheng L, Kushner PJ, Agard DA, Greene GL. The structural basis of estrogen receptor/coactivator recognition and theantagonism of this interaction by tamoxifen. *Cell.* 17. 1998;95:927-37.

17. Schwabe JW, Chapman L, Finch JT, Rhodes D. The crystal structure of the estrogen receptor DNA-binding domain bound to DNA: how receptors discriminate between their response elements. *Cell.* 1993;75:567-78.

18. Green S, Kumar V, Theulaz I, Wahli W, Chambon P. The N-terminal DNA-binding 'zinc finger'of the oestrogen and glucocorticoid receptors determines target gene specificity. *Embo J.* 1988;7:3037-44.

19. Pelzer T, Shamim A, Wolfges S, Schumann M, Neyses L. Modulation of cardiac hypertrophy by estrogens. *Adv Exp Med Biol.* 1997;432:83-9.

20. Pelzer T, Shamim A, Neyses L. Estrogen effects in the heart. *Mol Cell Biochem.* 1996;160-161:307-313.

21. Demirovic J and Myerburg RJ. Epidemiology of sudden coronary death: an overview. *Prog in Cardiovas Dis.* 1994;37:39-48.

22. Braunwald E ed. *Heart Disease: A textbook of Cardiovascular Medicine.* 5th ed Philadelphia, PA: WB Saunders Co. 1997.

23. Schactzkin A, Cupples A, Heeren T, Morelock S, Kannel WB. Sudden death in the Framingham heart study: differences in incidence and risk factors by sex and coronary disease status. *Am J Epidemiol..*1984;120:888-899.

24. Farb A, Burke AP, Tang AL, Liang Y, Manna P, Smialek J, Virmani R.Coronary plaque erosion without rupture into a lipid core: a frequent cause of coronary thrombosis in sudden coronary death. *Circulation.* 1996;93:1354-1363.

25. Burke AP, Farb A, Malcom GT, Liang Y, Smialek J, Virmeni R. Effect of Risk Factors on the mechanism of sudden coronary death in women. *Circulation..* 1998;97:2110-2116.

26. Johnson BD, Zheng W, Korach KS, Scheuer T, Catterall WA, Rubanyi GM. Increased expression of of the cardiac L-type calcium channel in estrogen receptor-deficient mice. *J Gen Physiol.* 1997;110:135-140

27. Cross HR, Lu L, Steenbergen C, Philipson KD, Murphy E. Overexpression of the cardiac Na+/Ca2+ exchanger increases susceptibility to ischemia/reperfusion injury in male, but not female, transgenic mice. *Circ Res.* 1998;83:1215-23.

28. Vaccarino V, Krumholz H, Berkman LF, Horwitz RI. Sex differences in mortality after myocardial infarction: Is there evidence for an increased risk for women? *Circulation.* 1995;91:1861-1871.

29. Stone PH, Thompson B, Anderson V, et al. For the TIMI III registry study group. Influence of race, sex, and age on management of unstable angina and non-Q-wave myocardial infarction. *JAMA.* 1996;275:1104-1112.

30. The GUSTO Investigators. An international randomized trial comparing four thrombolytic strategies for acute myocardial infarction. *N Engl J Med.* 1993;329:673-682

31. Mosca L, Judelson, D, King K, Limacher M, Oparil S, Pasternak R, Pearson T, Redberg R, Smith S, Winston M, Zinberg S. A guide to preventive cardiology for women: ACC/AHA Consensus Panel Statement. *Circulation.* in press

32. Wenger NK and Julian DG, ed. *Women and Heart Disease.* London, England: Martin Dunitz Ltd. 1997.

33. Rosenberg L, Palmer JR, Shapiro S. Decline in the risk of myocardial infarction among women who stop smoking. *N Engl J Med.* 1990;322:213-217.

34. Douglas PS and Ginsburg GS. The evaluation of women with chest pain. *N Engl J Med.* 1996;334:1311-1315.

35. Manson JE, Colditz GA, Stampfer MJ, et al. A prospective study of maturity-onset diabetes mellitus and risk of coronary heart disease and stroke in women. *Arch Intern Med.* 1991;151:1141-1147.

36. Oparil S. Cardiovascular risk reduction in women. *J Women's Health.* 1996;5:23-31.

37. UK Prospective Diabetes Study (UKPDS) Group. Intensive blood-glucose control with sulphonylureas or insulin compared with conventional treatment and risk of complications in patients with type 2 diabetes (UKPDS 33). *Lancet.* 1998;352:837-853.

38. UK Prospective Diabetes Study (UKPDS) Group. Effect of intensive blood-glucose control with metformin on complications in overweight patients with type 2 diabetes (UKPDS 34). *Lancet.* 1998;352:854-865.

39. Barrett-Connor E. Sex differences in coronary heart disease: Why are women so superior? The 1995 Ancel Keys Lecture. *Circulation.* 1997;95:252-264.

40. Wenger NK. Addressing coronary heart disease risk in women. *Cleve Clin J Medi.* 1998; 65:464-469.

41. Joint National Committee on Detection, Evaluation, and Treatment of High Blood Pressure. The sixth report of the Joint National Committee on Detection, Evaluation, and Treatment of High Blood Pressure (JNC VI). *Arch Intern Med.* 1997;157:2413-2446.

42. Colvin PL, Jr., Wagner JD, Adams MR, Sorci-Thomas MG. Sex steroids increase cholesterol 7alpha-hydroxylase mRNA in nonhuman primates. *Metabolism.* 1998;47:391-5.

43. Marsh MM, Walker VR, L KC, Banka CL. Protection against atherosclerosis by estrogen is independent of plasma cholesterol levels in LDL receptor-deficient mice. *J Lipid Res.* 1999;40:893-900.

44. Sudhir K, Chou TM, Chatterjee K, Smith EP, Williams TC, Kane JP, Malloy MJ, Korach KS, Rubanyi GM. Premature coronary artery disease associated with a disruptive mutation in the estrogen receptor gene in a man. *Circulation.* 1997;96:3774-7.

45. Walsh BW, Kuller LH, Wild RA, Paul S, Farmer M, Lawrence JB, Shah AS, Anderson PW. Effects of raloxifene on serum lipids and coagulation factors in healthy postmenopausal women [see comments]. *Jama.* 1998;279:1445-51.

46. Williams JK, Honore EK, Adams MR. Contrasting effects of conjugated estrogens and tamoxifen on dilator responses of atherosclerotic epicardial coronary arteries in nonhuman primates.*Circulation.* 1997;96:1970-5.

47. Scandinavian Simvastatin Survival Study Group. Randomised trial of cholesterol lowering in 4444 patients with coronary heart disease: the Scandinavian Simvastatin Survival Study (4S). *Lancet.* 1994; 344: 1383-1389.

48. Sacks FM, Pfeffer MA, Moye LA, et al. The effect of pravastatin on coronary events after myocardial infarction in patients with average cholesterol levels (The cholesterol and recurrent events (CARE) trial). *N Engl J Med.* 1996;335:1001-1009.

49. Lewis SJ, Sacks FM, Mitchell JS, et al. For the CARE Investigators. Effect of pravastatin on cardiovascular events in women after myocardial infarction. *J Am Coll Cardiol.* 1998; 32:140-146.

50. Downs JR, Clearfield M, Weis S, et al. Primary prevention of acute coronary events with lovastatin in men and women with average cholesterol levels. Results of AFCAPS/TexCAPS. *JAMA.* 1998;279:1615-1661.

51. Hulley S, Grady D, Bush T, et al. Randomized trial of estrogen plus progestin for secondary prevention of coronary heart disease in postmenopausal women (HERS). *JAMA.* 1998;280:605-613.

52. Schrott HG, Bittner VA, Vittinghoff E, Herrington DM, Hulley S for the HERS Research Group. Adherence to national cholesterol education program treatment goals in postmenopausal women with heart disease. *JAMA.* 1997; 277:1281-1286.

53. Calhoun DA, Oparil S: Gender and blood pressure. In: Hypertension Primer, American Heart Association, 1998.

54. Stassen J, Bulpitt CJ, Fagard R, Lijnen P, Amery A. The influence of menopause on blood pressure. *J Human Hypertens.* 1989;3:427-433.

55. Owens JF, Stoney CM, Matthews KA. Menopausal status influences ambulatory blood pressure levels and blood pressure changes during mental stress. *Circulation.* 1993; 88:2794-2802.

56. Nestel PJ, Clifton PM, Noakes M, McArthur R, Howe PR. Enhanced blood pressure response to dietary salt in elderly women, especially those with small waist:hip ratio. *J Hypertens.* 1993;11:1387-1394.

57. Tominaga T, Suzuki H, Ogata Y, Matsukawa S, Saruta T. The role of sex hormones and sodium intake in postmenopausal hypertension. *J Human Hypertens.* 1991;5:495-500.

58. Lee HW, Eghbali-Webb M. Estrogen enhances proliferative capacity of cardiac fibroblasts by estrogen receptor- and mitogen-activated protein kinase-dependent pathways. *J Mol Cell Cardiol.* 1998;30:1359-68.

59. Grohe C, Kahlert S, Lobbert K, Neyses L, van Eickels M, Stimpel M, Vetter H. Angiotensin 84. converting enzyme inhibition modulates cardiac fibroblast growth. *J Hypertens.* 1998;16:377-84

60. Dubey RK, Gillespie DG, Jackson EK, Keller PJ. 17Beta-estradiol, its metabolites, and progesterone inhibit cardiac fibroblast growth. *Hypertension.* 1998;31:522-8.

61. Nickenig G, Baumer AT, Grohe C, Kahlert S, Strehlow K, Rosenkranz S, Stablein A, Beckers F, Smits JF, Daemen MJ, Vetter H, Bohm M. Estrogen modulates AT1 receptor gene expression in vitro and in vivo. *Circulation.* 1998;97:2197-201.

62. Cui Y, Narayanan CS, Zhou J, Kumar A. Exon-I is involved in positive as well as negative regulation of human angiotensinogen gene expression. *Gene.* 1998;224:97-107.

63. Berman M, Gewirtz H. Acute effects of 17 beta-estradiol on the coronary microcirculation: observations in sedated, closed-chest domestic swine. *Coron Artery Dis.* 1997;8:351-61.

64. Minshall RD, Miyagawa K, Chadwick CC, Novy MJ, Hermsmeyer K. In vitro modulation of primate coronary vascular muscle cell reactivity by ovarian steroid hormones. *Faseb J.* 1998;12:1419-29.

65. Burt VL, Whelton P, Roccella EJ, et al. Prevalence of hypertension in the US adult population: Results of the Third National Health and Nutrition Examination Survey, 1988-1991. *Hypertension.* 1995;25:305-313.

66. Klungel OH, deBoer A, Paes AH, Seidell JC, Bakker A. Sex differences in the pharmacological treatment of hypertension: a review of population based studies. *J Hypertens.* 1997;15:591-600.

67. Royal College of General Practitioners' Oral Contraception Study. *Oral Contraceptives and Health.* 1974;Pitman, New York.

68. Chasan-Taber L, Willett WC, Manson JE, et al. Prospective study of oral contraceptives and hypertension among women in the United States. *Circulation.* 1996;94:483-489.

69. Narkiewicz K, Graniero GR, D'Este D, Mattarei M, Zonzin P, Palatini P. Ambulatory blood pressure in mild hypertensive women taking oral contraceptives. A case control study. *Am J Hypertens.* 1995;8:249-253.

70. Gueyffier F, Boutitie F, Boissel J-P, et al. Effect of antihypertensive drug treatment on cardiovascular outcomes in women and men. A meta-analysis of individual patient data from randomized, controlled trials. The INDANA Investigators. *Ann Intern Med.* 1997;126:761-767.

71. Jackson R, Barham P, Bills J, et al. Management of raised blood pressure in New Zealand: A discussion document. *BMJ.* 1993;307:107-110.

72. Lewis CE. Characteristics and treatment of hypertension in women: A review of the literature. *Am J Med Sci.* 1996;311:193-199.

73. Cauley JA, Cummings SR, Seeley DG, et al. Effects of thiazide diuretic therapy on bone mass, fractures, and falls. The Study of Osteoporotic Fractures Research Group. *Ann Intern Med.* 1993;118:666-673.

74. Israili ZH, Hall WD. Cough and angioneurotic edema associated with angiotensin- converting enzyme inhibitor therapy. *Ann Intern Med.* 1992;117:234-242.

75. Welch GN and Loscalzo J. Homocysteine and atherombosis. *N Engl J Med.* 1998;338:1042- 1050.

76. Oakley OP. Eat right and take a multivitamin. *N Engl J Med.* 1998;338:1060-1061.

77. Ridker PM, Cushman, Stampfer MJ, Tracy RP, Hennkens CH. Inflammation, aspirin, and the risk of cardiovascular disease in apparently healthy men. *N Engl J Med.* 1777;336(14):973- 979.

78. Ridker PM, Buring JE, Shih J, Matias M, Hennekens CH. Prospective study of C-reactive protein and the risk of future cardiovascular events among apparently healthy women. *Circulation.* 1998;98:731- 733.

79. Psaty BM, Heckbert SR, Atkins D, Lemaitre R, Koepsell TD, Wahl PW, Siscovick DS, Wagner EH. The risk of myocardial infarction associated with the combined use of estrogens and progestins in postmenopausal women. *Arch Intern Med.* 1994;154:1333-1339.

80. Grodstein F, Stampfer MJ, Manson JE, Colditz GA, Willett WC, Rosner B, Speizer FE, Hennekens CH. Postmenopausal estrogen and progestin use and the risk of cardiovascular disease. *N Engl J Med.* 1996;335:453-461.

81. Oparil S. Hormones and Vasoprotection: the Arthur C. Corcoran Memorial Lecture. *Hypertension..* 1999 in press.

82. O'Brien JE, Peterson ED, Keeler GP, Berdan LG, Ohman EM, Faxon DP, Jacobs AK, Topol EJ, Califf RM. Relation between estrogen replacement therapy and restenosis after percutaneous coronary interventions. *J Am Coll Cardiol.* 1996;28:1111-1118.

83. Matthews KA, Kuller LH, Wing RR, Meilahn EN, Plantinga P. Prior to use of estrogen replacement therapy, are users healthier than non-users? *Am J Epidemiol*. 1996;143:971-78.

84. Rossouw JE. Estrogens for prevention of coronary heart disease: putting the brakes on the bandwagon. *Circulation*. 1996;94:2982-2985.

85. The Women's Health Initiative Study Group. Design of the Women's Health Initiative clinical trial and observational study. *Control Clin Trials*. 1998;19:61-109.

86. PEPI Trial Writing Group. Effects of estrogen or estrogen/progestin regimens on heart disease risk factors in postmenopausal women. The Postmenopausal Estrogen/Progestin Interventions (PEPI) Trial. *JAMA*. 1995;3:199-208.

87. Gebara OCE, Mittleman MA, Sutherland P, Lipinska I, Matheney T, Xu P, Welty FK, Wilson PWF, Levy D, Muller JE, Tofler GH. Association between increased estrogen status and increased fibrinolytic potential in the Framingham Offspring Study. *Circulation*. 1995;91:1952-1958.

88. Miyagawa K, Rösch J, Stanczyk F, Hermsmeyer K. Medroxyprogesterone interferes with ovarian steroid protection against coronary vasospasm. *Nat Med*. 1997;3:324-327.

89. Williams JK, Adams MR. Estrogens, progestins and coronary artery reactivity. *Nat Med*. 1997;3:273-274.

90. Cerqueira, MD. Diagnostic testing strategies for coronary artery disease: special issues related to gender. *Am J Cardiol*. 1995;75:52D-60D.

91. Davis KB, Chaitman B, Ryan T, Bittner V, Kennedy JW. Comparison of 15-year survival for men and women after initial medical or surgical treatment for coronary artery disease: a CASS registry study. *J Am Coll Cardiol*. 1995;25:1000-1009.

92. Gianrossi R, et al. Exercise induced ST depression in the diagnosis of coronary artery disease: a meta-analysis. *Circulation*. 1989;80:87-98.

93. Clark PI, Glasser SP, Lyman GH, Krug-Fite J, Root A. Relation of results of exercise stress tests in young women to phases of the menstrual cycle. *Am J Cardiol*. 1988;61:197-205.

94. Tobin JN, Wassertheil-Smoller S, Wexler JP, et al. Sex bias in considering coronary bypass surgery. *Ann Intern Med*. 1987; 107:19-25.

95. Ayanian JZ, Epstein AM. Differences in the use of procedures between women and men hospitalized for coronary heart disease. *N Engl J Med*. 1991;325:221-225.

96. Steingart RM, Packer M, Hamm P, et al. Sex differences in the management of coronary artery disease. *N Engl J Med*. 1991;325:226-230.

97. Krumholz HM, Douglas PS, Lauer MS, Pasternak RC. Selection of patients for coronary angiography and coronary revascularization early after myocardial infarction: Is there evidence for a gender bias? *Ann Intern Med*. 1992;116:785-790.

98. Bickell NA, Pieper KS, Lee KL, Mark DB, Glower DD, Pryor DB, Califf RM. Referral patterns for coronary artery disease treatment: Gender bias or good clinical judgment? *Ann Intern Med*. 1992; 116:791-797.

99. Shaw LJ, Miller D, Romeis JC, Kargl D, Younis LT, Chaitman BR. Gender differences in the noninvasive evaluation and management of patients with suspected coronary artery disease. *Ann Intern Med*. 1994;120:559-566.

100. Weitzman S, Cooper L, Chambless L, Rosamond W, Clegg L, Marcucci G, Romm F, White A. Gender, racial, and geographic differences in the performance of cardiac diagnostic and therapeutic procedures for hospitalized acute myocardial infarction in four states. *Am J Cardiol*. 1997;79:722-726.

101. Bernstein SJ, Hilborne LH, Leape LL, Park RE, Brook RH. The appropriateness of uses of cardiovascular procedures in women and men. *Arch Intern Med*. 1994;154:2759-2765.

102. Weintraub WS, Kosinski AS, Wenger NK. Is there a bias against performing coronary revascularization in women? *Am J Cardiol*. 1996;78:1154-1160.

103. Tu JV, Naylor DC, Kumar D, DeBuono BA, McNeil BJ, Hannan EL. Coronary artery bypass surgery in Ontario and New York State: which rate is right? *Ann Intern Med*. 1997;126:13-19.

104. Boden WE, O'Rourke RA, Crawford MH, et al. Outcomes in patients with acute non-Q- wave myocardial infarction randomly assigned to an invasive as compared with a conservative management strategy. Veterans Affairs Non-Q-Wave Infarction Strategies in Hospital (VANQWISH) Trial Investigation. *N Engl J Med*. 1998;338:1785-1792.

105. Lange RA, Hillis LD. Use and overuse of angiography and revascularization for acute coronary syndromes (editorial). *N Engl J Med*. 1998;338:1838-1839.

106. The TIMI Study Group. Comparison of invasive and conservative strategies after treatment with intravenous tissue plasminogen activator in acute myocardial infarction: the results of the Thrombolysis in Myocardial Infarction (TIMI) phase II trial. *N Engl J Med*. 1989;320:618-627.

107. Williams DO, Braunwald E, Thompson B, Sharaf BL, Buller CE, Knaterund GL. Results of percutaneous transluminal coronary angioplasty in unstable angina and non-Q-wave myocardial infarction: observations from the TIMI IIIB trial. *Circulation*. 1996;94:2749-2755.

INDEX

Page numbers in *italics* indicate figures. Page numbers followed by "t" indicate tables.